THE KNEE & SHOULDER
HANDBOOK

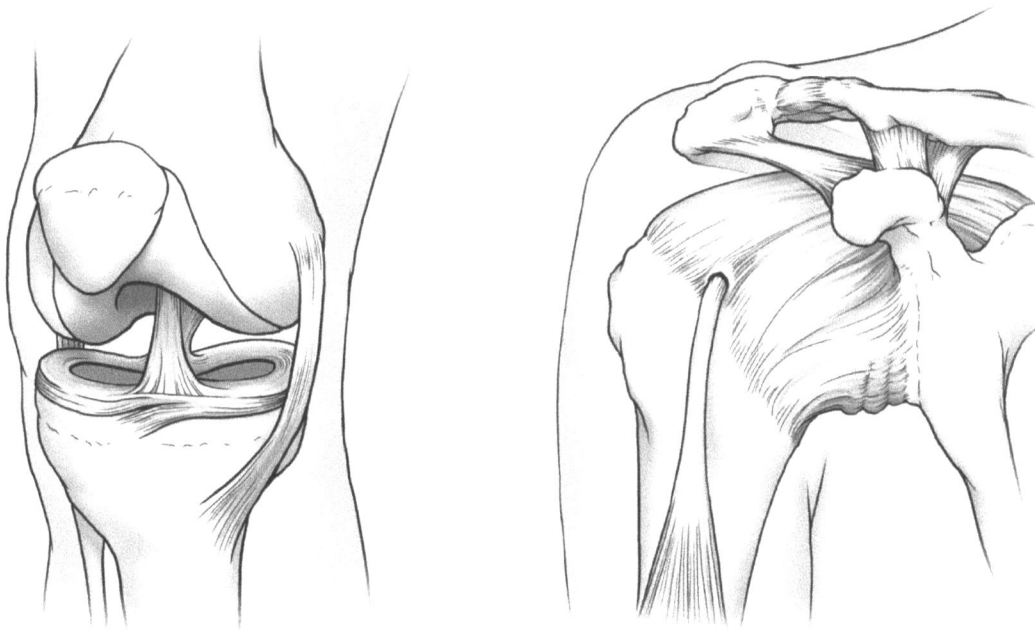

THE KEYS TO A
PAIN-FREE, ACTIVE LIFE

ALAN REZNIK, MD
MBA, FAAOS

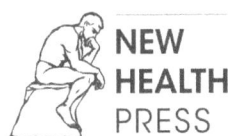

NEW HEALTH PRESS

Published by New Health Press

Printed in the United States of America
10 9 8 7 6 5 4 3 2 1

Photo and Art Credits:
Laura Kovalcin—Anatomy drawings of knee and shoulder
Elizabeth Reznik—Surgical and therapy photos
William Schreiber, MD—Sports photo
Aspaeris.com (ACL prevention shorts)—Valgus collapse diagram

Copyedit by Liz Crooks
Design and Layout by Libby Kingsbury
Proofread by Kelly Clody

ISBN: 979-8-9863472-3-3
E-Book ISBN: 979-8-9863472-4-0

The information in this book is the author's best representation of the top practices and includes many of the most accepted treatments for common knee and shoulder problems. Practices vary by surgeon's experience, location, facility, and the patient's individual medical condition. The information in this book cannot replace a good physical examination, a review of tests, and a full understanding of the medical history in each individual case. The author cannot be held responsible for errors or consequences from the use or misuse of the information presented in this book. The author makes no warranties, express or implied, with respect to the contents of this publication. The information presented here is not a substitute for advice, opinions, or instructions from a physician familiar with the specifics of the patient's condition. It is the sole responsibility of the treating physician, with the full respect of the presenting condition, medical history, and experience, to determine the best treatment options for any given patient or condition. Neither the publisher nor the author assumes any responsibility for any injury or damage to persons or property.

TABLE OF CONTENTS

Acknowledgments vi

Introduction 1

Part One: Injuries in Children 3
  1. Play It Safe! 5
  2. Overuse Injuries 7
  3. General Advice for Children in Sports 14
  4. Knee Pain in Young Children and Teenagers 19

Part Two: The Knee 27
  5. The Unreliable Knee 29
  6. "Water on the Knee" 34
  7. ACL: Anterior Cruciate Ligament Tears 42
  8. Deformities of the Knee and Osteoarthritis 56
  9. Meniscus Tears: Torn "Cartilage" in the Knee 61
 10. Other Cartilage Defects 70
 11. Kneecap Pain and Dislocations 76
 12. Injury to the Knee Extensor Mechanism 83
 13. Loose Bodies, Cartilage Defects, Bone Bruises, Stress Fractures, and Cartilage Loss 90
 14. Knee Replacements 95

Part Three: The Shoulder 97
 15. Frozen Shoulder (Adhesive Capsulitis) 100
 16. Shoulder Instability and Dislocations 105
 17. Torn Cartilage in the Shoulder: "SLAP" Tears 113
 18. Rotator Cuff Tears 117
 19. Biceps Tendon: Tendonitis, Partial Tears, Subluxation, and Ruptures 129
 20. The AC Joint 134
 21. Clavicle Fractures 139

Part Four: Sports Tumors, General Injury Prevention, and Bone Health 149
 22. What Are Sports Tumors? 151
 23. Bone Health and General Injury Prevention 157

Special Section: "Why Am I in Pain?" 161
 24. Why Am I In Pain? 163
 25. What to Tell Your MD and Why 165

Appendix IA: Knee Anatomy 169
Appendix IB: Shoulder Anatomy 170
Appendix II: Physical Therapy 171
Appendix III: Q&A with Dr. Reznik 177

Appendix IV: Making the Most of Your Office Visit 182
Glossary 185
Dr. Reznik's Pulications..197
Websites of Interest 201
Dr. Reznik's Patents 202
Index 203
Author Bio 209

This handbook was written with great appreciation for all the lessons my patients have taught me in 30-plus years of practice. I thank them for letting me into their lives, allowing me to help them navigate their medical problems and help restore their activity level as best as possible when injured. There is a great joy in healing people.

The book is also dedicated to all the teachers, mentors, colleagues, and friends who have shared their orthopaedic experience and knowledge with me. None of this would be possible without the kindness of those who taught me the art of being an orthopaedic surgeon. It is my wish that the information here will be a small part of paying it forward to the many students who will learn some hard-earned wisdom and help them help patients in the future. This book is also in recognition that successful treatments are a partnership between the doctor and the patient. The best-educated patient makes the best-healing partner.

Hence, this book is for those who need to know more about their knee and shoulder ailments and need to have their path to successfully treating those ailments explained by a friendly voice.

—AMR

ACKNOWLEDGMENTS

I am grateful to have been taught by very smart and caring teachers: the clinical faculty at New York's Mount Sinai Hospital during my orthopaedic residency; Professor Robert Duthie and everyone on the "top floor" at Oxford University's Orthopaedic Department; and Dale Daniel, Ray Sachs, Mary Lou Stone, Steven Shoemaker, and Don Fithian from the San Diego sports fellowship. They are the people who helped me shape my daily clinical practice and my zeal for teaching.

I thank my wife Elizabeth for her endless support for all my side projects and her role as a photographer, proofreader, and life partner. And with great pride, I thank my daughter Jane, who at age 18 thought it was a good idea to work with her dad on a project that may help people better understand orthopaedics. She was instrumental in getting the first edition of this book off the ground using language that she would find clarifying, not confusing.

A special thanks to my editor, Michele Turk, who was willing to take on this project. She guided the second edition and pushed me to expand the individual sections and add material. She continually asked the questions needed to bring the text up to date with the latest advances in the field. I also want to thank GMK Writing and Editing, Gary Krebs, Elizabeth Crooks, Libby Kingsbury, and Katie Benoit, who helped to polish this new and greatly improved final version.

This work is for my patients, who remind me each day how important it is for us to educate them. Through them it has become clear that the best-educated patient can participate in shared decision-making with their physician and become the most successful after treatment. It is my hope that this book will give patients outside my own practice the same advantage of knowing more about what ails them and help them participate in improving their own orthopaedic health.

INTRODUCTION

REMEMBER HOW IT SOUNDED WHEN THE ADULTS SPOKE TO THE FAMOUS CARTOON character Charlie Brown? To me, it is the same as listening to a doctor after he says, "It looks like you may need surgery." It is in my patients' eyes. The look down or at the wall. It's all a mystery and somewhat frightening. Just like in Charlie Brown, all they hear is "Wah-wah wah-wah. . . ." Nothing I say makes sense to them; they are instantly lost in a fog of all the bad stories they have ever heard, and they are scared.

Telling anyone that surgery was an option seemed to cause them both short-term memory loss and retrograde amnesia. It was worrisome. No one was listening to a thing I said. With this in mind, I started to write short information booklets for my patients. The "wah-wahs" become clearer when written down. To this day the booklets contain a summary of the problems they have, the possible treatments, and the care afterward. I ask my patients to read the information and write down their questions for the next visit. It is like surgery homework. I even encourage them to bring family members with them to go over the answers. Now there are my online videos to help explain the procedures. There is a list of frequently asked questions (with the answers) and even an article on how to make the most of your office visit.

It became clear to me that the common complaints of knees locking, buckling, and giving way were poorly understood and that too many children were being injured while participating in sports. Most of their injuries occurred because the adults around them lacked understanding of simple safety precautions for growing children or lacked appreciation for the special concerns we have for injuries to growing bones. Thus, this book was born.

Inside, you will find articles on a series of common knee and shoulder problems. They contain tips for understanding your diagnoses and many of the most preferred treatment options. There are sections on childhood injuries, injury prevention or "playing it safe," bone health, why we have pain, and "sports" tumors. Of course, this book cannot be a substitute for a good physical exam by an experienced physician nor can it give you an exact diagnosis. Once you have a diagnosis, the information here can help you understand your own knee or shoulder problem. In my experience, the well-informed patients can participate more fully in their own recoveries and get the best of all possible results.

It is my sincere hope that this understanding, along with expert treatment by your doctor, will help you avoid complications and improve your chances of an excellent outcome.

—**Alan M. Reznik, MD, MBA, FAAOS**

PART ONE

INJURIES IN CHILDREN

Children and their parents find that sports can be a great source of exercise and social interaction. They also provide a way to teach the young athlete team building, self-respect, and goal setting. Youth sports can deliver the rewards of gratification, local fame, a college scholarship, or even a professional career. Sports can have other benefits, too, such as physical fitness, the teaching of life lessons, and the ability to accept constructive criticism. More than this, they can help young people balance schoolwork, screen time, and playtime—something that is hard to do these days. Moreover, the health benefits of sports cannot be overemphasized. Nevertheless, concerns may arise when sports are taken to the extreme at a young age. This extreme can take the "fun" out of "fun and games," lower a child's self-esteem, and make happy children unhappy with, sadly, very disappointed parents.

In this section of the book, we will see tips on when to see the doctor as well as how to avoid injuries, improve some elements of sports performance, and help the growing young athlete avoid things that may alter their ability to play sports later in life.

1 PLAY IT SAFE!

OFTEN, SPORTS MEDICINE PHYSICIANS SEE PATIENTS WITH STRESS INJURIES from too much of one sport. When we are responsible for caring for child athletes, we need to remember that sports should always be fun for children, not unhealthy or dangerous.

Parents must be aware that they, coaches, and trainers can push children into year-round, single-sport activity, yet unsupervised sports, multiple leagues, and year-round participation in a single sport can cause frustration and athlete burnout. This type of overtraining has been proven to increase overuse injuries and sometimes leads to career-ending injuries among young athletes. More recently, college recruiters have noted that child athletes who play more than one sport are more attractive than those who play only one sport. These recruiters and coaches have come to appreciate and respect the overlapping of multisport skills in the "best of the best" athletes. This may make the single-sport focus, which has been popular for so many years, less desirable for future child athletes. For these reasons, the American Academy of Orthopaedic Surgeons (AAOS) launched an awareness campaign on single-sport injuries to help parents avoid falling into the single-sport trap with their children.

In the US alone, there are over three-quarters of a million emergency room visits each year by children under the age of 15. A major cause of this is the alarming rate of injuries that occur while children play sports. "Play It Safe," one of the first sports injury prevention campaigns, was created by the AAOS. The idea originated in the 1970s, with a campaign for powerline safety in the UK, which was followed by a similar water safety campaign for children in the late 1980s, and after that, a campaign for youth sports. In the US, the "Play It Safe" campaign was designed to increase awareness and to reduce injuries to children during athletic activities. It promoted the use of helmets when biking, the improvement of playground designs, and the awareness of dehydration and heat stroke.

This campaign and others have highlighted that most injuries in children occur in unorganized or casual sports, such as pickup games of basketball, baseball, and football. Still significant, though, is that organized league sports make up about one-third of injuries. As the "Play It Safe" campaign expresses, reducing the risk of injury in both organized and casual sports should be a goal of the parents, teachers, and coaches involved in youth sports.

Since the 1970s, there have been many more initiatives. These include the NFL's "Play 60" program, which promotes basic physical exercise to improve children's health, and in 2018, the AAOS launched its "OneSport" campaign to make doctors and parents aware of the dangers of overuse injuries.

Below are some **Facts about Overuse Sports Injuries** that appear on the AAOS's OrthoInfo website (See Websites of Interest, page 201.)

- Overuse injuries in children happen gradually over time but can have a lifelong effect on their athletic abilities, health, and quality of life.

- When a young child whose body is still growing and developing repeatedly participates in one type of athletic activity, their body does not have enough time to heal properly between sessions of playing.

- Intense and repetitive training can lead to pediatric trauma and may require surgery to shoulders, knees, elbows, and wrists.

- While most experts agree that some degree of sports specialization is necessary, there is much debate about how early intense training should begin.

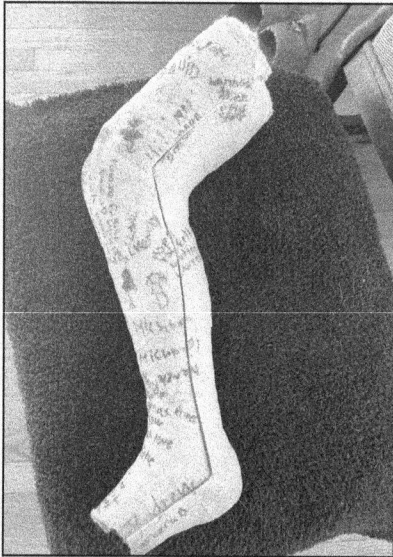

This is a photo of a cast used in treatment for a tibia fracture in a nine-year-old very active little leaguer. He fractured his tibia sliding into a base in a baseball game over 25 years ago. He returned to full sports within four months after injury. Since then, he served in the military and became a police officer. He remains fully active in many sports with no pain or limitations. This highlights the choice between casting and surgery. Young children, unlike adults, have the potential to completely remodel or reshape bones as they grow so healing fractures mend and straighten over time.

In many cases, a fracture allows it to heal without surgery and the fracture disappears as the child grows, leaving no deformity, deficiency, or abnormality on X-rays in adulthood. Parents may not like the cast, yet, in the right setting, surgery is avoided. The outcome can be the same or better with fewer complications, and a cast might be well worth the inconvenience.

2 OVERUSE INJURIES

OVERUSE INJURIES ARE MUCH MORE COMMON THAN MOST PEOPLE THINK. MORE often they are a result of increasing sports-specific training or heavy exercise at a rate that is faster than the rate the muscle, tendons, bones, and joints can adjust to the new loads. In increased activities or high-level competitive sports, there are physiologic changes that are needed for the more intense new exercise or sports activity. Most people think of gaining strength or increasing aerobic activity and forget the dynamic nature of the human body. Muscles require weight-bearing stress, rest periods, increased protein in the diet, and time to grow larger. Tendons may need to lengthen or shorten to the ideal length for the desired activity. Bones need to become stronger, and joints need rest periods to avoid cartilage failure.

If we don't pay attention to the needs of all the structures, muscles fatigue and tear; tendons develop tendonitis, partial tears, or rupture; bones develop stress fractures; and joints swell. This quickly causes a loss of all the muscle gains as the body shuts down. Overuse injuries frequently end seasons for young athletes or force them to change position or even sports. So, what are the most common ones and what can we do to prevent them?

Overuse Injuries Affect Many Young Athletes

Overuse injuries are seen among athletes between the ages of five and 14 in many common sports, often from overtraining in preparation for competition. Here are statistics showing the population of injured young athletes due to overuse, in order of most frequent to least frequent.

- 28% of football players
- 25% of baseball players
- 22% of soccer players
- 15% of basketball players
- 12% of softball players

The AAOS promotes the idea, "Youth sports should always be fun. The 'winning at all costs' attitude of coaches, parents, professional athletes, and peers can lead to injury." Remember, having unrealistic expectations can lead a child to continue to play despite warning signs of injury. This puts the child at increased risk. Lastly, the AAOS reminds us, "Coaches and parents can prevent injuries by fostering an atmosphere of healthy competition that emphasizes self-reliance, confidence, and cooperation, [leading to] a positive self-image, rather than just winning." See the AAOS website on OrthoInfo (see Websites of Interest, page 201).

Young Athletes Are Not Just Small Adults

Children are growing all the time. This gives them some advantages over adults when it comes to their risk of injury. To start, their bones have a little more spring and are more likely to bend before they break. Children are shorter, and hence, lower to the ground, which gives them a lower center of gravity and a shorter distance to fall. They also weigh less than adults, making most minor falls fairly inconsequential. At the same time, they tend to be less prepared for injury. All of these factors help to explain some of the injuries that are most prevalent in child athletes.

In addition:

- A child's sense of danger is far less than that of an adult.

- Children grow at differing rates and at different times during development.

- A sudden growth spurt or a change in limb length can create the gawky behavior that makes some children accident-prone.

For example, during times of rapid growth many things are happening at once. The bones in children grow in areas near each joint, known as the growth plates, and if this occurs more quickly than in the rest of the body, the rest of the body must catch up. The muscles can become tighter as they try to get longer, lagging behind the rapid growth of the bones. With the body's newly lengthened limbs, the brain does not know exactly where the hands and feet end. This is because the internal nerve systems for position, sense, and balance are out of tune with the child's longer limbs. It is as if their internal "GPS" of limb position loses its signal for a while. Coordination decreases and athletic skills that were excellent only a few months earlier seem to disappear. When this happens, there is a decrease in playing ability for almost all sports, which can be a source of embarrassment for the child, on top of their physical awkwardness. Injuries frequently follow as the parents and child try to rush Mother Nature's ability to catch up by overplaying or doing too much training.

Age-Size-Weight Mismatch

Adults must be aware of their children's limits, given their size and weight. Some kids are fully grown at 14, while others are not. I often hear stories of children in an age-based league playing against kids who weigh 50 to 100 pounds more than they do—especially in football. Worse yet, some parents hold kids back in kindergarten so that they will have an advantage throughout all future sports, stemming from being slightly older and larger. That may work fine for a while, but all the other kids catch up eventually, and this strategy only has limited value in the short run.

To "help" children with age-size-weight differences, many parents and young athletes have turned to hormones and supplements. Even though food supplements are very popular nowadays, as they are considered "safer" than hormones and steroids, they are still problematic. Creatine is one supplement that can increase muscle size and, possibly, strength, but it is not healthy for many athletes, especially those in need of agility. This supplement may not improve performance in some sports in which flexibility, reflexes, balance, and speed are more important than brute strength, yet it may in other sports. Moreover, creatine involves certain risks, as well. It can pull water into the muscle cells, indirectly resulting in dehydration; it can cause muscle cramps; and in rare cases, it can lead to kidney problems (renal insufficiency).

In my practice, I frequently see young athletes pursue the goal of pure strength over agility and balance. They use steroids, creatine, and growth hormones inappropriately. All of this ends up reducing their performance in skill-based sports. Most often, it is a pitcher, basketball player, or tennis star who has huge quadriceps from doing leg presses but cannot stand on one leg for more than 30 seconds or do a one-legged squat without tipping to one side or the other. It turns out that, during heavy weight training, the larger weights do not train the smaller muscles needed for hip control and balance. Furthermore, a weakness in the force chain, which passes from the arm to the ground through the hip, combined with weak balance control, can lead to elbow and shoulder injuries or falls when certain athletes, such as lacrosse, soccer, basketball, or football players, have even low-impact collisions.

Many coaches and parents take children's performance to an extreme level from very young ages. They lie about a child's age or weight to give them an unfair advantage, which is simply wrong. Worse yet, studies have shown that since the late 1990s, up to 500,000 male and female young athletes in the US were using black market steroids to increase muscle mass each year. Today, many of these same substances are banned in professional and Olympic sports for good reason. The risks they pose are serious and, in extreme cases, potentially life-threatening for children.

On rare occasions children are deficient in hormones that prevent normal growth, and specialists prescribe growth hormones to help correct for delayed growth. Occasionally, misguided parents or teenagers who feel pressured to excel think that these same drugs will enhance both growth and performance even when there is no reason to give these hormones to a healthy child without a documented deficiency. They have risks of causing premature maturation and early growth plate arrest. The result could be wider, shorter bones, and children can end up shorter than they would have otherwise been because of a loss of long-term growth. These "performance-enhancing" or "growth" products should be completely avoided in otherwise typical, active, growing children.

Injuries in Growing Children Create Special Concerns

I have operated on adults many times for problems that were caused by childhood injuries that were neglected many years earlier. That's why it's important to be aware of injuries in the growing child that may cause a bone deformity in adulthood that can lead to loss of use of a joint or premature arthritis. We all need to remember that children's growth plates are softer than calcified bone in the middle of the limbs and, therefore, are more susceptible to injury in the active child. When an injury to a growth plate occurs, both future growth and alignment of the limb are at risk if the injury is not recognized and treated properly.

Children's growing bones can buckle and bend without breaking all the way. This creates fractures in the middle of the bone, which are often known as "greenstick" fractures since they resemble what happens when you try to break a growing tree branch. These greenstick fractures break, deform, and stay deformed, even though part of the bone (branch) is still intact. Both growth plate and greenstick fractures affect bone growth.

At the very same time, the good news is that because the child is growing, he or she can remodel some deformed or broken bones and often overcome minor disturbances in growth. In my orthopaedic practice, we use many ways to decide if a given fracture in a growing child is a cause for alarm or can correct itself. The child's age, the fracture location, the bone's angulation (amount of bend), and the fragment's displacement (separation) are important factors in determining how well a fracture will heal without orthopaedic surgical intervention.

For example, if an eight-year-old breaks his collar bone, we can accept a good amount of angulation (bending of the fracture). We know the body will remodel it as it heals and grows back to its natural shape without surgery. Typically, for a fracture in the middle of straight bone in a growing child, we can accept up to twenty-five degrees of angulation, minus the age at the time of the injury. For an eight-year-old, that would be seventeen degrees. In figure 2, we see three

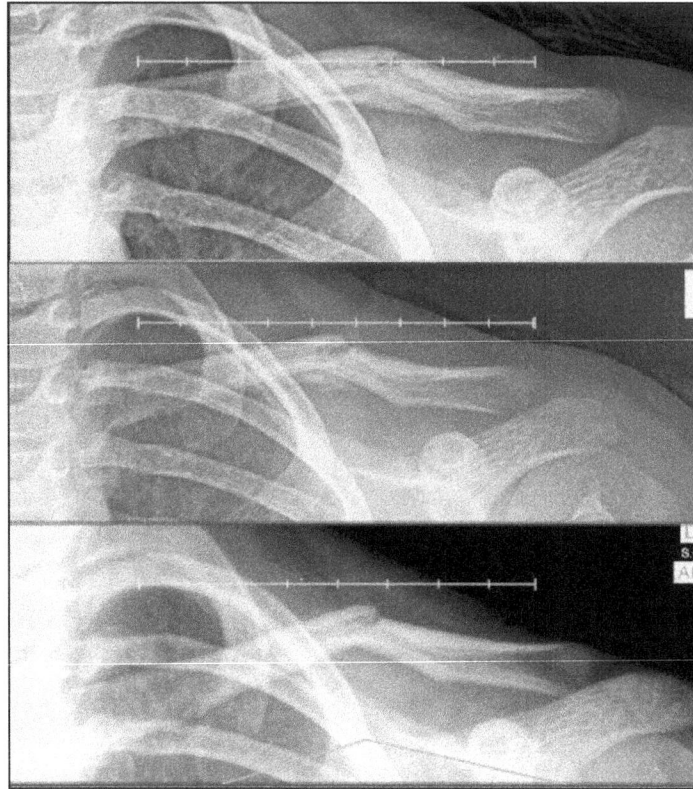

2 Clavicle fracture in an eight-year-old child.

views of the same fracture of a period of eight weeks. The lower image is the first x-ray, then the middle image is approximately three to four weeks later, and the top image is at eight weeks. The bone is healing and "growing straighter" than the original broken alignment. The deformity is correcting itself as expected.

Understanding the position, deformity, energy of impact, and age of the patient can also help us to determine and make a "prediction" of the outcomes with no treatment, cast reduction, or surgery. After a growth plate injury, if a deformity will result without treatment, prompt treatment by an orthopaedic surgeon is necessary.

Children can also develop special injuries from sports or repetitive use, including pitcher's elbow, jumper's knee, Osgood Schlatter's disease, stress fractures, and osteochondral fractures. These can all cause issues into adulthood if allowed to persist untreated and will be discussed in more detail later in the book. For the most part, these injuries are unique to growing children and are frequently overlooked, although many of the problems resulting from these injuries are not fully appreciated until adulthood.

Unique Diagnoses and Treatments Only Seen in Children

"Children are not small adults," my Yale Medical School professors used to say. This is true in so many ways. Their bones are actively growing. The area of growth is softer than the rest of the bone. Their bones have more flexibility. They are more like a young tree branch than a mature oak branch. Their muscles are getting longer all the time. Their coordination changes as they go through growth spurts. Because they grow quickly, they just don't know where the ends of their limbs are. They lose sports skills until they can retune their muscle memory for a specific sport. These factors together help explain injuries only seen in growing children.

Growth Plate Injuries: A Tricky Diagnosis in Children

As children grow, their growth plates add new cells. These young bone cells have no calcium so they cannot be seen on an X-ray. So, when the calcified bone does not line up correctly after an injury or there is a deformity, we must assume there is a growth plate injury. In these cases, a precise history of the injury (the force involved, the position of the limb, the direction of impact, and the anatomic location of the injury) helps to ensure a correct diagnosis. Therefore, there is no substitute for an examination by experienced hands because many of the findings we may see on an X-ray are often only seen once new bone is being made and the healing process is well underway. Many times, when we see X-ray changes as a result of a growth plate injury it is too late to easily correct the damage to the growth plate.

In young children, many injuries can be treated with a sling, splint, or cast. Other injuries absolutely require a perfect realignment of the broken pieces to avoid a loss of growth or a long-term deformity. This means that sometimes a missed diagnosis becomes a missed opportunity for a simpler treatment. In practice, the goal of all treatments should be to provide the least invasive treatment that allows a child's bones to heal with the lowest risk of future deformity and loss of future growth. This may require special techniques that would not be used in adults. Many of the adult repair methods are not useful in children. Some of these techniques can injure the growth plate and should be avoided. In general, orthopaedic surgeons are the most experienced in these issues as well as how to avoid them.

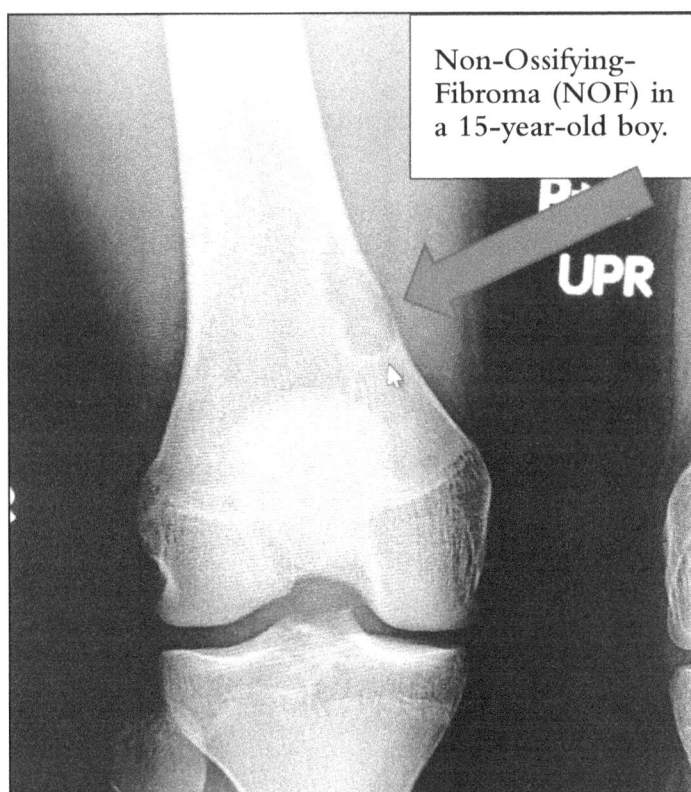

Non-Ossifying-Fibroma (NOF) in a 15-year-old boy.

3 Benign bone lesion common in children. NOF, non-ossifying-fibroma. Occurs in early teens and often self-resolves through skeletal maturity.

Noncancerous Bone Lesions

In children and adolescents, we sometimes see bone abnormalities that are present but not cancerous. These are often found after an injury and are frequently not related to the injury itself. An NOF (non-ossifying fibroma) is one such lesion (see Image 3).

NOFs are thought to be remnants of the growing cartilage and usually self-resolve (disappear) when the bone is fully mature. Simple observation can make everyone feel happier, as often they slowly go away. If they change in shape, enlarge, or persist, then further evaluation may be needed.

Understanding Proper Nutrition

It is well-known that during periods of rapid growth, the growth plates enlarge by making new cartilage that later in the growth process become calcified and then turns into new hard bone. During rapid growth, the new cartilage forms faster than the calcification. Therefore, the fast-growing growth plates are softer than bone, and they are more prone to injury. It is important to remember that a growing child needs protein, calcium, vitamin D, vitamin C, and a good diet with calories to make new bone. Furthermore, good nutrition and vitamin intake, including calcium, vitamin D, and vitamin C, are important for proper bone formation and bone health.

Without the calcium and vitamins C and D, the bones don't mature as fast and can even become deformed. Vitamin D deficiency causes a disease called rickets, a malnourished state that occurs when the soft growth plates bend under daily use. The most notable change is seen in the knees, which become bowed as the child grows. Vitamin D has been added to milk products in many countries around the world for this very reason. Before vitamin D was added to milk, we saw vitamin D deficiency and rickets far more often than we do today.

Obesity in children is another concern. It is well-documented that a child can be overweight and still be malnourished if they eat an unbalanced diet with inadequate nutrition. It is also possible for a person to eat a healthy diet and become overweight if they have other medical problems, like low thyroid function. When the thyroid does not function properly, or there is a lack of iodide in the diet, a child's metabolism is slowed, and they gain significant weight. Children who are gaining weight, lethargic, and always tired should have their thyroid function checked. Between the ages of eight and 12, these children are prone to a special growth plate injury called a slipped capital femoral epiphysis (it's a tongue twister, so we say "skiffee" for short, using the initials SCFE). When a SCFE occurs, the growth plate at the ball of the hip starts to crack and slip.

The quicker a physician attends to this type of injury, the better, because the less slip, the better. If the growth plate is slipping, it needs to be pinned in place to prevent it from falling off the shaft. If it does, the chance of advanced arthritis later in life is much higher than normal. At the same time, this typically occurs in overweight children, so they must have nutritional checks (like vitamin D level and protein level in the blood as well as thyroid testing).

Dos and Don'ts of Injury Prevention in the Child Athlete

More children are competing in youth sports than ever before, and they are starting at younger ages, which may increase the risk of injury. Understanding the risks to children are different than adults. There are some specific tips for injury prevention in young athletes. These are some of the more important dos and don'ts.

Do:

- Young athletes should be encouraged to play in organized or supervised sports.

- Be an organizer and participate as an adult to make sure your child is safe. Organized sports can offer the protection of adult supervision, safety rules, and lessons in good sportsmanship.

- Children should have training, specific stretching, and exercise programs to prepare them for sports. They should also warm up and stretch before participating in sports.

- Children should drink plenty of fluids.

- Children should have appropriately fitting equipment.

Don't:

- Don't forget that coaches and parents should consider the child's age, height, and weight before matching them in sports based on age alone.

- Don't be an absent parent. The parent should be sure the coaches have appropriate training and qualifications to coach their children.

- Don't forget that safety starts with the field and equipment. Children must have access to a safe playing area and appropriate, well-maintained equipment.

- Don't forget to check the conditions every time your child participates in a competition. Field conditions, weather conditions, and available supervision should always be factors when deciding to have a competition.

- Don't forget that children have less control over how much they sweat and their fluid intake than adults. Smaller bodies have a higher surface area per body weight. They sweat more water in the heat per pound than adults, and they also get cold faster in the winter. In hot weather, parents should be sure that their children are well-hydrated and be aware of the risks of hyperthermia on very hot and humid days.

- Don't forget that single-sport children have higher injury rates. A single sport itself, with or without preparation, should not be a child's only form of exercise. A good balance of different activities (for example, biking, swimming, and hiking with the family in the off season) offers different exercise value and lower injury rates than an extra tackle football practice.

3 GENERAL ADVICE FOR CHILDREN IN SPORTS

THERE ARE SIMPLE GUIDELINES TO FOLLOW FOR CHILDREN IN SPORTS. THESE INCLUDE using appropriately sized gear and ensuring safe settings for safe sports. There must be enough adult supervision and an understanding of the safe physical limits for the growing child at each stage of development. Here are some tips on appropriate gear, field conditions, weather conditions, available supervision, pitching limits, and improving quality exercises for young athletes.

Use Appropriate Gear

Protective gear is important and sport-specific. The correct size equipment should always be used. Hand-me-downs should also be checked for proper fit and function. Older, broken protective equipment like helmets and shoulder pads do not prevent injury. Due to our increased awareness of the serious long-term effects of concussions and possible brain injury, using the proper sport-specific helmets for biking, skiing, and roller-skating are no longer optional. Mouth guards, shin guards, and plastic face guards have helped to reduce injuries and should always be used. Face shields have dramatically reduced permanent eye injuries. Elbow pads and wrist protectors should be worn for in-line skating, even on pathways designed for skating. Binding releases for skis should be tested and calibrated to the child's skill level, height, and weight each and every season.

Consider Field Conditions, Weather Conditions, and Available Supervision

These three factors should always be considered when deciding whether to have a competition.

Monitor Field Conditions

At the start of each season, the fields themselves need to be inspected. AstroTurf does not last forever (max is 8–10 years), and aging artificial fields are dangerous and sometimes require repair or updating. Artificial turf fields do develop hard spots, seams split, areas become matted, and drainage becomes poor, causing slippery puddles. These are warnings the field is becoming unsafe for use. Indoor turf on concrete also increases injury risk. Large cleats should be avoided, especially for young players. If cleats are properly used, they should match the surface on which the athletes are playing. Sharp grass cleats should not ever be used on artificial turf. The feet stick to the ground, the leg twists with a higher force, and knee injuries skyrocket.

Monitor Weather Conditions

In hot weather, parents should be sure that their children are well-hydrated and be aware of the risks of hyperthermia on very hot and humid days. There are specific play rules for heat and humidity. Each year children and young adults die of heat stroke because they are not hydrated enough, or they are playing with too much equipment for a very hot day. Likewise, there are days when the heat and humidity make it impossible to sweat normally. Heat builds up in children, leading to heatstroke and deaths on "no-play days" every summer. Playing football in full equipment in preseason summer camps is the most common cause. However, heatstroke is preventable. Many football camps in the summer don't allow children to "suit up" and only play flag football during practice until the weather cools down. On the days when the temperature and humidity are both high and normal sweating is not enough to cool an active child, no one should be on the field. It is just too dangerous.

Have Available Supervision

Appropriate supervision is a more complex issue these days. It is rare that coaches have professional training or are fully aware of many sports-related safety issues. For example, many Little League® coaches are parents and don't know or, worse, don't follow the pitch and throw count rules. Many have personal conflicts of interest. Some have a child on the team and are willing to bend the rules for their own child to pitch or to give their own child more playing time than others. This has its own implications for their child's safety. Some feel a win or loss is their own personal triumph and will push kids past the point of fun.

Youth sports are for gaining skills in the sport itself, learning social norms, experiencing the importance of teamwork, and learning the ability to be a good winner, not a sore loser. It is a place where bullying can occur and should be handled by the adults in a positive, corrective light. Parents should not be helicopters and yet should have some clear understanding of the lessons to be learned by fair sporting competition. The interest of the parents and coaches in a win should never override the safety of all involved. Competition should have some element of fun for all involved.

Coaches should know basic first aid, what to do and not do if a child injures their neck, and basic up-to-date cardiopulmonary resuscitation (CPR) training. They should also know the signs of cardiac events and when someone may have heat exhaustion, heat stroke, and/or dehydration.

Observe Pitching Limits for Growing Children and Young Adults

We have all heard the expression, "Be careful, or you might throw your arm out." What is this all about? In a young athlete, a "thrown out arm" can be a result of "overthrowing." This most often occurs when an overzealous coach, parent, or even the athlete themself tries to get around the pitch count rules. Sadly, this practice is widespread. After all, who doesn't want to win a tough game? Everyone thinks, "Why not use your best pitcher in a pinch? How can it hurt?"

Yet, it can literally hurt the young pitcher.

All young athletes are growing, and there are very delicate areas of the bone that provide this growth. Immature cartilage expands and swells, and these cells are eventually replaced by new bone. This special area of bone is called the growth plate. It is vulnerable to stress and repetitive motion. If damaged, growth can be stopped or stunted. The soft cartilage around the growth plate can also crack and fail, causing loose bodies to form in the elbow (for similar issues of locking and swelling, see chapter 13 on loose bodies in the knee). These injuries can ruin even a bright pitching future, and in most of these cases, overthrowing or ignoring pitch counts are major culprits (see Images 4 and 5 on the following pages).

Everyone likes to believe that their child will become the next Tom Seaver, Serena Williams, Roger Clemens, Mariano Rivera, Tom Brady, Shaquille O'Neal, Tiger Woods, or Roger Federer. The coaches know this and are taking their cue from the excited parents who truly believe that their kid is Superman (or some other invincible comic book character). The result is that they all want to skirt the rules, even when the leagues are highly supervised. So, coaches and parents let ball players pitch year-round, "forget" the date of the last full game they pitched, or worse, neglect to press the pitch counter button in the middle of a game, so the count can be "accidentally" extended (this last one I would not have believed if I had not seen it myself during a heated game between two local rival teams when the parent/coach just wanted his kid to stay in the game and be the "hero" that day).

Parents and coaches need to know that the average age when most professional pitchers start pitching was at one time as high as 17 years old, and many players don't even pitch before the end of high school or early in college. Overpitching and injuring a promising 10-year-old's elbow, shoulder, knee, or growth potential has never resulted in a Major League star. Knowing this, dual seasons and multiple additional travel teams should be avoided. Safety rules for growing athletes, such as pitch counts (see the box below), should be strictly followed, and children should not be played in multiple leagues in the same sport in the same season to get around these rules, no matter how great an athlete the parents think their child is. The rules are designed to protect growing children from injury; ignoring the rules will risk serious growth injury and only shorten their playing careers.

The eligibility of a player to pitch in a Little League® baseball game is governed by a pitch count that is related to the number of pitches throw in a given game. The pitch count also

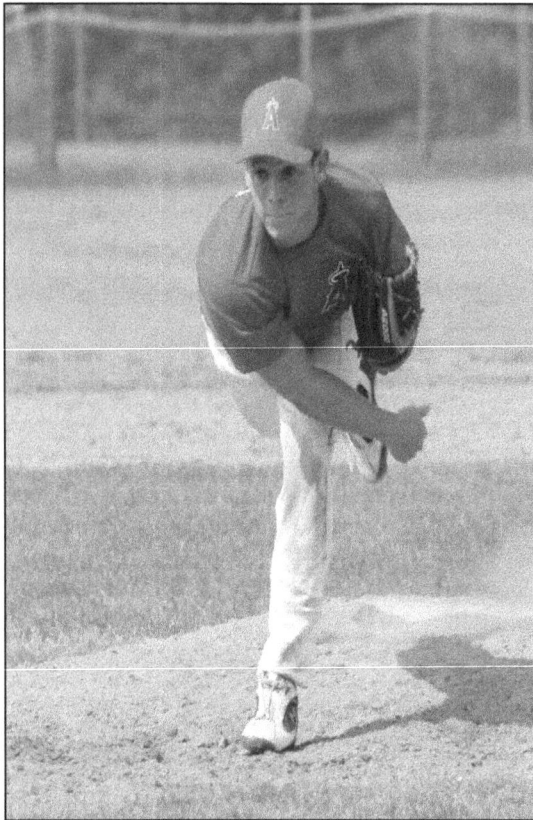

4 Single leg stance in fastball pitching. Power is generated through a ground reaction force on the supporting leg. Hip strength and balance are very important in pitching well.

What are some basic pitching rules?

- No curve balls before age 14.
- For younger players, a good rule of thumb is no more than 5.5 pitches per year of age per game.
- In young players, no more than 1,000 pitches per full season.
- For older players (with more mature bones), no more than 75 pitches per game, and no more than 2,000 pitches per full season.
- No more than 8 months of pitching per year.
- No dual season (pitching for more than one team in the same season, which is much more common than one may expect).

determines how many days of rest are required before that player may pitch again in a Little League® game. These are nationally accepted standards. Beware of the parent that thinks these are "stupid rules" and has a young child pitch in multiple leagues to "make the pitcher better" because they think they are not getting enough innings of play. These parents rarely get away with it; shoulder and elbow grow plate injuries occur, and those children rarely pitch in higher level leagues.

Little League® Baseball	
Ages 6–8	50 pitches per day
Ages 9–10	75 pitches per day
Ages 11–12	85 pitches per day
Ages 13–16	95 pitches per day

RESTING RULES

Age 14 and younger

Pitch count	days of rest
1–20	0
21–35	1
36–50	2
51–65	3
66–85 (age 12)	4
66–95 (age 13-16)	4

Official Pitch count for Lesser-Known Catcher Rules

Any player who has played the position of catcher in four (4) or more innings in a game is not eligible to pitch on that calendar day.

A player who played the position of catcher for three (3) innings or less, moves to the pitcher position, and delivers 21 pitches or more (**15- and 16-year-olds:** 31 pitches or more) in the same day may not return to the catcher position on that calendar day and must follow the pitch count rest rules.

(Adapted for this book, data from the Little League® official web site 2023.)

5 Pitch Count: pitching safety rules for adolescent pitchers to prevent growth plate injuries.

Monitor Exercise and Form

Parents need to remember that a season off gives the growing areas of bone time to recover. In more mature players, above age 14, light lifting in season helps strengthen other muscles and prevent some injuries. They also need to know that repetitive lifting of very heavy weights can crush the new growth cells and indirectly stunt growth. Lifting very heavy weights creates more strong, slow-twitch fibers that can crowd out the body's fast-twitch muscle. This will make muscles heavier, less flexible, and slower. In turn, more slow-twitch muscle fibers will decrease throwing speed. Yes, you can overdo it with weight lifting and lose pitching velocity!

Core and balance exercises are key to good form and help transfer force from the ground to the ball. **The ability to transfer force from the legs to the arms is the key to throwing harder and faster.** If the hips and core are weak, a child is forced to throw with only the force of the arm. Small children can get away with this in low-demand leagues, but in adolescents and teens this quickly becomes a weakness that cannot be overcome without throwing or burning the arm out. A combination of great core strength, hip control, and balance takes stress off the arm, elbow, and shoulder.

Parents of pitchers should find out if their child's pitching form is an issue. It is more helpful to have a pitching coach check it and make the needed corrections than to add weight training to bad form. Always pull pitchers from a game if a pitch hits the ground in front of the plate or they throw over the backstop. These are warning signs that the star pitcher is getting tired and an injury is right around the corner.

Children should be encouraged to tell a supervising adult when they are hurt instead of trying to play through painful injuries. Last, children should never be given performance-enhancing drugs or supplements.

4 KNEE PAIN IN YOUNG CHILDREN AND TEENAGERS

PAIN IN THE FRONT OF THE KNEE IS ONE OF THE MOST COMMON PROBLEMS SEEN in young children and adolescents. The symptoms of possible knee injuries range from constant pain to pain only with heavy activity. The potential causes range from tendonitis to a growth plate injury. In this chapter, we will look at a number of these problems and treatment options.

Osgood-Schlatter's Disease

Osgood-Schlatter's disease (OS) is one of the more common causes of anterior knee pain in a growing child. It is likely to occur in children who participate in sports that involve running and jumping. It is most common in basketball players because of the fast starts, quick stops, and frequent jumps. These repetitive motions put weight on the kneecap (patella), the tendon attached to it (patella tendon), and its attachment to the tibia (the tibial tubercle).

In children, the tibial tubercle is directly above the growth plate. The constant traction provided by some sports on this area can injure the growth plate under the tubercle. Repetitive injury causes the growth plate to stretch or enlarge, leading the bone at the tendon attachment to enlarge as well (see Image 6). When the growth plate is injured, the enlarged bone can be tender, and the growth plate itself can hurt when weight is placed on it. This explains why going up or down stairs, kneeling, running, or jumping can increase knee pain. The problem is caused by microscopic fractures in the growth plate. Furthermore, on rare occasion and with enough force, the tubercle can break. Sometimes a small part can break off, causing a separate piece of bone to form within the patella tendon. This can also create a painful limp that prevents play.

If the growth plate is injured and a piece has broken off, continued activity will worsen the condition. When the individual is running or squatting, the tendon pulls on the tibial tubercle growth plate exactly where the tendon attaches. A gap forms in the growth plate itself, a traction fracture of the soft growing bone, and will enlarge as it tries to heal. A boney bump will form at the top of the tibia exactly where the tendon pulls on it. This bump can be painful and be hard to kneel on in adulthood. It is a cause of chronic tendonitis in adults as well. I have operated on a good number of adults who had OS as a child that was ignored. In many of these cases, I have had to remove the bone spur because of daily pain and loss of function.

Treatment for Osgood-Schlatter's Disease

In general, early treatment for this problem is based on the level of symptoms present. If there is no boney bump, and the area over the tibial attachment (tibial tubercle) is only mildly tender, then rest, ice, and nonsteroidal anti-inflammatory drugs (NSAIDs) may work well. The patient can safely return to sports when the symptoms are gone. While the area is tender, the patient should avoid all activities that cause pain. This includes squatting, kneeling, running, stair climbing (particularly as an exercise), and jumping. The adage "no pain, no gain" does not apply here.

In moderate cases, a bump and gap (or a widening of the growth plate) can be seen on an X-ray. In these cases, the patient may benefit from immobilization with a knee immobilizer, then a period of rest, and a slow return to sports. In severe cases, when walking is painful, the fracture in the growth plate may be unstable or getting worse with activity. When that happens, X-rays of the knee must be taken and reviewed to be sure that there is no significant displacement of the growth plate fracture.

The exam should focus on the injury to the patella tendon's attachment to the bone. If this is broken or separated, it may need to be fixed, although, in the youngest patients, repair runs the risk of an early closure of the anterior growth plate. If this happens, there is a risk of a back bowing of the tibia (so-called recurvatum of the knee, meaning bowing backward). This deformity can be problematic in that the leg is bowed backward when standing and will behave as if the whole limb is shorter than that on the other side. Sometimes surgery is needed to stop the progression of the deformity or correct it after growth stops (see Image 7).

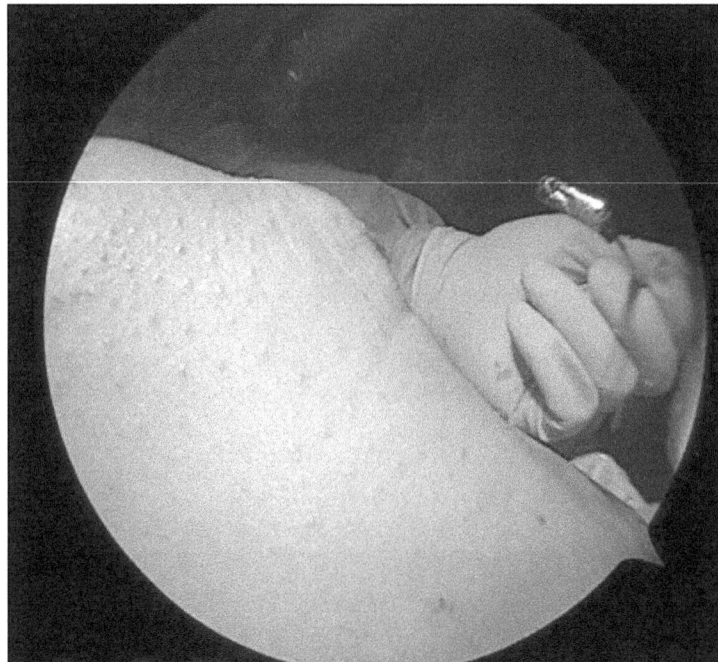

6 Osgood Schlater's disease: elevation of the tibial tubercle from stress on the growth plate. Overuse and overgrowth of the bone.

Jumper's Knee

This problem is very similar to Osgood-Schlatter's, but it occurs on the patella side, as opposed to the tibial tubercle side, of the patella tendon. In this case, the traction causes the lining on the patella (its growth plate) to pull off the bone, resulting in pain and weakness. The traction causes new bone to form, just as it does in OS disease, only on the tip of the knee cap (see Image 8). It is treated according to the symptoms as explained previously. In rare cases, it can also be associated with a "sleeve fracture," which occurs when a small fragment of bone with a sleeve of periosteum (membrane that lines the outer surface of the bone) pulls off the kneecap, weakening the attachment of the tendon and making use of the knee impossible. Operative repair is needed in severely displaced cases.

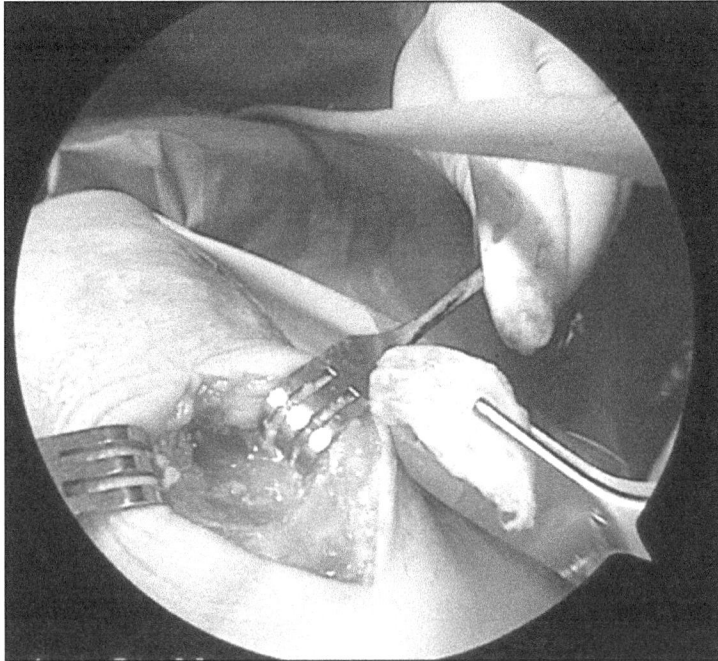

7 Removal of the tibial tubercle fragment when causing symptoms.

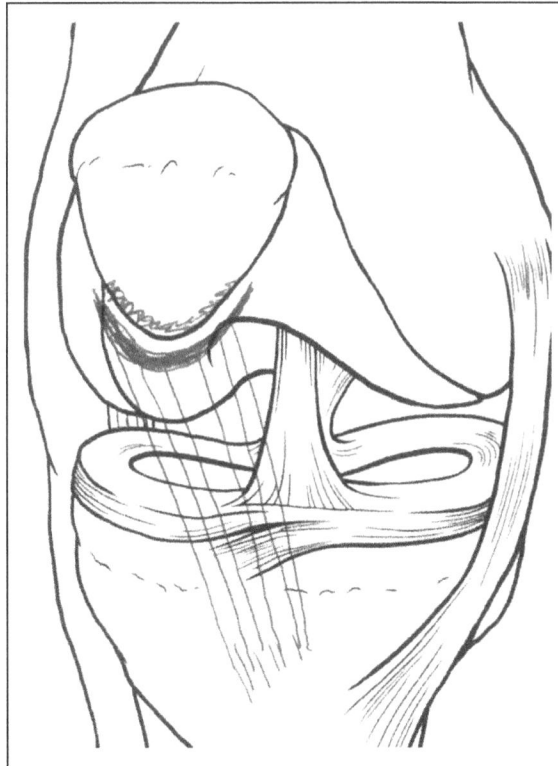

8 Jumpers Knee: stress and stretching (causing tendonitis) of the attachment of the patella tendon to the patella. If severe, the growth of the patella is altered by pulling the growth plate off with the tendon and causing elongation (lengthening) of the bone.

Patellar Tendinitis

When this problem arises, the tendon that connects the tibial tubercle and the patella is inflamed. When the patella tendon becomes inflamed or injured repetitively (from jumping, performing squats, kneeling, crawling, or being a baseball catcher), pain may persist or even become chronic. The tendon hurts when pressed, stretched, or loaded with activity. Fortunately, this is the lesser of anterior knee pain problems and, most often, can be treated with simple measures. Once again, rest, ice, and NSAIDs may be the best treatment, and patients can safely return to sports when their symptoms are gone.

On rare occasions, the tendon can become thickened, tight, or stiff. In some cases, scar tissue forms in the tendon itself (so-called fibrosis of the tendon). The tendon can even develop partial tears or cystic degeneration over time. Immobilization may be needed in patients with more difficult cases involving partial tears. In cases that fail to improve with immobilization through fibrosis of the tendon, or when there are cysts in the tendon on an MRI, partial tears, or activity-limiting pain, surgical exploration may be required. At the time of surgery, the removal of cysts and scar tissue, followed by a period of protection and therapy, often heals the tendon and solves the problem.

Growing Pains

This is the term used by many people to explain any knee pain in children. However, it is not just an old wives' tale. Since rapid bone growth can cause pain as the soft tissues, tendons, and ligaments around the knee try to catch up, particularly during a growth spurt, children may complain of pain with activity or at night after activity. Frequently, it wakes them from sleep. However, this diagnosis should only be used after a complete exam, including X-rays, yields no concrete findings, like those mentioned in this chapter. NSAIDs, local application of ice or warm compresses, rest, and gentle stretching can help ease the pain. Growing pains can also be an indication of bone weakness or poor calcification from metabolic issues like thyroid deficiency, vitamin D deficiency, lack of calcium in the diet, or general malnutrition.

Kneecap or Patellafemoral Pain

This problem is more common in teenage girls than boys and is often due to maltracking (poor alignment) of the kneecap, or simply from softening of the cartilage from overuse. When maltracking or malalignment occurs in the kneecap, it indicates that it is not staying in the groove, which can cause uneven wear or pressure on the kneecap and pain over time. This is discussed in more detail in Part Two, Chapter 11, "Kneecap Pain and Dislocations."

Osteochondritis Dissecans

In osteochondritis dissecans (OCD), a fragment of bone below the joint surface loses its blood supply and, along with the cartilage covering it, separates from the rest of the bone. The bone fragment with its cartilage cover is referred to as an osteochondritis lesion. Without blood flow, the bone under the surface is not viable. Fluid produced by the lining of the joint (the synovium), called synovial fluid, can continue to nourish a broken fragment, and it may enlarge. The fragment can cause locking of the joint, pain, and swelling. Treatment of this problem depends on several factors: the age of the patient, the size of the lesion, its location, the condition of the bone base it came from, and the extent to which the lesion is still attached to the bone.

The most common place children experience OCD is the knee. The bottom of the femur is

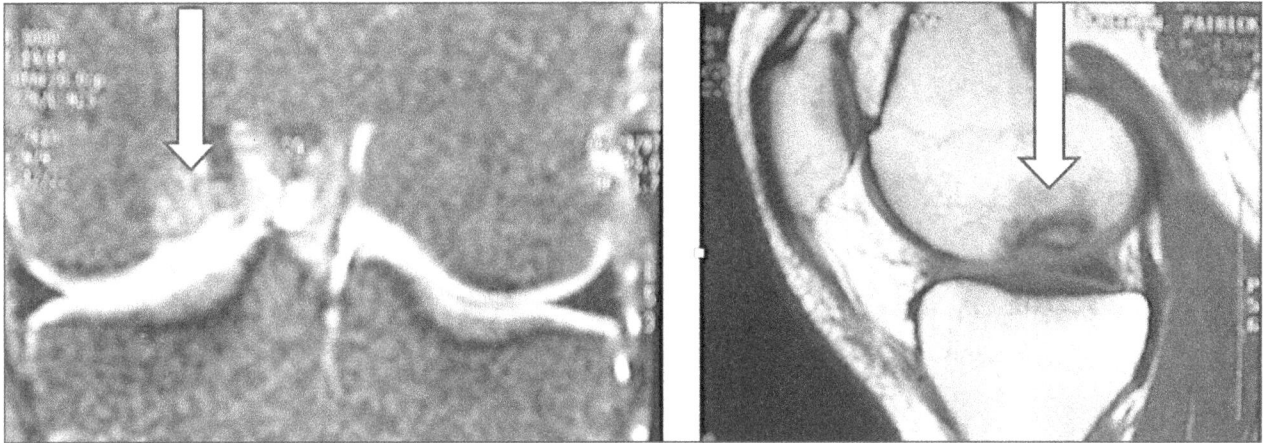

9 OCD, Osteochondritis Dissecans: a defect in the bone with or without a loose fragment of bone just below the surface.

made up of two matching curved surfaces with a notch for the anterior cruciate ligament (ACL) and posterior cruciate ligament (PCL) between them. These surfaces are called the medial and lateral femoral condyles. The medial condyle is on the inner side of the knee, and the lateral is on the outer side. The condyles are covered with a type of cartilage called articular cartilage to ensure the smooth movement of the joint. OCD can occur in the lateral condyle or on the patella. However, the most common place in the knee for it to occur is on the lateral side of the medial femoral condyle, toward the middle of the joint (see the MRIs in Image 9 above; the arrows point to the defect).

This is because the inside of the knee bears more weight. The involved area is near a raised spot on the tibia called the tibial eminence. Loading and twisting cause the tibial eminence and femur to hit each other and microscopic fracturing to occur. If the injured area is under constant stress from weight-bearing activities, running, or repetitive trauma, it won't have time to heal. The blood supply to the area fails, the body walls off the dead piece of bone, and the fragment loosens, which can cause more mechanical symptoms like locking and swelling.

The exact causes of this disease and the associated bone breakdown in any specific individual are often unknown. Most doctors believe that it is due to repetitive trauma, but an underlying vascular problem in the local bone under the lesion may also play a role. It could also be caused by an unnoticed injury, steroid use, elevated blood fats, or a genetic predisposition. It occurs commonly in older children and adolescents who participate in sports. Doctors also believe that the repetitive motion of sports can cause a small segment of the bone to fatigue and fracture under the surface. If there is continued microtrauma from repetitive loading (for example, running on an already injured knee), it will prevent the defect from healing and, again, loosen the bone fragment. This loose fragment causes swelling and pain. If the fragment comes off completely, it's called a loose body. Loose bodies can get trapped between the joint surfaces and cause the knee to lock. The defect, without the cartilage present, is not smooth, so the bones rubbing against each other can cause arthritis over time.

How Will I Know If My Child Has OCD?

A child with OCD will feel pain in the knee, especially after being active, and will experience some swelling in the knee or a tight feeling inside the knee from fluid buildup. They may experience catching or locking and difficulty with full extension of the leg. If the fragment breaks free or enlarges, symptoms will get worse over time. Eventually, it may become too painful to put any weight on the leg at all.

OCD is usually diagnosed with X-rays (including those with a special notch view). To assess a lesion and determine if there is any bone damage or if there is fluid under the lesion itself, an MRI may be ordered. If there is fluid present under the bone fragment, it's a sign that the cartilage is loose, and surgery is required. Sometimes OCD is recognized when a person is being tested for something else. In growing children, an early lesion that is not loose can heal with the use of crutches, rest, and a brace or cast. Again, in children as in adults, if the defect is displaced or loose, or if an MRI shows fluid under it, surgery may be necessary.

Treatment Options for OCD

If the bone and cartilage aren't completely detached from the bone, nonsurgical treatment may be appropriate and necessary (see Images 10 and 11). The younger the patient, the more normal bone growth remains (this is known as being "skeletally immature"—that is, when a child is still actively growing) and the more likely this approach will be successful. The treatment may require up to six weeks of immobilization while using crutches, so the patient doesn't put any weight on the injured leg. It can take three months to heal fully, so a brace can also be helpful. After casting, patients should avoid any activities that cause pain. Remember, after long periods of immobilization, a good physical therapy program to build up the muscles around the knee is always important (see Appendix II, Physical Therapy).

If conservative treatment is unsuccessful, the fragment is unstable, or the patient is older, surgery is the best choice to restore the smooth surface. There are several options for surgery, depending on the state of the fragments. First, if the cartilage hasn't broken loose, it can be drilled to stimulate new blood supply, and it can be fixed in place using pins or screws, which are sunk

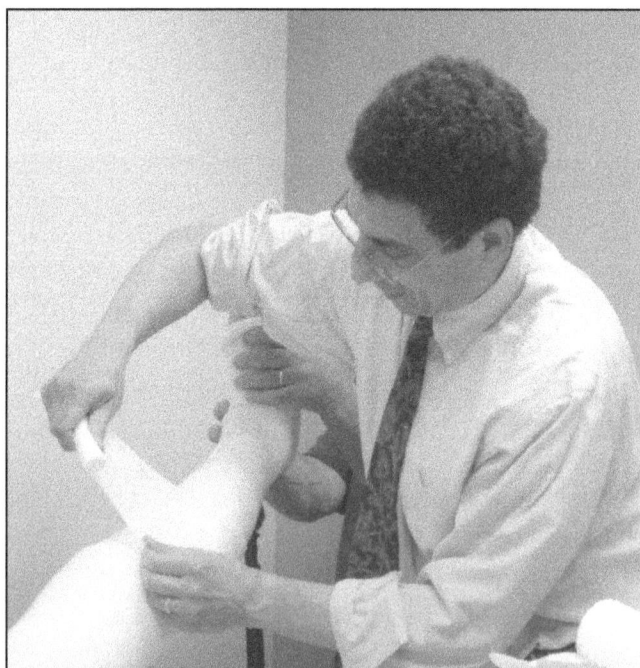

10 Nonoperative treatment for OCD of the knee in a growing child. Application of cast to protect the bone and allow the defect to heal.

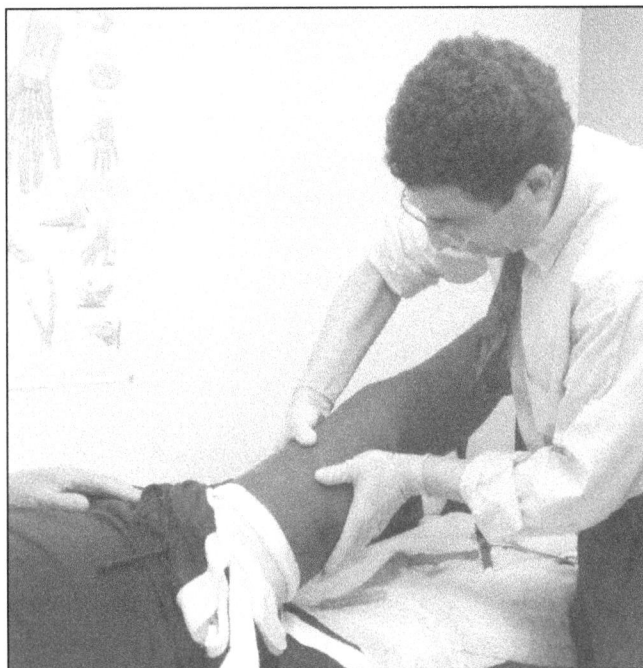

11 Application of fiberglas casting material.

into the cartilage to hold it in place while it heals. If biodegradable pins are used, they do not need to be taken out.

Sometimes the damaged fragment may not fit perfectly back into place. The bone around the defect may have also changed, and the surgeon will, therefore, need to recontour it, rebuild it, or graft it. If the fragments are completely loose, fragmented, or missing altogether, the surgeon may clear the cavity to reach the fresh, healthy bone and attach a bone graft into position with screws or pins. If it is loose and can be replaced, the piece should be put back and fixed in place.

When there is complete bone loss, a surgical procedure may be necessary to replace the bone. It will usually be done using a local autograft (from one's own body), an allograft (from a donor), or a scaffold material. An autograft works well, but there may be concerns about the loss of cartilage at the donor site.

The doctor will try to pick a non-weight-bearing donor site that won't cause any pain or further problems. Finally, fragments from smaller, shallow defects that cannot be mended are cleaned, and the bone is drilled to stimulate new growth of cartilage, a procedure called the "microfracture technique." This approach offers the advantage of not requiring a graft and has good clinical outcomes overall. The only downside is that the cartilage that forms after microfracture is fibrocartilage (scar cartilage), as opposed to true hyaline cartilage (joint surface cartilage), and it has different properties than the natural joint surface.

Another option is to replace the damaged area by harvesting bone that's covered with undamaged articular cartilage from a less weight-bearing part of the knee. During surgery, a plug of bone and cartilage is removed (like hair plugs in a hair transplant) and moved to the new location. Lastly, cartilage cells can be harvested and grown in a laboratory to make healthy cartilage, which is then implanted. If the cartilage defect is very large and is severely damaged, the knee may need to be replaced later in life. This is not an option in children. In these cases, allograft cartilage from an organ donor that is frozen after harvesting may be needed.

There are also other procedures being developed, such as a biological knee replacement. In these procedures, the body's articular cartilage and bone are harvested, mashed into a paste, and put onto the part of the body without cartilage to grow a new piece of cartilage. This last option is very experimental and not generally available as of now. These last few options are intended for larger defects, yet the first option (bone plug grafting), along with microfracture, are considered most frequently.

As of this writing, I have started to use a newer procedure called MACI (matrix-induced autologous chondrocyte implantation). During this procedure, we take a very small sample of one's own cartilage cells, grow them in a lab (creating thousands of times more cells), and place them in a matrix. This matrix is then glued into the knee and the patient's own cells grow to fill the defect. It is an amazing procedure but it's only indicated in younger patients (age 18 up to age 55) for larger defects (pending insurance coverage, they must be at least 1.5 square centimeters or over 1 square inch of surface loss). That means a good amount of cartilage loss from the inside surface of the knee is required for this procedure to be of value.

It must be noted that even if it's treated well, initial joint damage from an OCD lesion can still lead to future joint problems (e.g., degenerative arthritis or osteoarthritis). The goal is to restore function, reduce the damage, create a good knee surface, and decrease the patient's risk of needing a knee replacement at a younger age. Most children can return to normal activities if the corrective surgery repairs the cartilage and the bone heals completely.

Osteonecrosis in Children (Rare)

Osteonecrosis (also known as avascular necrosis, or AVN) means "bone death." It is very similar to osteochondritis dissecans except that the cause is most often vascular in nature, instead of repetitive trauma; it involves the bone more than the cartilage surface, at first. Osteonecrosis, like OCD, is most often located in the medial femoral condyle. AVN can also occur on the outside of the leg (the lateral femoral condyle) or near the upper end of the tibia.

Osteonecrosis starts when a piece of bone loses its blood supply and starts to die. If untreated, loss of joint space or support for the cartilage occur over time as the body reabsorbs the dead bone. This can end up involving the cartilage, as in a case of OCD. If the area collapses, it will mimic the symptoms of severe arthritis and be treated in the same way. In children, the most common causes of osteonecrosis are high-dose steroids for other illnesses, sickle cell, or genetic, very high cholesterol (congenital hyperlipidemia) in somewhat rare situations. When it does occur in children, it is very painful. In my own practice, I treated an active 18-year-old patient with spontaneous AVN in the knee, and it turned out that he did have the sickle trait.

Early Treatment Is Best

In all cases—in OS, jumper's knee, patella tendonitis, kneecap pain, OCD, and the rare case of AVN—early treatment is best because it often affords a simpler treatment. As discussed earlier in this chapter, during the initial evaluation the patient's vitamin and calcium intake should be reviewed as part of their history. Supplements should be given if either of these intakes are poor. Look for other medical conditions like poor nutrition. Thyroid conditions, kidney failure, and intestinal problems can interfere with bone health and the absorption of vitamin D from the gut and/or the ability to use calcium from the diet. All medical issues should be addressed when the child has them to best help the bones heal.

Medical conditions aside, chronic recurrent cases of each of these injuries may require immobilization or even casting to completely rest the tissues and allow them to heal. In chronic cases, a small piece of bone may have broken off and embedded in the tendon. When the individual is an adult, this fragment may become even more problematic and may need to be removed.

PART TWO

THE KNEE

To propel the body forward, the leg muscles move the hip, the knee, and the foot in a coordinated way. The knee is in the middle of the force chain and must then balance all of the forces required to move the body forward in a stable way. It is the motion of the knee and its connection to the hip above and the foot below that gives us the ability to run, jump, negotiate stairs, hit a ball with a bat, ski, play ice hockey, or throw a ball, all while keeping perfect balance. The knee is controlled by the muscles around it and held in place by four major ligaments. These structures must allow for bending, twisting, and pivoting motions required for all our physical activities. At the same time, the knee's cartilage is smooth enough to lower the energy needed for work, exercise, and sports. In short, it is our knee's amazing design, good health, and excellent function that is key to an active life.

In this section we will review all the issues in and around the knee's function. This includes injuries to the meniscus, articular cartilage, ligaments, bones, and bone alignment. We will discuss what makes the knee lock, buckle, and/or give way. I will also explain other conditions like water on (and in) the knee, inflammatory conditions, gout, Lyme disease, and the things that will heal with immobilization, medications, or just rest. We will see the differences between what can be treated medically without surgery and which injuries require surgical repair.

5 THE UNRELIABLE KNEE

THE FUNCTION OF THE KNEE DEPENDS ON THE KNEE'S SPECIAL DESIGN AND ITS unique combination of flexibility and stability. The knee's function may be lost if it becomes painful, locks, buckles, gives way, or swells. Then when its flexibility fails or the knee is unstable, it becomes an unreliable knee.

The unreliable knee results in the inability to perform sports, work, and sometimes even the ability to walk short distances. It can have a negative impact on your quality of life and is a frequent cause of a doctor's visit, most often after an injury.

What Are Locking, Buckling, and Giving Way?

"Standing still, I turned to get something off a shelf behind me, and bam, my knee just went."

"Every time I get up from a squatting position, my knee won't straighten."

"Going down stairs, my knee gives out. I just don't trust it."

Statements like these are often the first clue that a patient has an unstable knee. The examples above are stories in which patients describe locking (the knee gets stuck in one position and won't move), buckling (the knee is made unstable by a twist or a turn), and giving way (the force of a routine activity causes the knee to stop supporting the body's weight).

The knee is the joint connecting the femur (the thigh bone) to the tibia (the shinbone) (see Image 12). In the knee joint, the end of the thigh bone is rounded, and the top of the shin is relatively flat. The two bones are very much like a rolling pin sitting on a narrow table. Given even a small push, the rolling pin will fall off. That's why the knee's cartilage and ligaments are so important. They hold the two together and still allow the knee to bend and straighten smoothly. Without the ligaments and the cartilage, we wouldn't be able to run, jump, twist, turn, squat, or pivot, and problems occur when they are injured or not working properly.

So why are knee injuries so common, and what should be done to prevent and treat them?

Locking

Locking is often caused by a piece of torn cartilage (the meniscus) stuck between the bones. Until this piece is moved out of the way and pushed back into place, the knee remains locked. A locked knee is difficult, if not impossible, to straighten; this can be painful and disabling. Many patients also have joint line tenderness directly over the meniscus on either the inside or the outside of the knee. Locking can also occur when a loose body (most often a loose piece of cartilage or bone) gets stuck between the bones. Loose bodies and their causes are discussed later in Chapter 13.

There are several tests your doctor can do in the exam room that can help make a diagnosis. These include the "flick" test (flicking the knee in short, quick rotations to either side), McMurray's sign (twisting the knee while bent in a direction that may catch the tear and seeing

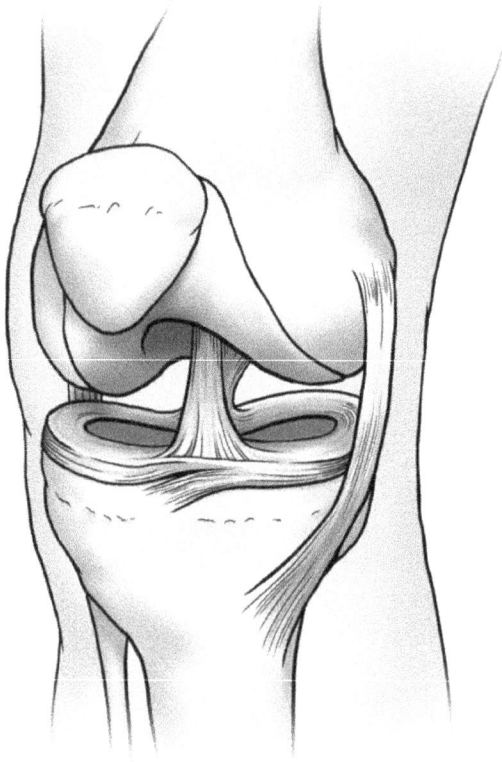

if straightening it causes a pop or pain), and Apley's compression test (twisting the knee when loaded with the patient's weight to see if there is pain). Sometimes a locked knee can be unlocked by a doctor who performs an unlocking maneuver in the exam room. This will often acutely relieve the pain and unlock the knee while confirming the diagnosis. If there are signs of injury to the cartilage during an examination, a tear is the most likely reason for the problem. Knee swelling may also be present.

A locked knee can also be caused by a ligament tear with a fragment of the ligament caught in the middle of the knee. A loose body can also become stuck between the bones of the knee. Both conditions may be seen with a torn meniscus. An X-ray may show the loose body, and the knee may be unstable if the ligaments are torn. Many times, the knee is too painful at the time of the injury to sort this out. A thorough examination and a plain X-ray of the knee go a long way in helping your doctor make an accurate diagnosis.

12

Buckling

Buckling can be caused by cartilage surface problems (surface defects, small flap tears, or softening), meniscus tears, ligament injuries, or kneecap problems like poor tracking of the kneecap or the kneecap slipping out of place. Buckling can also occur when pieces of cartilage get stuck and quickly move between the bones, so the knee gives way but does not "lock." Finally, buckling can be caused by issues with the kneecap. To treat these problems, it is important to understand the different causes of buckling.

Kneecap-related buckling is a result of pain under the kneecap, which causes a reflex release of the quadriceps (quads) muscles. The body is trying in its own way to protect your knee by turning the quadriceps muscles off. The loss of muscular control of the knee causes a sense of instability. The quads turn off, and the hamstrings fire to keep you from falling. Sometimes we don't feel pain in the kneecap when this happens.

To understand this better, keep in mind that the kneecap is part of the quads' mechanism. This muscle and tendon unit allows us to squat, jump, and kick. It also prevents us from tumbling forward when walking, jogging, running, and going downhill or down stairs. Without the quadriceps muscles, patella, and patella tendon, we could not stand on one leg. During any of these activities, the body can sense when the kneecap or the knee joint is going to hurt; frequently this causes the quads mechanism to release or give to protect the knee—and your body—from pain (hence the term "give way"). Unfortunately, it can occur at inopportune times. It's a bit like when you touch (or get near) a hot stove; your body pulls your hand back quickly, or, in this case, "recalls" that the current movement of the knee will cause a sharp pain. The quads turn off as a reflex to protect the knee from that pain. This self-protection action of the knee is just like pulling your hand off the hot stove to avoid the painful burning sensation. The quads shut down to unload the knee and avoid the potential pain in the knee, which can cause an instant sense of buckling.

Giving Way

Giving way is the sense that the knee is suddenly not able to support the body's weight during an activity. You can give way on stairs, going downhill, or twisting from one side to another. Giving way implies the person is applying body weight to the knee and the knee does not support it. The knee may buckle or the patient may fall. Giving way can also be caused by a cartilage tear, a ligament problem, a torn ligament, or loose bodies trapped inside the knee. It's difficult to tell the difference between the different diagnoses, which is why a physician's examination of the knee is key. This is especially true if the knee is swollen or painful, both common symptoms after almost all recent injuries of many types.

Clinical Exam and Tests

Fortunately, there are clinical tests that should be included in a routine knee exam, which help us find the causes of injuries. For torn ligaments, a Lachman, or anterior draw test, is helpful. This shows an abnormal movement between the femur and the tibia. Abnormal movements on this test are signs of an ACL or PCL tear. More movement than normal is an important finding when the injury is a torn ligament. The looser the knee is after an injury (meaning the more abnormal movement between the two major bones of the knee joint, namely the femur and the tibia), the more unstable it will be when someone participates in sports.

The other test is called a pivot shift, which is harder to explain. The goal is to reproduce the shift that occurs when the knee pivots in sports or twisting motions, the so-called pivot-shift. This test reproduces the movement when the knee gives out or buckles because the ACL is not working. If there is a shift when the knee moves, the test is positive for an ACL tear.

In addition, I always check for swelling inside the knee. If it's very swollen, taking the fluid off can help to control pain. Seeing the fluid is also helpful in making a diagnosis. If it is clear, it is more likely to be a cartilage injury or meniscus tear. If there is blood in the fluid, it is more likely that there is a ligament or muscle tear. If there are fat droplets in bloody fluid, it is more likely that there is a fracture. If it is cloudy, it could be inflammatory, like gout, Lyme, or infection.

Special instruments, like the KT-1000, can also help physicians decide if one of the major ligaments, like the ACL, is damaged. The KT-1000 is a very sensitive knee-testing device that allows us to confirm a tear. It can measure small movements between the femur and the tibia. More than 3 millimeters of a side-to-side difference in the test is usually diagnostic of an ACL or PCL tear (see Image 13).

Diagnosing the Problem: X-ray and MRI

After taking a thorough history and conducting a physical exam, plain X-rays of the knee are always needed to determine if there are loose chips, calcifications, loose bodies, a fracture, a dislocation, a bone tumor, or arthritis. Many patients want to jump to an MRI first, even though it is a very expensive first-line test and not indicated. Many insurance companies will not pay for it and wisely so! Can you imagine the health-care costs if every knee sprain had an MRI first before trying ice, rest, an anti-inflammatory medication, being examined by a qualified doctor, and getting a plain X-ray?

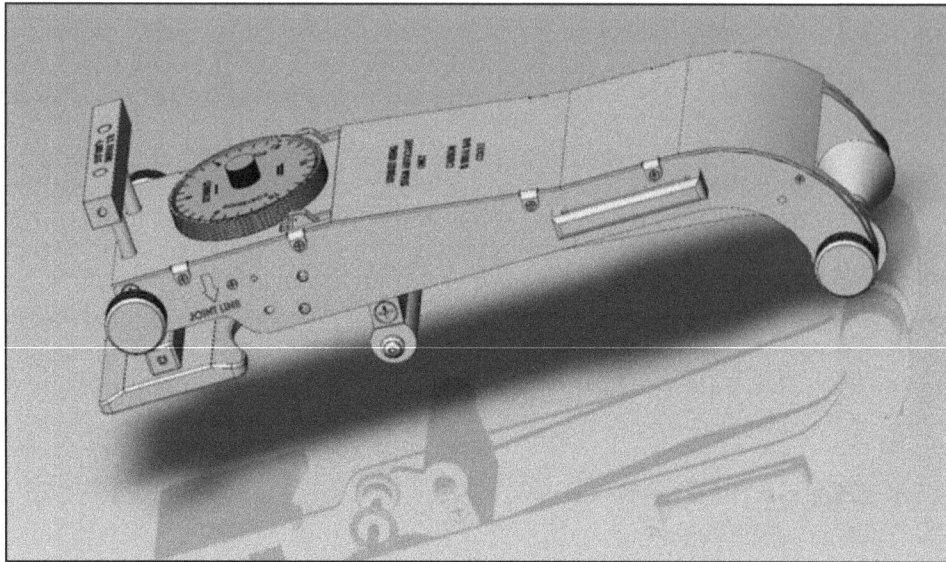

13 KT 1000 Knee Arthrotomer: Knee tester that measures the movement of the knee and helps decide if the ligaments are working properly. It can be used for making a diagnosis of a ligament tear and assessing if a surgical repair is working properly.

KT-1000 Testing

The gold standard in most scientific studies of ACL tears and reconstructions is the KT-1000, which was invented in San Diego by Lawrence L. Malcom and Dale Daniel (US patents 4868471A and 4583555). The device can measure side-to-side differences between the two knees and, based on the numbers, gives us a sense of whether the injured knee is unstable compared to the uninjured side.

For example, if there is less than a 3-millimeter difference between the two knees when tested with the KT-1000, there is an excellent chance the ACL is working well, and many times an MRE (Magnetic Resonance Image) is not needed (saving a good deal of money). If the test is positive (a difference of more than 3 millimeters), there is a 95% chance there is a tear. Provided the patient is relaxed and not guarding or protecting the knee with muscle spasms or tension, the KT-1000 values are as follows:

< 3 mm	no tear
3–5 mm	a tear that may only affect the highest levels of physical activity or sports
5–7 mm	a tear that causes problems for recreational sports, heavy labor (the working athlete), and weekend warriors
> 7 mm	a tear that most likely will adversely affect activities of daily living in most patients

The KT-1000 help predict who needs ligament reconstruction. In the operating room, it helps confirm the extent of the injury. After the repair, I use it in the operating room a second time to prove the repaired knee matches the good knee. This is very helpful in assuring both an anatomic and accurate repair.

If the knee is painful and an exam confirms a possible injury, an X-ray is the first-line test to check alignment, see the joint space, look for calcium deposits, see signs of arthritis, diagnose a fractured bone, or see a loose body in the knee. In short, the most common diagnoses can be made with a good history, a physical exam, and plain X-rays. A KT-1000 test is also a helpful tool in making a diagnosis of an ACL tear or a PCL tear.

What surprises many of my patients is the fact that an expensive test like an MRI is last on the list. So many of my patients think it is the first test that should be done if they are hurt. But it's just not so. When your doctor can make a clear diagnosis with your history, exam, and X-ray, an MRI is not needed and is a waste of highly valued medical resources.

If surgery is needed, many insurance companies require a confirmation of the diagnosis by an MRI. This "knee jerk" requirement has, over time, confused many people who think that their doctor needs it to know what is wrong. In my practice, I have a very good idea what the MRI will show 90% of the time before it is done. The MRI helps doctors determine the extent of the injury.

For example, if I suspect a loose body is causing locking, the MRI will show me how big the loose body is or if there are three of them instead of one. Sometimes the knee giving way can be from an ACL tear, a meniscus tear, and/or a loose body, and an MRI will show all three. An MRI can also show us if the bone is bruised after an ACL tear, if the damage to the bone is big or small, and other details that can help with surgical planning. Sometimes the nature of the bone bruising is helpful in deciding whether the injury is old or new. Sometimes it tells us a story about the severity of the injury or the mechanism of the injury.

Less often, if a patient has enough findings to warrant surgery and needs an MRI for pre-op planning, and they cannot have an MRI for medical reasons (like metal clips or fragments in the body, or a pacemaker), a special CT scan (CT arthrogram) may help. Another option is looking into the knee with a fiberoptic telescope (an outpatient diagnostic arthroscopy), which can show whether there is a meniscus or ligament tear, and the problem can then be treated properly at the same time.

Treatment

Once your doctor makes the diagnosis, the treatment varies, depending on the diagnosis and the cause of the injury. Treatment can include simple exercises, physical therapy, bracing, and arthroscopy, along with the removal of the loose bodies or meniscus tear, repair of a defect, reconstruction of a ligament, and other restorative procedures described in this book. The early correction of these mechanical problems can lead to a speedy recovery with the hopes of greatly reducing the risk of recurrence, future injury, long-term problems, and early degenerative arthritis. These issues are discussed individually, in much more detail, in the chapters to follow.

6 "WATER ON THE KNEE"

PATIENTS OFTEN SHOW UP IN MY OFFICE WITH SEEMINGLY UNEXPLAINABLE SWELL-
ing of the knee. When asked, they can't recall a fall or a twist that may have caused an injury.
There was no trauma and no history of sports participation. In short, there is no mechanical
reason (e.g., a ligament tear, unstable kneecap, torn cartilage or meniscus tear, trauma, or fracture)
for the swelling. In these cases, we must look elsewhere for the cause of the problem.

To better understand the other sources of knee swelling, we must consider what makes the
knee, or any joint, move so smoothly. The knee is well-lubricated by the constant production
of small amounts of fluid made by the lining of the joint. The lining is called the synovium, and
the fluid is called synovial fluid. Synovial fluid helps lubricate the knee and enables the smooth
motion of the joint. Conditions of the knee that irritate the lining cause it to make more fluid.
When extra liquid accumulates in the knee, it will swell, hence the expression "water in the
knee" (see Images 14 and 15). So, what causes the lining to be irritated and make fluid, and more
importantly, what can we do about it?

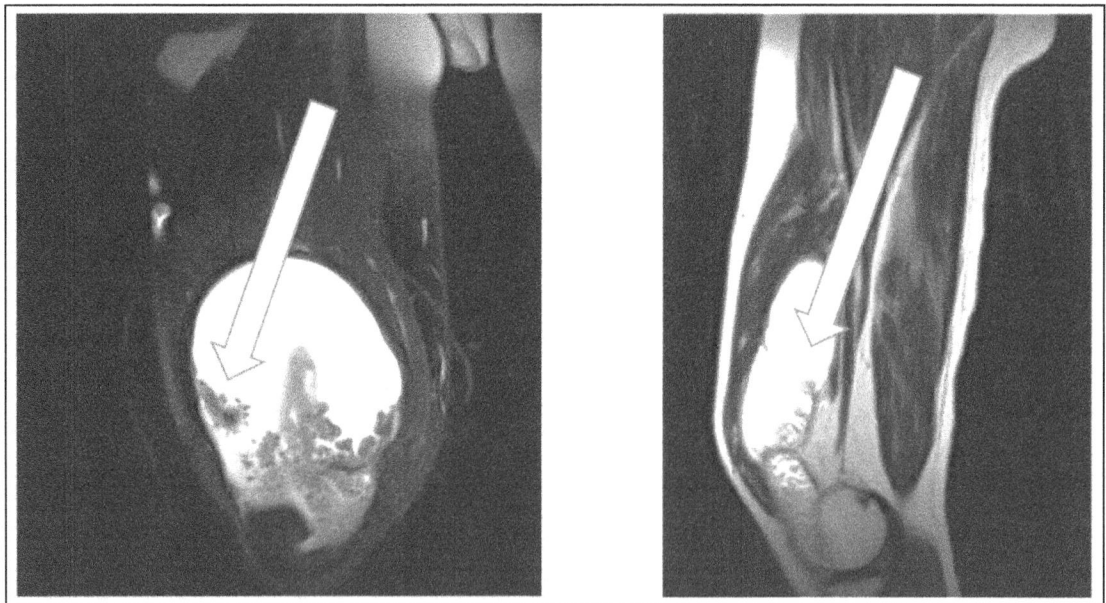

14 MRI images of a large amount of fluid in the knee, a large "knee effusion." In the image of water in
the knee, you can see the thickened knee's synovial lining that makes the knee fluid.

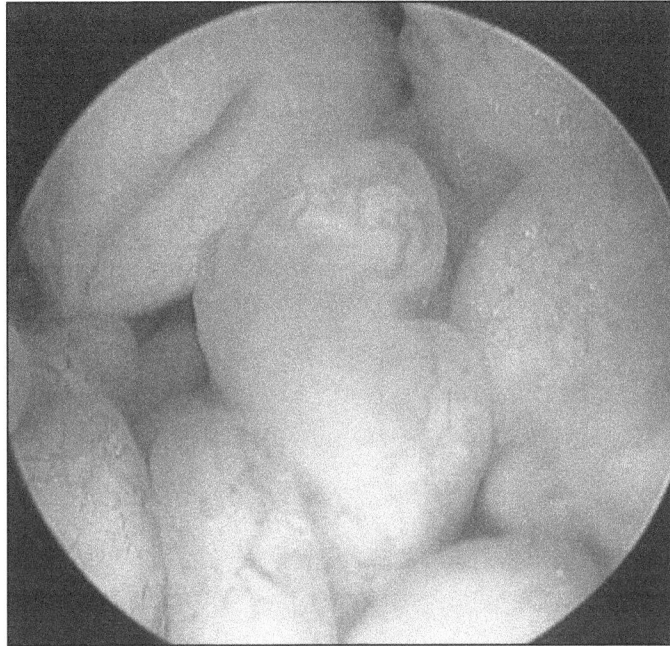

15 Arthroscopic view of the swollen synovial tissue (knee lining) shown in the MRI of Image 14.

Why Does My Knee Make Fluid And Swell?

Most commonly, the knee makes fluid after an injury to "solve" the problem. Likewise, if the knee is arthritic for any reason, it tries to fix the lack of smooth motion by making fluid. Therefore, the first cause of water in the knee in the absence of trauma can be just simple wear and tear. With trauma or an injury, a torn ligament or a meniscus tear is more likely, as previously discussed in the section on buckling in Chapter 5. Removal of some of the fluid can help decrease the symptoms of water in the knee and yield important clues to its cause. In simple wear and tear, the fluid is clear or a bit yellow, and a little like a very light syrup in consistency. In other conditions like gout, Lyme disease, infection, or trauma with a fracture or torn ligaments, it may appear to be cloudy, white, or even bloody (see sidebar on pg. 37 for information about Lyme disease). It may contain a high number of white blood cells, altered sugar and protein content, flecks of cartilage, crystals, or bacteria. Sometimes, when the fluid is not clear, a diagnosis can be made by sending a sample of the fluid to a lab for testing.

The lining itself can also be a direct cause of swelling. For example, when a patient has gout, the knee accumulates crystals. The crystals will cause the lining to become inflamed and make fluid, and it makes knee movement painful; it's like having sand in your car's gearbox (see Image 16 on following page).

In patients with gout, there is a significant inflammatory response as the white blood cells try to digest the crystals. Unfortunately, they cannot digest them, and in the process, the white cells release destructive enzymes in vain. If the gout is not treated, the powerful enzymes will slowly destroy the joint.

In patients with rheumatoid arthritis, the swelling is caused by the body's own immune reaction to cartilage, and the knee makes fluid. The lining in the patients with rheumatoid arthritis and those with other inflammatory arthritic conditions can grow, make enzymes, and worsen the situation.

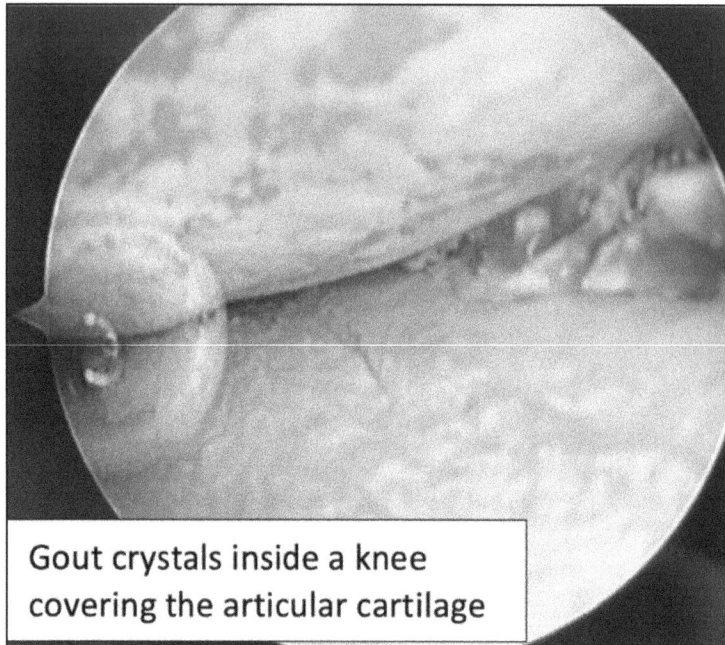

Gout crystals inside a knee covering the articular cartilage

16

There are several diseases like this, including psoriatic arthritis, Reiter's syndrome, ankylosing spondylitis, and pseudogout (calcium pyrophosphate crystals instead of calcium urate), to name a few. They can all be painful, cause swelling, and, like gout, if not treated, can ultimately destroy any joint that has an active inflammatory response.

Infection is another cause of swelling. After a viral infection, there are syndromes associated with transient swelling of a joint. This is called a viral synovitis, which is often self-limited, meaning that it goes away on its own when the viral illness ends. Arthritic conditions like Lyme disease can be associated with infection. Gonorrhea can also cause a joint infection that can be hard to diagnose, but it is extremely rare these days.

Another type of infection is bacterial. Bacterial infections can occur after the joint is punctured with a small object like a nail, needle, splinter, or piece of dirt. It can happen after a fall on the ground. It can also be the result of an infection in another part of the body or of other factors that increase the risk of infection, like being treated with chemotherapy for cancer or being diabetic. These can be urgent problems and are associated with fever, loss of motion, painful motion, significant swelling, and redness. If you think you have an infection, call your doctor.

Bleeding into the joint can also be another cause of knee swelling. In rare situations, bleeding can happen after minor trauma. People prone to this reaction may be on blood thinners, have bleeding disorders like hemophilia or sickle cell disease, or have low platelet counts or poor platelet function. Sometimes, chronic use of NSAIDs in high doses or cancer chemotherapy can inhibit platelet function as well.

Pigmented Villonodular Synovitis

Recurrent bleeding into a joint without one of these problems can be the only sign of another disease of the knee lining, called pigmented villonodular synovitis (PVNS). PVNS has MRI

Lyme Disease

Lyme disease often presents as a swollen knee or joint in a patient who cannot recall a tick bite. The swollen joint is, in fact, the second phase of Lyme disease, a three-part infection that starts with a local rash near the bite of a tick.

The tick linked to Lyme is the very small deer tick (the black-legged tick), not the bigger dog tick (see Image below). That's why most people miss this bite. The tick infects the host with the infective agent, a spirochete called Borrelia burgdorferi in the US. In Europe and Asia, there are two different Borrelia, called garni and afzelli, and the disease is similar in the US and Europe. The symptoms usually occur in phases, sometimes many months apart; some patients don't know what to look for and miss the early signs of Lyme disease. The first stages are often missed completely. Lyme disease doesn't inevitably start with a tick bite, because not all people with tick bites get the disease.

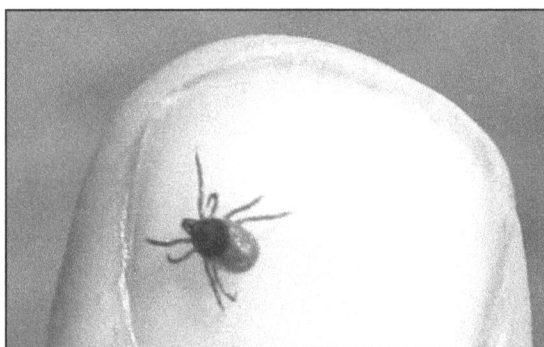

(My) Phase Zero: Maybe you spot a tick on an arm or leg and you have it tested for Lyme. If it's positive and the tick was not embedded in you for a long time, you most likely will not get the rash and may not be infected. If it's positive and the tick was embedded for a long time, you most likely will get the rash and may become infected. You should be treated if the tick tests positive even if there is no rash. Preventing the next phases of the disease is always better than treating Lyme later on. Remember, if the tick tests negative for Lyme, there is no treatment needed.

Phase One: The first stage is a tick bite and rash. The tick may be off of your body already, but the rash is there, frequently a ring with a bite mark in the center when you look very carefully.

Phase Two: In time, the spirochete infection can move to a joint and is associated with a relatively painless swelling. The rash is gone, and the joint swells weeks or months later. The swelling may resolve without treatment, but that doesn't mean the infection is cured! It may become dormant before it returns in the far more serious phase three. It is important to recognize potential Lyme cases and treat them in one of the first two stages.

Phase Three: If left untreated in phases zero, one, or two, Lyme disease will return in its third phase. This last phase is very serious and often occurs months to years later without warning or a clear connection to the joint swelling or a tick bite. The infection involves the central nervous system and the brain, heart, and other organs. In this form, it can include seizures, heart rhythm abnormalities, coma, and even death. Sometimes the presentation of heart issues and seizures is so strange that the diagnosis is not made easily because the history of a bite, rash, and joint swelling is long forgotten. So, treatment early on can be important, and the telltale signs of Lyme should not be ignored. If there is an unexplained knee effusion (swelling) without trauma or inflammatory disease, a Lyme test should be included in the workup, especially if you live in an area of the country known for Lyme infections, like New England.

findings like the nodules seen in the example of psoriatic arthritis already shown, except for the additional finding of hemosiderin deposits. The deposits are iron-containing synovial (knee lining) nodules caused by recurrent bleeding.

The iron in the blood stains the synovium a characteristic rust-orange color. Sometimes it is a small single nodule or part of the lining. This variety is treated with a simple arthroscopic removal. Occasionally, the area is bigger, and a total synovectomy (removal of the entire lining) is needed. Again, this can be done with the arthroscope. Lastly, there is a malignant version. This is very rare and occurs in one in two million of the general population. This requires an arthroscopic total synovectomy and local radiation treatment. (See sidebar on page 40.)

Cortisone Injections

If a doctor has recommended a steroid injection for your condition, there are several things you should know about the use of these injections. There are many myths about their use, and the rumors are so common that many of my patients have an unwarranted fear of them. In most cases, the proper use of these injections is both safe and effective.

When there are no signs of a bacterial infection, for the most part, a steroid injection is a safe, reliable method for reducing inflammation and swelling and decreasing the pain in an affected area. Cortisone is a powerful anti-inflammatory drug that is a direct relative of the natural substances produced by your own body. When injected into the affected area, the irritation and inflammation can be reduced dramatically. This can promote both short- and, more importantly, long-term healing. A misconception is that the injection is simply for temporary pain relief. Our goal is long-term relief and, combined with the other recommendations, curing the condition.

A steroid preparation, as used in our office, is mixed with a short- and sometimes long-acting local Novocain-type anesthetic (Marcaine). The injection, therefore, may bring immediate relief to your symptoms and last for at least six to eight hours after it is administered. The cortisone itself takes seven to 10 days to achieve its full effect. Therefore, it may take time before your symptoms start to respond. There also may be a few days when your symptoms worsen before they improve. For that reason, we recommend the use of ice and NSAIDs along with the injection and for several days afterward.

Local injections of cortisone, in general, have limited side effects on the body, and mostly affect the area injected. Still, people with diabetes may see a transient rise in their blood sugar; therefore, you should monitor your blood sugars, and if there is a change, please let your orthopaedic surgeon or your diabetes doctor know. Less commonly, some patients can see an increase in appetite, heart rate, flushing of the face, or energy level.

Side effects of cortisone injections are rare. One-third of people experience discomfort several hours afterward when the Novocain wears off and before the cortisone begins to reduce the inflammation. Usually, this will subside by the next day. Some people can get thinning of the skin or a change of pigmentation at the injection site; these side effects occur in less than 5% of our patients, though more often with patients with olive, brown, or very dark skin. The cortisone can affect the pigment cells in a small zone around the injection, and they may stop making their pigment near the site.

Patients often ask me if they should limit the number of cortisone injections to a given area of the body. In general, I do not recommend more than three injections to the same area in one year. If a third injection is being contemplated, your doctor should consider other treatments and conduct further investigations (like more X-rays and bloodwork to check for systemic disease or an MRI). Infections are extremely rare after an injection, but even though the area will be prepared in a sterile manner, they can still occur. If there is any concern that an infection might have developed after an injection, look for the symptoms noted previously and contact your doctor's office. If there is redness and swelling that spreads from the involved area, it's painful to move, hot to touch, or you develop a fever, infection is on the list of concerns.

A cortisone injection is just one component of your overall treatment, which may include NSAIDs and physical therapy. After your injection, you may resume light activities, but you should avoid strenuous activities or exercise for at least seven to 10 days after the injection. Ice can help diminish discomfort from the injection or the underlying inflammation. Use it for 15–20 minutes on, 15–20 minutes off, and then on again with some type of thin cloth between the ice and your skin. Caution: Ice left on too long may cause frostbite.

Again, if there is any increased redness, swelling, or pain at the injection site, or if you have a fever or chills or other concerns, please call your doctor's office. **When infections do occur, they MUST BE treated with antibiotics, and acute joint infections (septic arthritis) may require emergent drainage as well as intravenous antibiotics.**

How Do We Treat Non-traumatic Knee Swelling?

Many arthritic conditions are treated with medication. In mild cases, the inflammation is often controlled with NSAIDs like Motrin, Advil, or Aleve. Swelling from mild to moderate degenerative arthritis due to wear and tear of the knee can also be treated with NSAIDs, glucosamine-chondroitin supplements, injections of cortisone, and/or a synthetic lubricant injection called hyaluronan (the same substance that normally lubricates the joint, in a concentrated injection). Platelet-rich plasma, better known as PRP, when given by injection has also helped patients with early arthritis and joint pain. With PRP we draw the patient's own blood, separate their own platelets from the red and white cells, activate the platelets to release their growth factors, and inject the activated platelets and factors into the knee.

In cases where extra weight is an issue, the extra load on the knee can be an underlying cause of the pain, and a weight-loss program can become crucial to decreasing the stress on the joint and the pain associated with the problem.

Gout

Acute gout attacks are treated with prescription anti-inflammatories (like indomethacin, colchicine, or in several cases, oral steroids), aspiration, or an injection of cortisone (see Image 16). Long-term gout is treated primarily by lowering uric acid levels in the blood. This is usually done with a medication called allopurinol.

Also, some dietary restrictions may be recommended, such as eliminating red wine and foods high in protein (like a big steak or big shellfish meal—for example, at an all-you-can-eat shrimp bar). This is why gout was known as a rich man's disease in the late 1700s. Most of the average population could not afford to include enough protein in their diet to get it.

In more severe cases, when there is a synovial disease or a systemic inflammatory conditions, like active rheumatoid arthritis, psoriatic arthritis, Lyme disease, anklyosing spondylitis or gout, nonsteroidal anti-inflammatories may not be enough to stop the progression of the inflammation, and cortisone immune system modulating drugs (like methotrexate, Enbrel, anakinra, Remicade, and Humira) or disease-modifying antirheumatic drugs (DMARDs, like Azulfidine, Plaquenil, and Arava) are the most effective treatments. When this occurs, it's best to consult a rheumatologist to manage these treatments.

Blood clotting disorders like hemophilia or platelet abnormalities are most often treated with clotting factors or platelet replacement by transfusion. Recurrent bleeding in the joint can be a cause of PVNS. (See sidebar on page 40.)

*Hemarthrosis means blood is found in the joint when drained.

Pigmented villonodular synovitis (PVNS) is a thickening of the lining of the joint. It can occur in any joint, but most commonly appears in the knee. It is seen equally in men and women and most frequently occurs between young adulthood and age 40.

It is most often seen in one of three forms:

✓ The first is a single nodule of abnormal lining that has hemosiderin (the remains of hemoglobin from blood cells).

✓ The second involves a larger area of the lining.

✓ The third is considered a locally malignant form that can extend past the joint and into the local tissue. It is very rare (one in two million people) but can be destructive if not treated early and aggressively.

Treatment ranges from simple arthroscopic removal of the nodule, to arthroscopic total synovectomy (removal of the entire diseased lining), to total synovectomy with local radiation. (This is only for the very rare malignant form, and I have seen only two cases since I started medical school in 1979.)

When Is Surgery Helpful?

Arthroscopic removal of the lining (a synovectomy) has been helpful in treating some inflammatory conditions with persistent recurring synovitis. In patients with synovitis, the lining is thickened and continues to make fluid containing destructive enzymes that digest the cartilage. When medications fail to work or the risks of the drug treatment are not acceptable to the patient, an arthroscopic synovectomy can be done as an outpatient procedure. A biopsy of the lining may also help make the diagnosis, like in PVNS. Removing the diseased lining is often enough to cure this type of PVNS. Removing all the lining tissue (a total synovectomy) can be required in the treatment of chronic, active Lyme arthritis. A total synovectomy can also reduce recurrent swelling and pain when conditions such as rheumatoid or psoriatic arthritis are resistant to medical therapy.

Knee replacement can be considered in the final stages of the arthritic condition because of ongoing arthritis, no matter what the cause. When the cartilage has worn away and quality of life is decreased because of loss of knee function, a knee replacement may be the best option. When the inflammation cannot be treated and pain and swelling continue, a knee replacement can remove the diseased tissues. With modern knee replacement surgery, the surfaces are replaced with metal or ceramic prostheses, most often with a plastic liner. These procedures have very high success rates. Patient satisfaction after knee replacement is among the highest of all surgical procedures.

Prepatellar Bursitis ("Nursemaid's Knee")

There are many different bursae in the body. These are very thin sacs that normally have a tiny amount of natural lubricant in them. They are like flat, sealed plastic bags, each one with a tiny drop of lubricating fluid in it. The "plastic sides" slide around easily with very little friction. As such, they serve as sliding surfaces between body parts to help them move smoothly. Bursae are commonly located between a tendon and a nearby bone, particularly near joints like the elbow and knee, which have a large range of motion.

When a bursa gets inflamed, it rubs against the bone and swells. When this happens to the bursa located between the skin over the kneecap and the kneecap itself, there is a bump or lump in front of the knee with thickened skin over it. This is truly what is meant by "water on the knee," as opposed to water in the knee, as described in an earlier section (also called "water on the knee" by many.) They are really two different things. With fluid in front of the knee, it really looks like there is something wrong inside of the knee.

When the fluid is in front of the knee, there is often nothing wrong inside the knee joint. In this case, the water is in a bursa (sac) in front of the patella and not in the knee at all. Most of the time, this bursa swells from continued kneeling and repeated mild trauma to the front of the knee while the individual is at work or doing repetitive motions. It is also seen in carpenters, plumbers, carpet layers, and other laborers. Activities like kneeling to get under a car, laying tile, or gardening act on the front of the knee. The bump in front of the kneecap is commonly known as nursemaid's knee. This is because nursemaids spent a lot of time kneeling (while washing the floor), and the swelling was caused by constant trauma to the bursa.

Treatment

Nursemaid's knee is treated first with rest, ice, and NSAIDs. If those treatments fail, your doctor may try to aspirate the knee and inject it with cortisone. In chronic cases, removal of the bursa may be necessary. I have had patients whose bursa had become infected after being punctured by a sharp object (like a splinter, tack, or sewing needle) left on the floor. In one rare case, a few grains of sand were imbedded in the bursa after a fall in the dirt. Years later, the painful swelling refused to clear. This was due to an infection that was mild, but chronic because the bacteria that caused it lived on the grains of sand and could not spread elsewhere. Naturally, this was cured only after the foreign bodies (the grains of sand) were removed.

Patients with occupations that require kneeling, like carpet installers and tile masons, should always wear kneepads to avoid these issues. Even those who wear the pads may still have bursitis from overuse. It is very hard to treat the swelling because the patient continues to traumatize the area daily at work.

7 ACL: ANTERIOR CRUCIATE LIGAMENT TEARS

THE ANTERIOR CRUCIATE LIGAMENT, OR ACL, CONNECTS THE FEMUR (THIGH BONE) to the tibia (shinbone). It is in the center of your knee. It is called a "cruciate ligament" because there are two ligaments that cross each other in the middle of your knee: one in the front, the ACL, and one behind it, the posterior cruciate ligament (PCL). There are two other main ligaments: one on the inside edge, the medial collateral ligament (MCL), and one on the outside edge, the lateral collateral ligament (LCL). Together, the four ligaments control the forward and backward motion of the knee bones on each other (ACL and PCL) and the side-to-side motion (MCL and LCL).

The ACL helps control front-to-back translation of the knee bones and rotation of the knee. It is frequently injured in pivoting sports like soccer, basketball, volleyball, skiing, lacrosse, and football (see Image 17). Any hyperextension injury or pivot injury with a steady onset of swelling within a few hours of the injury followed by instability of the knee with any twisting or pivoting motion is suspect for an ACL injury. The ACL helps make the knee stable and keeps the tibia from moving too far forward on the femur. Many times, it is injured in a fast shift in direction and often without contact with another player.

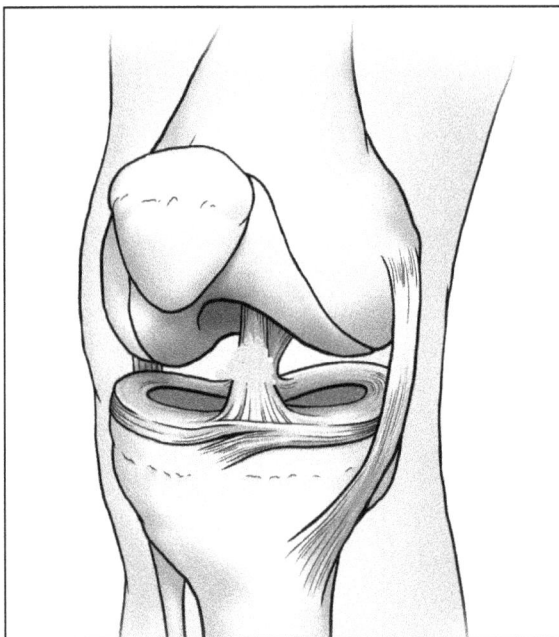

17 Knee with depiction of a torn ACL.

How Do You Diagnose an ACL Tear?

At the time of injury, you will feel a pop, or it may feel like something has snapped. It is usually not that painful. The knee will often swell within two to four hours. The ligament is vascular (meaning it has many blood vessels), so the small vessels in the torn ligament will slowly bleed into the joint, causing a hemarthrosis, or blood-filled swelling of the joint. Once the knee is swollen, you may experience pain from the joint being tight inside. You may also experience an inability to walk, an inability to full bear weight on the leg, or the knee giving out or buckling. The tibia twists and shifts forward without warning. If left untreated the shifting can further damage the knee over time.

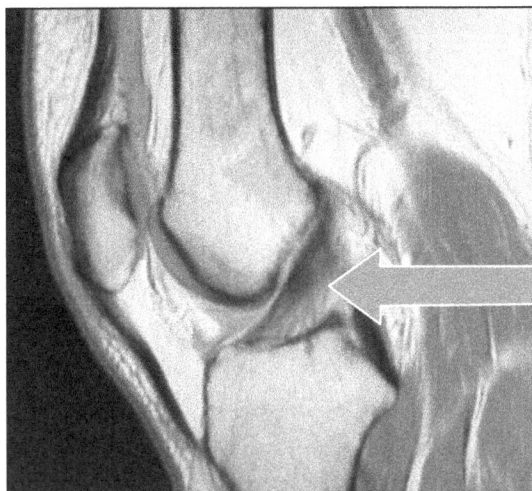

18 MRI of an intact ACL.

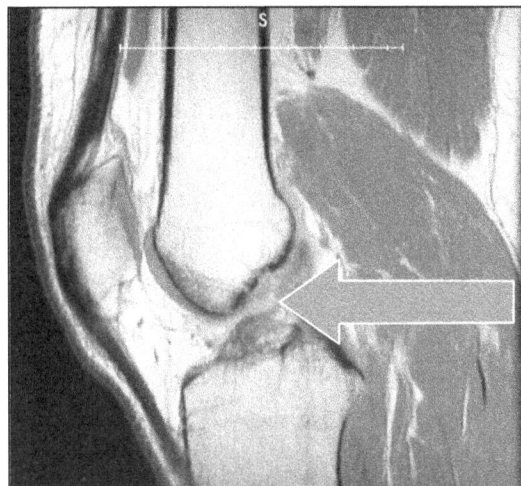

19 MRI of a torn ACL.

Your doctor can often make the diagnosis by taking a medical history and performing a physical exam, which may include a Lachman test and a pivot shift test. In a Lachman test, the anterior movement of the knee is tested by pulling forward on the tibia while holding the femur in place. In a pivot shift test, the doctor will test the knee's rotation as it bends. Both tests are meant to simulate what happens when the knee gives out. An X-ray showing a small fracture at the lateral edge of the tibia would confirm the diagnosis. In addition, a special instrument called a KT-1000 can perform an instrumented Lachman test. It can also be used to confirm the diagnosis of an ACL or PCL tear and help determine the best treatment choice. Furthermore, an MRI can confirm the tear in the ligament and reveal any other damage to the cartilage or bone (see Images 18 and 19).

Different Levels of Instability After an ACL Tear

Some patients have good secondary restraints (other ligaments that help control the knee, namely the PCL, LCL, and MCL). Even if your MRI shows an ACL tear, the knee may be stable (in other words, the knee is functioning as if the ACL was not torn even though it is seen as damaged on the MRI) based on an examination with a KT-1000.

In patients who have low demand for twisting and pivoting activities, nonsurgical treatment may be best. In other patients, if the knee has poor or weaker secondary restraints, instability can occur with most activities, and they will need an ACL reconstruction.

A second group of patients may have a middle level of instability when tested. They will have difficulty with twisting, jumping, heavy work, and recreational sports. These patients need their knee repaired and ligament reconstructed to return to sports, recreation, or work activities at their prior level.

A third group of patients will have a small amount of instability. They will not have too much difficulty with regular activity. If they are not in higher-level sports or a work environment requiring lots of physical activity, many do not need an ACL reconstruction and can be treated using a brace and physical therapy. The patients with high activity levels who play competitive sports (varsity high school, competitive college, or higher levels—semipro and pro) cannot compete.

In my practice, the ACL ligament is reconstructed with minimally invasive arthroscopic techniques on an outpatient basis. It requires placing a tendon graft into the patient's knee to

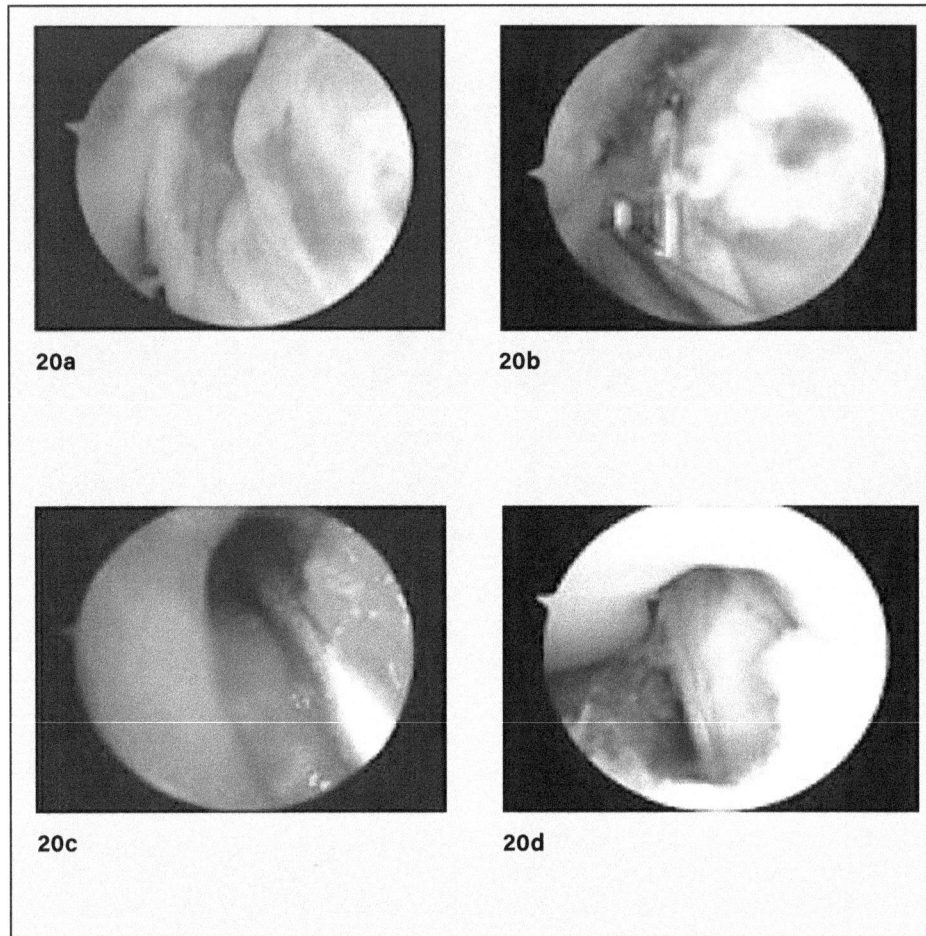

20 a, b, c, and d Arthroscopic view of (a) ACL tear, (b) ACL guide in place during reconstruction of the ligament, (c) guide pin in place to drill ACL tunnels for graft placement, and (d) new ACL graft in place.

replace the ligament since those fibers are destroyed at the time of injury. I use special instruments to drill bone tunnels in the tibia and the femur at the location of the natural ACL. The graft is guided through the tunnels using fine wires and sutures until it sits in the correct position. (This is very much like building a ship inside a small bottle.) The graft is then anchored in place with a titanium screw on one side and dissolving pins on the other. The knee is also checked for damage or tears to any other structures at the time of surgery. If there are meniscus tears, cartilage tears, loose chips, or other issues in the knee, they are repaired at the same time (see Images 20a-d above).

The knee is then tested again with the KT-1000 to be sure the ligament reconstruction has recreated the same stability as the patient's other knee as much as possible before the patient leaves the operating room.

Once the graft is secured in place, the knee has been fully inspected, and all issues have been treated, the knee is injected with local anesthetic for pain relief, the wounds are dressed, and a cooling pad (to control swelling and reduce any discomfort) is placed inside the dressings. A knee immobilizer is placed over the dressing and cooling pad to protect the knee. This stays on until the patient's first physical therapy appointment.

Female Athletes and ACL Tears

Muscle control in women is not the same as in men. It turns out that women's and men's muscles react in different ways when they are playing sports. Video footage of high school athletes during competition has taught us that men and women have different ways of jumping and landing; women tend to bend their knees less, landing with their knees straighter, and they use their quadriceps muscles to a greater extent than their hamstrings. This causes them to be more flat-footed when they land, increasing strain on the ACL, particularly at the end of a quick move. The muscle pattern difference, plus the anatomic factors, explain why many of the injuries occur as noncontact events.

What Can Be Done About This?

Since the anatomic factors are unchangeable, a woman can decrease her risk of injury by trying to improve her muscle balance and landing style. By studying video footage, we know that practicing two-legged landings has the potential to reduce the risk of injury for female athletes. Keeping their knees bent while jumping and landing on the balls of their feet while using their hamstrings (back of thigh) and glutei (buttock) muscles will help protect their knees. In fact, studies have shown that preseason and in-season balance and jumping programs provide some protection, although not all authors agree on how much. Rehab can help, and the leg muscles will compensate for some of the loss, but they cannot replace the mechanical protection that a healthy ACL gives in high-level sports. The result is often a recurrent injury that leads to the tearing of the meniscus or other cartilage damage, which can be the start of arthritis and is associated with knee locking (getting stuck in one place). With a repetitive injury, the knee can become completely locked, and the athlete will not be able to extend the knee or even walk on it. To avoid these long-term problems, most injured athletes opt for surgery.

Valgus Collapse

It has also been noted and research has shown that female athletes are at an increased risk for valgus collapse, also known as "knocked-knee." When athletes jump and land, the knee falls into a knocked-knee position, which increases stress on the ACL. Along with the other factors mentioned in this chapter, the knee is at risk for injury. Some data shows that training can decrease the tendency to land with valgus collapse and reduce the risk of ACL injury.

Image 21 demonstrates common postures observed while female athletes are in motion. From left to right, the figures shown increasing degrees of valgus collapse. This type of motion is called "dynamic valgus collapse." It sometimes happens more often with increased activity and muscle fatigue. The weakness in the leg, if not corrected with training exercises, may also hinder performance and cause injury in a competitive sports environment.

ACL Brace

ACL bracing has some pros and cons (see Image 22). Many patients, athletic trainers, and physicians today don't believe that braces are needed or worth using and that the graft is stable enough in the early post-op period to tolerate normal activities of daily living within six to eight weeks. About 10 to 15 years ago, so-called advanced, rapid, or "quick" rehab programs with an early return to sports were very popular. They often returned many young athletes to full sports at four months after a reconstruction of the ACL. These programs almost always failed and caused many retears. The idea gets some momentum from "newer" and maybe "better" surgical techniques, but no matter how clever your surgeon may be, Mother Nature likes to have her own timetable. It is clear that most patients have very different opinions of what are normal activities, what are

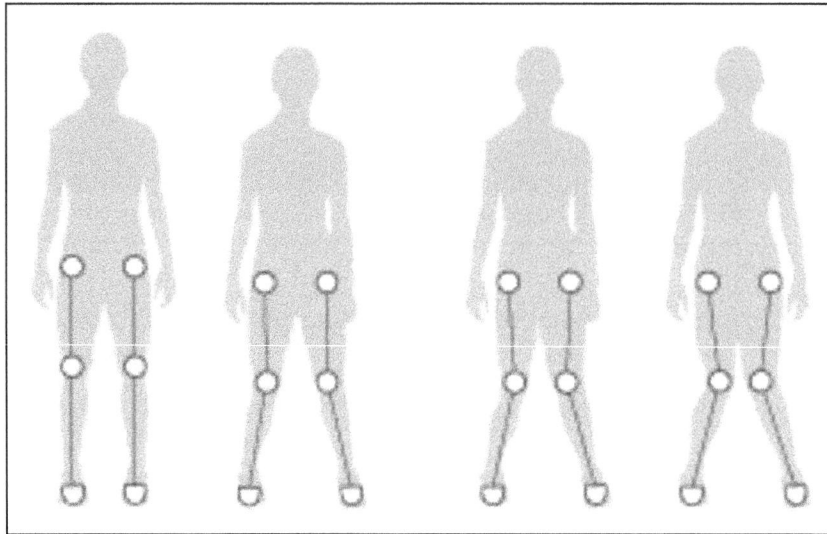

21 Graphis showing the knee alignment typically seen in female athletes at high risk for ACL tears. Left: normal alignment, moving to right, increasing knocked-knee positions (valgus knees) that increase loads on ACLs during sports and are responsible for so-called "valgus collapse" with jumping and pivoting that frequently ends with a tear of the ACL. Training can alter the jumping style and reduce risks.

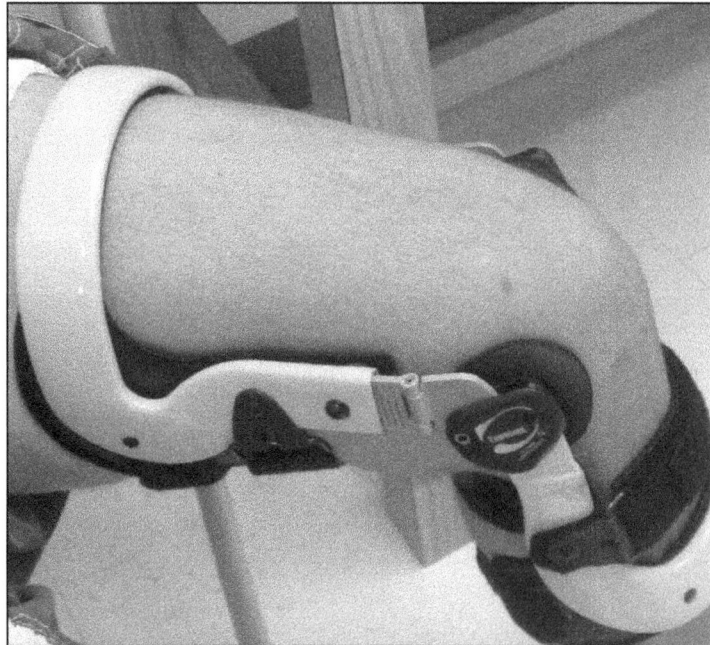

22 Custom ACL sports brace.

safe activities, and what are not safe activities. Often these are not based on science or fact and many times are a result of bad information posted on the Internet. Asking what people think is their normal activity level is important. It can really help the doctor to understand what the patient is willing to do and not do postoperatively. We can then council them appropriately.

That understood, bracing is one way to slow patients down, reminding them that the biology of an ACL repair requires revascularization of the ligament, and this means the graft gets softer at three to six months postoperation as new blood vessels grow in. It then gets stronger over the next six months up to one year after the surgery. I like to use braces to protect my patients when they feel the best and the graft is most weak, between six months and one year after surgery. Most importantly, the data does support brace use when first returning to pivoting sports, especially at the highest levels of competitiveness. The data shows that athletes are concerned and nervous about reinjury. This apprehension causes constant guarding. This makes normal reactions delayed during competition. As a result, bracing can prevent reinjury to the surgery side as well as an unwanted injury to the other leg. The newer data showed that post-op apprehension (fear of reinjury) occurs up to two years postoperatively and that it increases risks of reinjury or injury to the other knee when the patient is back at full strength (up to 20% to 25% of the time). I feel the brace gives the patient more confidence and decreases the apprehension that may be the cause of a second injury. So, I always recommend bracing the operative knee when back at full strength for the first full year of competition even though there is a lot of literature that states clearly bracing after surgery is not needed.

KT-1000 Testing

The KT-1000 helps us decide whether people need surgical repair. It has an advantage over an MRI since it's a physiological test and measures the ACL's actual function. Sometimes an MRI shows swelling in the ACL or a cyst in the ligament, but the ligament fibers are intact. Conversely, if a patient has a locked knee, where the meniscus is trapped in the middle, the KT-1000 test may appear normal even if the ACL is not working. Combining an MRI and a KT-1000 exam helps determine the best treatment plan for all patients when the ACL is injured. (See sidebar on page 48-49.)

Nonsurgical Treatment of the ACL

The knee is often bruised internally after an ACL injury. Therefore, the patient should use crutches for a few days or even weeks after the injury. Ice and compression will help relieve the swelling and help the patient to regain the full range of motion. Wearing an ACL brace can pre-vent reinjury. When the measured KT-1000 differences between the healthy and injured knee are small, the knee is stable enough to consider nonoperative treatments plus physical therapy with or without an ACL brace. If treating ACL tears without surgery, wearing an ACL brace for heavy sports may help prevent further injury to the knee.

In some cases, if the knee is stable, a brace may not add any stability, but it may add another way for the body to be able to feel the knee's position (the sense called proprioception), protect-ing it from further injury. When your body knows better where your knee and foot are, it will be able to prevent you from falling by using the correct muscles during activity. Physical therapy is important to help strengthen the muscles around the knee. For a return to sports, patients might also consider special conditioning and bracing (see "Female Athletes," page 45).

If the knee continues to give way after nonoperative treatment, the meniscus can become damaged. This is one of the main concerns when an ACL is not reconstructed shortly after an injury. Instability and subsequent meniscus tears can lead to more damage to the knee over time. In addition, locking and swelling can occur with activity. Recurrent swelling is a sign of increas-ing damage. Repairing the knee before more damage happens is important to some very active patients.

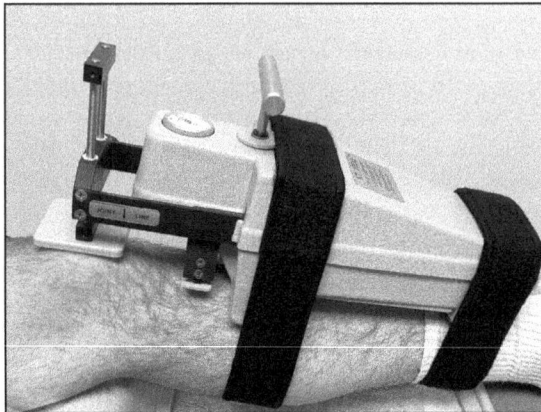

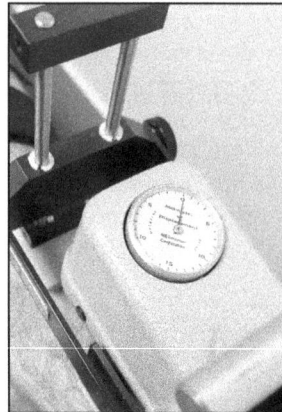

23a and 23b KT-1000 Knee Arthrotomer: Knee tester that measures the movement of the knee and helps decide if the ligaments are working properly. It can be used for making a diagnosis of a ligament tear and if a surgical repair is working properly.

What Is a KT-1000 Test and How Does It Work?

A KT-1000 is a small machine that is strapped onto the tibia and is used to diagnose ACL injuries. One pad touches the tibia and the other touches the kneecap. These pads are used to measure the range of motion in the leg, testing the ACL by pulling up the tibia. A typical reading for a normal leg in this test would be around 6–8 millimeters of anterior displacement. In addition to testing the ACL, when the KT-1000 is in place, the patient is asked to contract their quads. This causes displacement that is small when the PCL is working well and larger when it is not. This test is called the "quads active test," and it can be done from different angles to help determine if the PCL is torn. The healthy leg will be tested first, and then the injured side is tested to gauge the difference. This comparison is called the "side-to-side" difference. If the ACL is torn, the displacement measured for the injured knee will be larger than the reading on the normal side. A side-to-side difference greater than 3 millimeters is diagnostic of an ACL tear. If the PCL is torn, the test will be positive and the quads active test will be positive, too.

The KT-1000 can help decide if surgery is required for knees that have a torn ACL but the remaining uninjured ligaments keep the knee relatively stable. At times it is stable enough that the patient may not need surgery to fix the ligament. Those patients with an isolated ACL tear on MRI, no meniscus tears, and a KT-1000 side-to-side difference of 3 millimeters or less will do well with therapy alone.

Dale Daniel (one of the inventors of the KT-1000) and other researchers have shown that the level of instability in the knee can predict the risk of future injury with respect to activity level. For example, a patient with low demand (meaning that he or she plays cards for fun, doesn't play contact sports, or has a desk job) and a nonathletic lifestyle may have very little difficulty with an ACL tear and less than 5 millimeters difference between the two knees. The injured knee will tolerate daily activities and light exercise. However, a high-demand athlete may have difficulty with this same side-to-side difference. Furthermore, patients with more than a 7-millimeter difference will have problems with activities of daily living. This instability has been shown to increase the risk of a cartilage tear in the knee, recurrent swelling, and, because of the cartilage injury, subsequent arthritis. They typically need their knees repaired.

Training the Brain to Prevent ACL Tears

Research has shown that the best method to prevent an ACL tear may be to train your brain to respond better to stressful movements like a fast cut, a jump, or a pivot. However, when athletes are tired, their reactions to unanticipated commands become slower, making tears more likely to occur. Additional research shows that this is also true when only one leg is fatigued. The tired brain (from the fatiguing activity) reacts slower, and even the non-tired limb exhibits poor muscle reactions. The researchers proposed that this is because the brain cannot react well even though the muscle is healthy. Therefore, in this case, both limbs are at risk even though only the muscles on one side are fatigued and are too tired to react properly.

The researchers concluded that training a person's brain for sports jumps, pivots, and landing correctly on both legs may be the best way to counter this issue. Exposing the athlete to many controlled movements and training their responses for good balance and muscle control can improve reaction time in sports. In other words, sharpening an athlete's anticipatory skills could reduce the risk of injury. When mentally prepared, the athlete can avoid dangerous actions.

Surgical Repair of the ACL

ACL surgery is suggested if people don't respond to nonsurgical treatment, or it is initially recommended based on the relative instability of the knee. Although not perfect, and not a measure of full rotation control, the KT-1000 side-to-side difference can help predict a person's risk of more damage in the future. The level of demand the patient places on the knee and other injuries present (e.g., associated meniscus tears) may also make it clear that the knee needs repair (see Images 24 and 25). Most recently we have refined these concepts to add rotational control as well as anterior motion; these are finer technical points for your surgeon to consider during surgery.

Of course, the age and activity level of the injured patient are important considerations. I have reconstructed knees in patients as young as 10 and as old as 72. The 10-year-old patient was a competitive youth soccer player with knee instability and the 72-year-old was a high-level international skier. Although these are rare indications for surgery, both patients were at high risk of reinjury without reconstruction, even at their respective ages.

It must be noted that if a repairable meniscus tear is present after the initial injury, surgery is recommended since the outcome of a meniscus repair is improved when the ACL is reconstructed at the same time. The ACL tear repair surgery is done as an arthroscopic outpatient procedure. A tendon graft can be taken from the patient's patellar tendon, quads tendon, or hamstrings (called an autograft), or it can be taken from a donor's patellar tendon, hamstrings, or Achilles' tendon (called an allograft). Bone tunnels will be drilled into the tibia and femur, and the graft is then guided through the tunnels and can be anchored with titanium or bioabsorbable screws, buttons, pins, and other devices. After the graft is in place, the small incisions are closed.

There are a few different options for surgery. The most common is an autograft from the patellar tendon, and some doctors choose to use a hamstring tendon (a semitendinosus or gracilis) autograft. Because of past complications with synthetic grafts, most surgeons do not use synthetic substances for reconstruction anymore, although some new experimental grafts are being tested (that are not currently FDA-approved). Many inventors have tried these. Most have failed the test of time. The latest innovation is ACL repair with a special mesh and a clot. This method

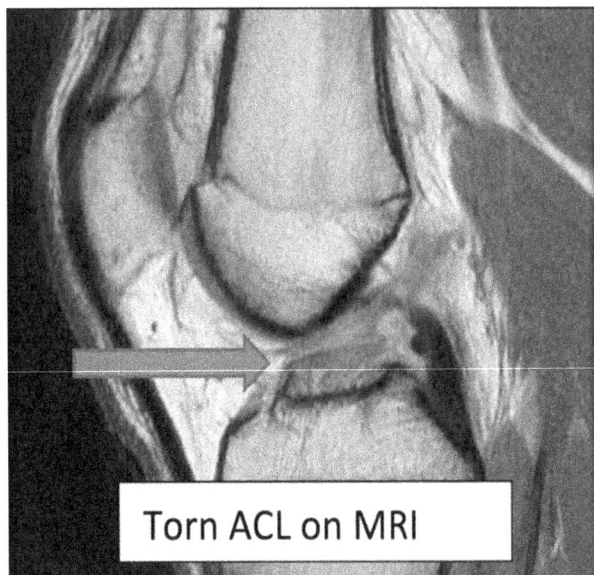

Torn ACL on MRI

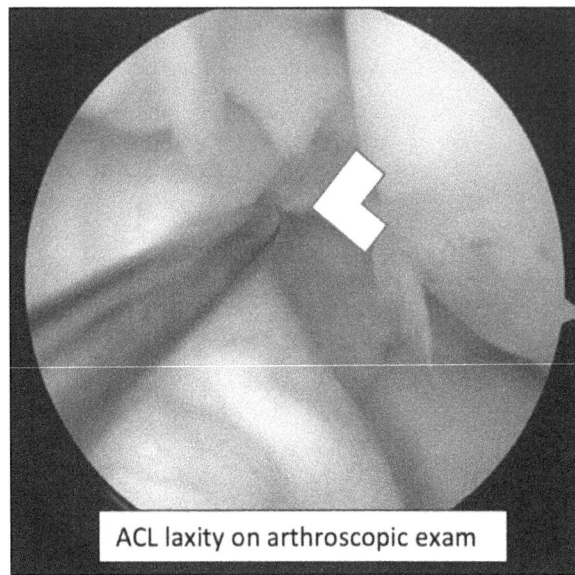

ACL laxity on arthroscopic exam

24 Torn ACL on MRI.

25 Arthroscopic of laxed or stretched ACL (that is not functioning based on KT-1000 exam).

would be for a few special cases where the ligament has torn off the bone more directly. The jury is out on the long-term effectiveness of this method when indicated.

The *New York Times* reported this as a viable option in July 2019, yet most of these procedures do not have long-term results, and some of these repairs have failed already. In a very select group, younger patients with specific types of tears like those located very close to the femoral attachment site of the ligament—a very small number of the people with ACL tears—may benefit from this type of repair, but there is no five- to 10-year data. Just the same, newer "repair" methods aside, I regularly repair tears in young patients when the ACL is torn off with a small piece of bone from the femur or the tibia and have been doing so for 30 years. In these cases, the idea is to put back the bone fragment with the ligament. When this type of repair is possible, these patients do well, and, despite the recent press, it's not a new idea.

There have been several reports of the effects of losing the donor site tissue and complications related to the healing process. There are known complications from graft harvest in autografts, including pain in front of the knee when the patella tendon is used and an inability to kneel after a patella tendon graft. When the hamstrings are used, there is residual hamstring weakness after the graft. For that reason, allografts have gained in popularity. More modern preparation of the grafts has made them stronger and the clinical outcomes of allograft vs. autograft are not significantly different, according to the most recent clinical criteria guidelines from the AAOS. Using a frozen tendon to fix the torn ACL causes less trauma to the knee, and the patient and does not sacrifice the normal structures around the knee (see Images 26a–c).

At the same time, there may be a small increase in the rerupture rate in younger patients when allografts are used. So, when it comes to using your own tendons for the graft or the frozen tendons, there is a trade-off of donor harvest site complications and long-term weakness at the graft donor site versus increased risk of reinjury in the younger age groups for the frozen tendon.

In general, patients age 25 and older have a harder time recovering from the graft donor site, and hence allograft may have some advantages for those cases. Some doctors prefer one type over another and will, therefore, favor that type of surgery. If they are more skilled in one area with

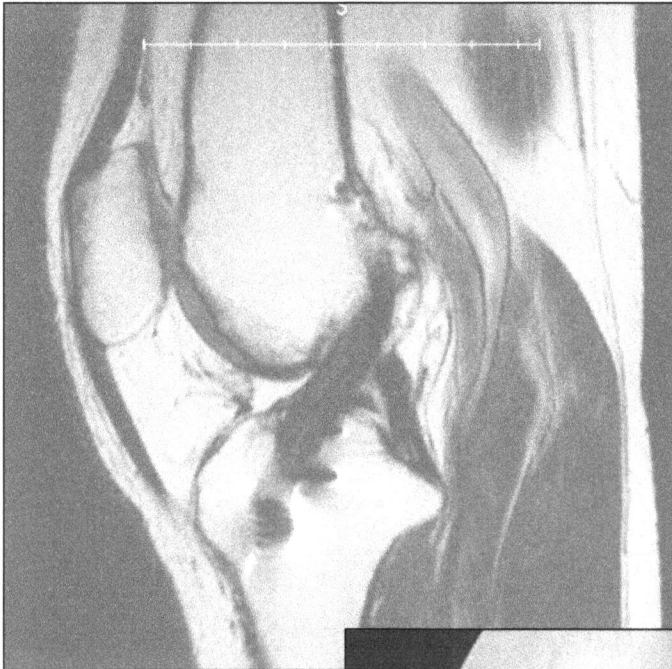

26a Solidly healed ACL graft on MRI. Note the normal position and the dense fibers of the new ACL.

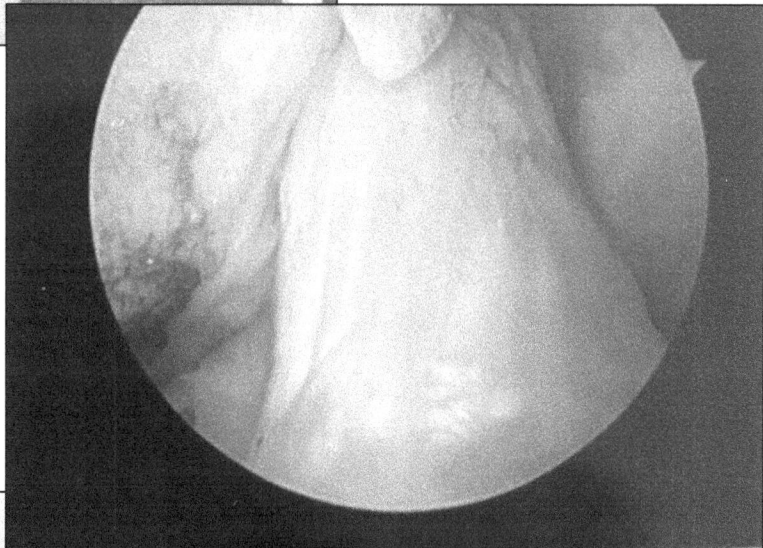

26b Arthroscopic view of an intact, fully functional ACL graft. Five years after Arthroscopic reconstruction with bone patella tendon bone allograft. Note anatomic tunnel placement and full healing of the allograft tissue.

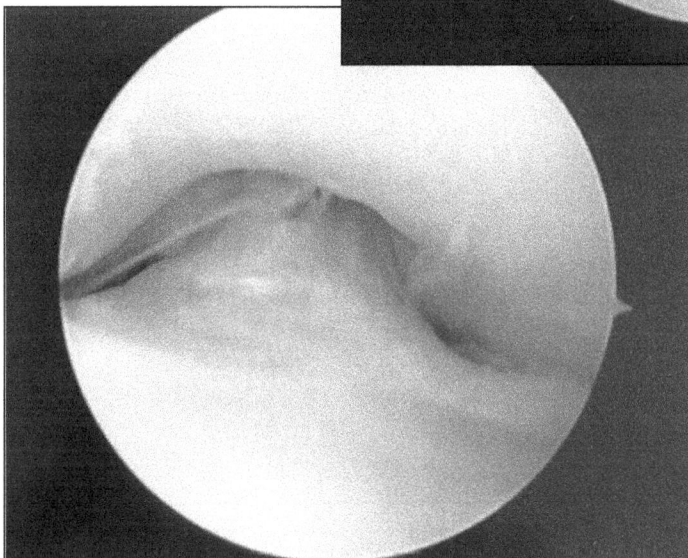

26c Arthroscopic view of ACL graft centered in the notch with the knee in full extension and anatomic in position.

a track record of good outcomes, it is wise to pick the option in which they have seen the best results in patients with the same injury. Patient choice is also important, as some patients don't want to use a healthy tendon to fix a torn ligament, while others don't like the idea of using a frozen tendon. Again, this is a personal decision with pros and cons on both sides of the equation.

ACL Tears in Very Young Athletes

The American Orthopaedic Society for Sports Medicine conducted a review study of the risks and benefits of repairing the ACL in a child under 14. In the past, doctors usually waited a long while before operating, for fear of creating a growth problem. This study shows that it is more prudent to perform the surgery sooner rather than later. Since the first writing of this book, new data shows that waiting six months or more puts the unstable knee at risk for more damage and meniscus tears. So, the patients who wait for surgery are much more likely to have additional injuries and knee problems because the knee is left unstable. More specifically, these problems include irreparable meniscus tears, chondral injuries, and kneecap (patella-trochlear groove) injuries. With more evidence from the current studies, it appears that delaying an ACL repair in young patients may create more risks than benefits.

When the ACL is repaired in a growing athlete, care must be taken to protect the growth plates in the knee. Studies in young athletes have shown that special techniques that avoid the femoral growth plate (by having the graft over the top of the back of the femur) can spare growth and protect the knee from instability. In rare cases when this is needed, this is my preferred approach.

Injuries to Other Knee Ligaments (MCL, LCL, PCL)

The ACL gets so much press that other ligament injuries seem much more mysterious and far less common. From New York Jets star quarterback Joe Namath (one of the first athletes to have a major knee reconstruction in the 1960s) to golf's Tiger Woods (who underwent surgery in 2008), as well as other athletes in soccer, basketball, and football, the ACL still gets all the headlines—after more than 50 years. The truth is, the knee has four major ligaments, two menisci, and a curved shape, and they each play an important role in its function. The four ligaments, the ACL, PCL, LCL, and MCL, all help to stabilize the two bones of the knee while allowing for full motion. It is a marvel that this joint works as well as it does.

Knee ligament injuries vary widely. As we have already discussed, the ACL can be injured with hyperextension, pivoting, and quick cutting motions. Next, I will discuss some problems that affect the other ligaments.

Medial Collateral Ligament

Of all the knee ligaments, the MCL is the most frequently injured and least frequently reported in the sports world. This may be due to the little-known fact that it is the strongest of all the ligaments, and it has two layers, so that partial injuries or sprains heal quickly and leave little functional deficit while healing. The ligament is located on the inner side of the knee, outside the synovial lining of the joint. Still, it can be sprained, partly torn, or completely torn (Grades 1, 2, and 3).

An examination of the patient will show little or no laxity in Grades 1 and 2 when a sideways (valgus) stress is applied. In other words, there is no movement on stress tests of side-to-side movement of the knee. Pain during stress testing and palpation over the femoral or the tibial insertion sites of the MCL help to make the diagnosis. Grade 3 sprains are far more unstable, as they are complete disruptions that leave the knee unstable (see Image 27). Grade 3 injuries often will heal with immobilization and protection. Once healing has started, motion is allowed in a protective brace. Grade 3 injuries require bracing for six to eight weeks and even more time to regain full strength. When torn, the proximal MCL injuries heal better than the distal MCL.

Occasionally, a severe Grade 3 sprain fails to heal. When a Grade 3 tear does not heal and instability persists, reconstruction or reefing (pulling the ligament onto the bone to tighten it) is needed. Sometimes reconstruction with a tendon autograft or tendon allograft is used to reconstruct the loose structures.

Children present an added concern since an injury to the growth plate can masquerade as an MCL injury. If an MCL is suspected in a growing child, X-rays, including stress views, or possibly an MRI, are mandatory to make certain that the growth plate is not injured. Growth plate injuries in children require complete cast treatment or other strict immobilization.

If there is an ACL and MCL combination injury, fixing the ACL alone will usually allow the MCL to heal.

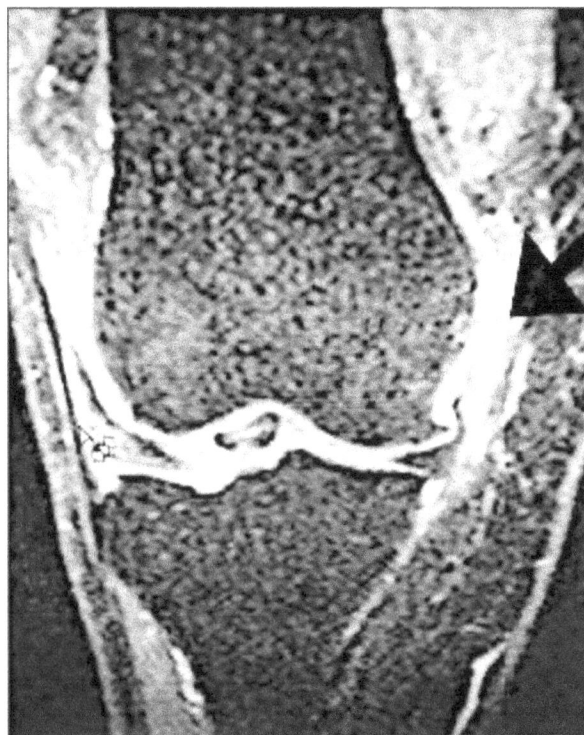

27 MRI view of a complete Grade 3 MCL tear (arrow).

Lateral Collateral Ligament

The LCL tears less often than the MCL, even though it is a weaker ligament. In fact, the LCL is the weakest of all four ligaments. The strength of the knee ligaments in order is MCL > PCL > ACL > LCL. Imagine how easy it is to be hit on the outside of the knee while playing sports. A blow to the outside of the knee is what stresses the MCL. Injuring the LCL requires the opposite stress, a blow to the inside of the knee. This injury is far less likely to occur in all sports than a blow to the outside of the knee. Therefore, even though the LCL is far weaker, it is much harder to injure. When the LCL is torn, it is often associated with tears of the lining of the knee joint on the same side (the posterior lateral corner of the knee). This causes rotational instability, and, on examination, the foot will turn out more on that side when compared to the uninjured side. This extra rotation is called a positive "dial sign." If the lateral side of your knee is injured and unstable, your doctor may be looking for the dial sign during an exam.

When the LCL is completely torn or partially torn and does not heal, it must be repaired. When a doctor repairs the LCL, research suggests that they augment the repair with a graft to help reinforce it. This will give the ligament the best chance of healing with good stability and solidly correct the instability that an LCL tear causes. I agree with this approach except when the ligament is avulsed with a piece of bone; in those cases, the ligament is intact and attached to the fracture, and repairing the fracture with the ligament on it may be strong enough without the addition of a graft.

Posterior Cruciate Ligament, or PCL, Tears With Other Ligament Injuries

The PCL, like the ACL, is inside the knee joint (see Image 28). It is stronger than the ACL, and injuring it takes a higher level of trauma. The trauma is often to the upper tibia and occurs in a collision during sports; a fall on the bent knee; or trauma like a car, ATV, or motorcycle accident. The injury results from a direct blow to the shinbone, a fall on the leg with the foot pointed down, or a dashboard injury when the shinbone hits before the kneecap. In the past, non-break-away bases were the primary cause of PCL injuries in baseball players who bent their knee while sliding. This has improved with the newer bases that "break away" when hit too hard.

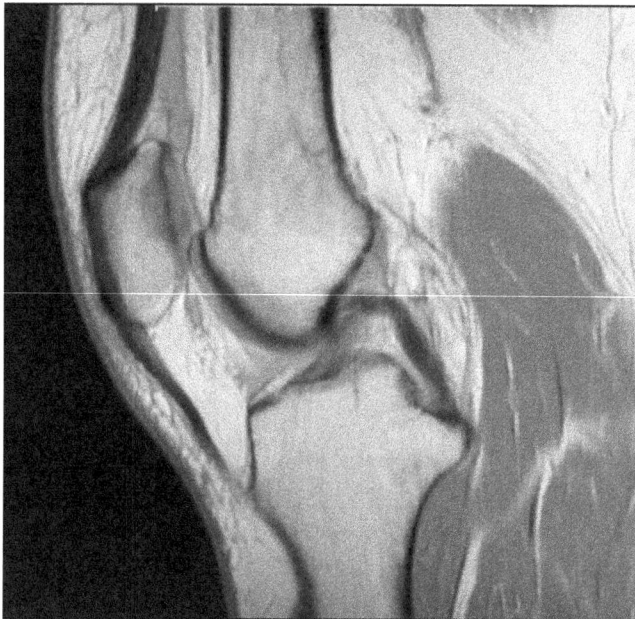

28 Normal view of an intact PCL on MRI (image at left).

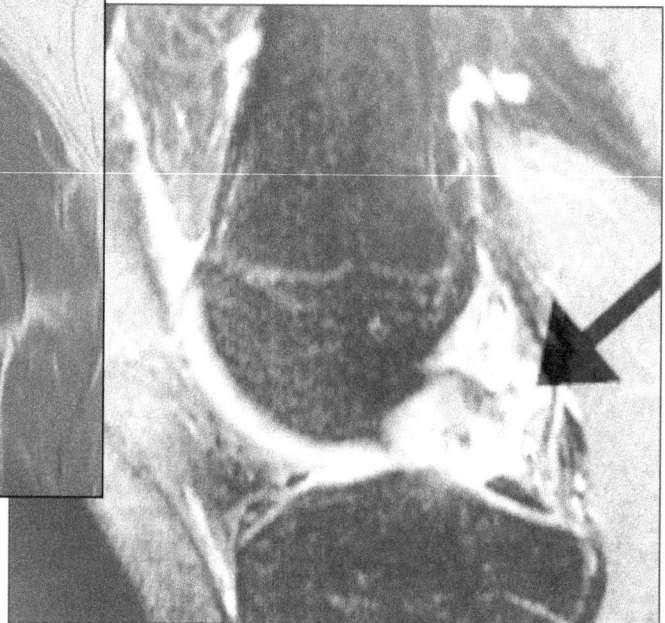

29 Complete tear of the MCL on MRI (arrow).

The initial symptom in a patient with a PCL tear is a swollen knee that improves with time. In addition, with an isolated PCL tear (when all the other ligaments are intact), people do not complain of knee instability or the knee giving way like ACL patients do. They usually have a slow onset of increasing kneecap pain or medial knee pain. This is primarily because of increased stresses seen by the kneecap and medial knee as a direct result of the loss of the PCL's main function (holding the tibia forward with knee motion).

When the PCL is torn, the tibia slips back under the femur (see Image 29). When the quads muscle pulls on the kneecap of the injured knee, it forces the tibia to slide forward and back into place. This sliding back and forth is a problem for the knee. The extra force needed to hold the tibia forward when the PCL is not working adds load to the quadriceps and, as a result, increases pressure on the kneecap. The constant shifting back and forth wears on the medial knee, too. Often PCL injured knees don't "feel" unstable, but the forces on the knee cap go up. Over time the kneecap wears out and becomes arthritic. As a result, PCL tears can be a relatively silent destroyer of kneecap cartilage.

Your doctor can test the knee for PCL instability and, pending the level of damage, figure out if it will need repair or reconstruction to help prevent future damage to the knee. In many cases, when instability is low, bracing and exercise may be the best treatment, but in others, reconstruction is best.

Note: When there is increased movement (the extra front-to-back sliding) of more than 10 millimeters (using the KT-1000), it is important to check for other injuries. In other words, when the knee movement after an ACL or PCL injury is larger than 10 millimeters, there are other ligaments torn or stretched. The second torn ligament can explain this level of abnormal motion. The extra motion is a tip-off to your doctor that there may be unrecognized ligament injuries or meniscus tears along with the ACL or PCL tear. The other ligament injuries are often the major reason for the increased instability seen in these patients.

In an LCL and PCL combination injury, the knee is very unstable, and both ligaments need to be repaired and reconstructed. As one would expect, with each additional ligament and more trauma to the knee, the more challenging it is to put the knee back together.

When the PCL is torn at the same time as other ligaments, the knee may have been dislocated at the time of the injury and gone back into place. No matter how they occur or how simple the injury mechanism sounds, knee dislocations are associated with severe trauma and are serious injuries. When the PCL is torn with other injuries, even if it looks well-centered or even normal on an X-ray, the knee can still be very unstable. We evaluate each ligament separately and often add information from an MRI to figure out the best treatment. Some of the ligaments need repair, while others need reconstruction.

Of course, more severe PCL injuries, along with other ligament tears, can cause significant functional instability. Knee dislocations that present with the bones out of place can also cause injury to important blood vessels and nerves. The most important of these is the popliteal artery since it supplies blood to the rest of the lower leg. When the popliteal artery is torn, it is a major concern; a special test is needed (an angiogram), and if the artery is torn or damaged, and circulation to the foot is lost or at risk of being lost, repair is mandatory.

8 DEFORMITIES OF THE KNEE AND OSTEOARTHRITIS

WE OFTEN SEE PEOPLE WITH BOWED LEGS OR KNOCKED KNEES. MANY OF THESE patients don't understand what happens to those knees over time. Likewise, physicians don't talk about why it occurs and what happens to those knees over time. The "normal" leg has a perfect mechanical balance. The knee joint is at the center of a straight line that connects the hip to the ankle. This is how the forces on the hip are shared equally on each half of the knee and balanced directly over the ankle, which puts the least amount of stress on each joint. It sounds simple and logical that we are built this way. So why do we see bowed legs and knocked knees?

Bowed Legs and Knocked Knees

When there is a mechanical deformity of the knee like bowed legs (a "varus" knee) or knocked knees (a "valgus" knee) (see Image 30), orthotics and braces have been shown to help improve function and decrease pain in some patients. Yet other researchers have debated the usefulness of braces and orthotics. In my practice, many patients have enjoyed relief by using unloader braces, and others have found corrective orthotics less cumbersome yet still helpful in reducing daily pain. This does not mean that braces and orthotics help everyone. They don't. Still, the patients that do get relief see improvements in function and are happy to use these devices.

In patients where part of the knee is in good health and another part is wearing out, who have significantly bowed legs or knocked knees, surgery to correct the problem is helpful. In

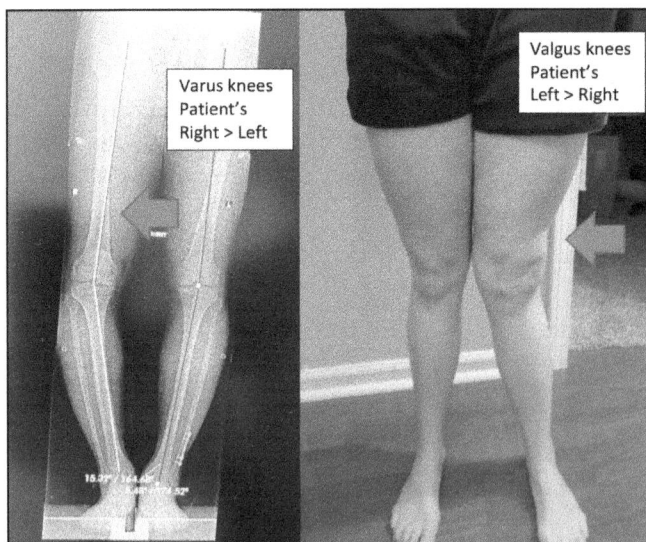

Varus knees
Patient's
Right > Left

Valgus knees
Patient's
Left > Right

30 Standing X-rays (left) showing bowlegs (a varus deformity) and photo (right) showing knocked knees left knee (a valgus deformity).

these patients, the repair is accomplished by cutting the bone and correcting the bowed or knocked knee deformity. This is done by straightening the bent bone, adding some bone grafting materials to fill the gap, and then fixing the bone in proper alignment with a special implant or metal plate with screws. Once completely healed, this correction can balance the loads on the knee and reduce the pain dramatically. Surgically the bone is premeasured and a plan for the needed correction is made (see X-rays in Image 30 of varus knees, or bowed legs, and the photo of valgus, or knocked, knees). The bone is repositioned to be in line with the loads on it and fixed in place with a plate. This moves the load back to the healthy side of the knee, which can improve function and potentially buy years of pain relief. (See Images 31a–d of a valgus knee being corrected with an opening wedge osteotomy of the distal femur.)

The truth is that some of us are born with a tendency to either have bowed or knocked knees, and then the forces of weight-bearing and growing help reshape our legs to a more

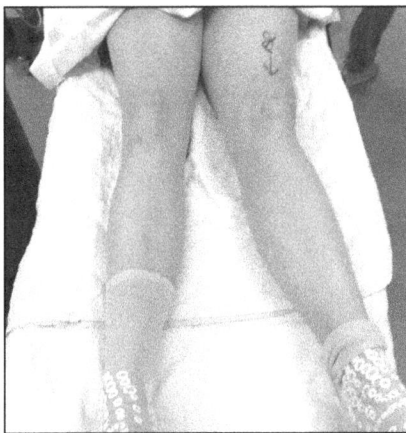

31a Photo of a. left valgus or knock knee prior to correction.

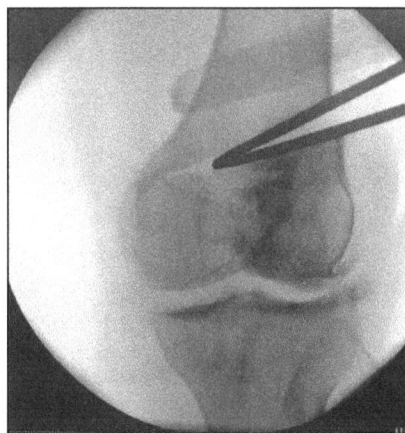

31b Intra operative X-ray image of correction.

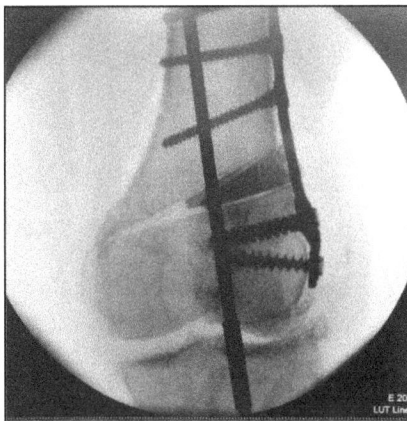

31c Plate holding correction in place with an X-ray alignment rod (held over the limb) showing the line between the hip, knee, and ankle.

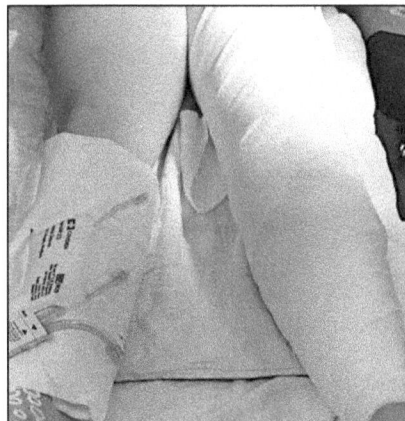

31d Final leg correction with post-op dressings on.

normal alignment. Sometimes it is seen in the parents as well as all the siblings. When the childhood bowing is excessive, and the body does not fully reshape the knee as it grows, we need to look for other causes of bowed legs. Sometimes nutritional conditions cause the bone to not grow properly or weaken the growth plate at a critical time and bowing gets worse. One example is vitamin D deficiency. When D is low during periods of growth, we get the disease called rickets. Early vitamin D replacement will correct this problem, but if you correct the deficiency too late, the deformity will remain.

Other conditions, like Blount's disease (a genetic recessive disorder, worsened by obesity and damage to the growth plate on the inside of the knee during growth) and trauma to the knee while growing will also cause a knee deformity. Adult fractures that heal incorrectly can also cause bowed or knocked knees. Patients who develop knocked knees and are overweight also tend to see this worsen over time. Medically, we call the deformity associated with bowed legs a "varus" deformity and the deformity associated with knocked knees a "valgus" deformity.

Bowed or Varus Knees

When the knee is bowed, more of the body's weight falls on (in other words, passes through) the inside part of the knee. This can become painful with activity or prolonged standing. The inside half of the knee will often wear faster than the outside, forcing the knee to bow more and more over time. This increases the stress on the inside of the knee. The cycle worsens until the inside (medial side) wears out. There are some tip-offs when this is happening. We often can look at a person's shoe and see the heel of the shoe wearing on the outside edge first. This is a result of the bowing at the knee and how it changes the person's gait.

Before this happens, weight loss (if the individual is overweight), activity modification, like working on softer surfaces, and soft shoe inserts help to decrease pain and can delay progression of the deformity. NSAIDs can decrease bone pain but do not change the knee mechanics. Increasing bowing of the leg also increases stress on the inside of the knee. In theory, tilting the foot the other direction with lateral wedges may help reduce pain. Wearing proper shoes with a good flat heel that is not worn unevenly matters; the more worn the heel the more force on the inside of the knee. Some doctors feel that going one step further by adding a lateral wedge to orthotics shifts some more weight off the inside of the knee. Studies have shown mixed benefits of this type of foot orthotic placed in the shoe for unloading the knee. In general, people who try orthotics with or without the lateral wedge and find they reduce pain should use them. Be aware that a very rigid orthotic may indirectly stiffen the foot and take away some of the foot's natural movement that also cushions impact on the knee. So others feel that soft, "bouncy" orthotics like the "back savers" also have some use in painful knees.

Medial unloader braces (see Image 32) also shift load off the medial knee and have been shown to give good pain relief. In some patients, they work well and can be well tolerated. Some heavy laborers also find them very helpful. The same is true for lateral unloading braces for knocked knees. In patients with deformity, pain, and limited arthritis who are relatively young for knee replacement, the deformity can be surgically corrected. When the knee is bowed outward (bowed legs) or inward (knocked knees), a corrective osteotomy that corrects the alignment shifts the weight and realigns the hip, knee, and ankle. With bowed legs the cut is usually in the tibia, and the correction can be made with an opening wedge. For knocked knees, the bone is cut in the femur and an opening wedge is made. In each case, the goal is to center the foot on a line that passes from the center of the hip through the center of the knee.

When the knee joint is worn out and the patient is older, a knee replacement may be the preferred operation. In slightly younger patients where the other two parts of the knee are clear of arthritic change, there is not a large deformity to correct, and the patient is not overweight, a partial knee replacement may be the best choice. In general, the realignment procedures (osteotomies) are very popular in Europe and less used in the US. In Europe, osteotomies are favored over partial knee and total knee replacement, and the opposite is true in the US. The truth is most likely in the middle, that we in the US underuse this bone correction operation, and Europeans may use it too much. The final answer is very debatable.

In my practice, I perform a correction for the angular problem in younger patients who are too young for replacement surgery. I have a few patients whom I performed this procedure on more than 20 years ago and who still have good results. Most have not required knee replacements since the correction of the deformity. The correction for varus knees can be done as a closing wedge just below the knee on the outside or an opening wedge on the inside. For several technical reasons, my preference is an opening wedge correction.

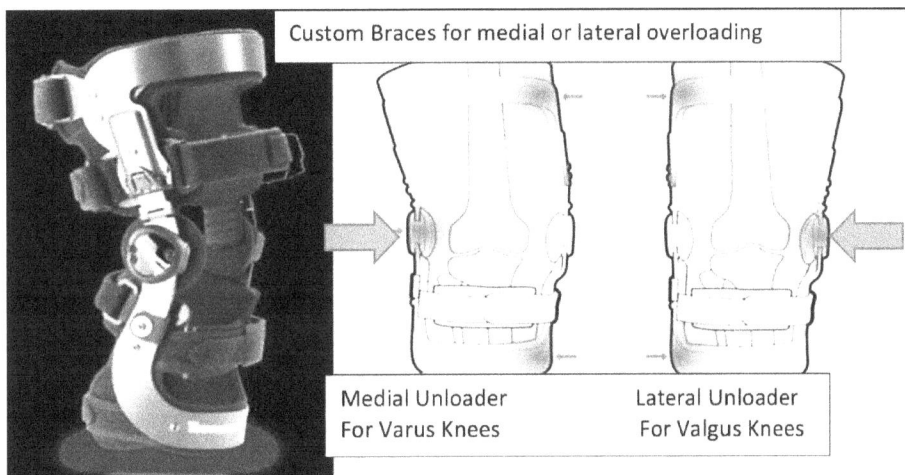

32 Brace for unloading the knee: medial unloader for varus knees, Lateral unloader for valgus knees.

Knocked or Valgus Knees

For valgus knees, when one knee is "knocking" against the other knee, the feet are not centered under the knees. The line through the center of the hip, knee, and ankle is not straight, so more of the weight falls on the outside part of the knee. This is also the case with a bowed knee, where the load is mostly on the inside of the knee. With knocked knees, the hip-knee-ankle line is also not straight but in the exact opposite direction. So, in knocked knees the knee can become painful on the outer side with activity or prolonged standing.

Worse, in knocked knees, the overloaded outside edge of the knee will wear faster than the inside, forcing the knee to bend in or become more "knocked" over time. This further increases the stress on the outside of the knee. The cycle worsens until the outside wears out, a problem caused by overloading on one side of the knee that is far worse in overweight patients. It also happens more quickly if there is a lateral cartilage tear in the knee or prior surgical removal of the lateral meniscus.

Before the knee wears out completely, weight loss (if overweight), activity modification, working on softer surfaces, and soft shoe inserts all help decrease stress on the knee. Just like in the varus knee, NSAIDs can decrease bone pain but do not change the knee mechanics. Lateral wedge orthotics are occasionally helpful; a good soft arch support may also help. Lateral unloader braces give some relief and are often well-tolerated.

Older patients will eventually need the knee replaced. Younger patients may have a partial knee replacement or a corrective osteotomy. In the case of knocked knees, we do the correction above the knee. Just like the corrections for bowed legs, these realignment procedures are very popular in Europe and performed less often in the US. In my practice, I offer and perform the correction for the angular problem in younger patients. When this operation works well, the leg is straight again, the gait is improved, and the pain is decreased, and these are some of my happiest patients (see Images 33–37).

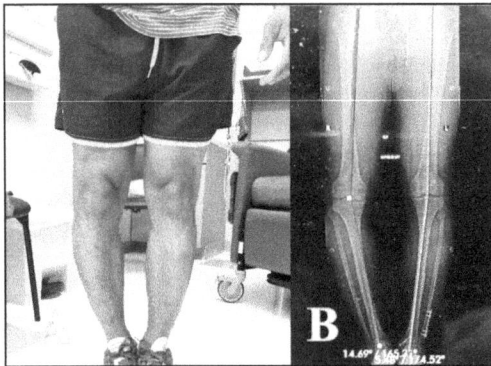

33 Left bowed leg with standing long leg X-ray for preoperative osteotomy planning.
Five years after Arthroscopic reconstruction with bone patella tendon bone allograft. Note anatomic tunnel placement and full healing of the allograft tissue.

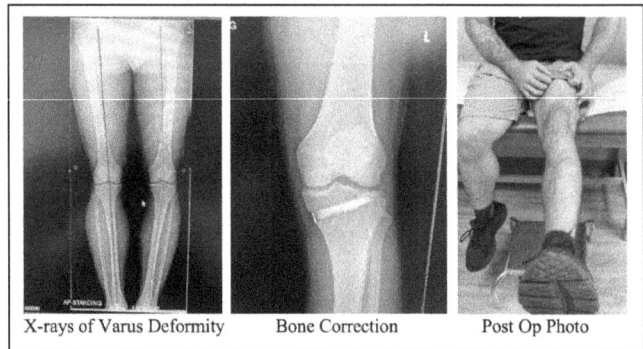

X-rays of Varus Deformity   Bone Correction   Post Op Photo

34 Bowleg correction, and post-operative photo after the osteotomy is healed.

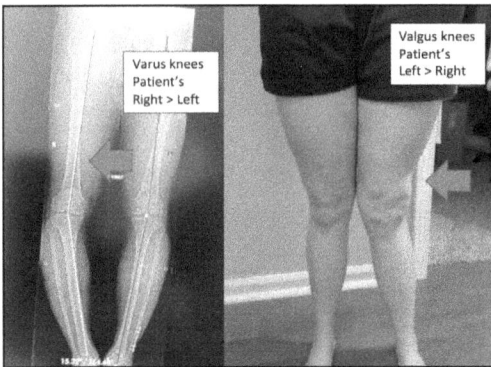

Varus knees Patient's Right > Left

Valgus knees Patient's Left > Right

35 Comparison of varus and valgus knees.

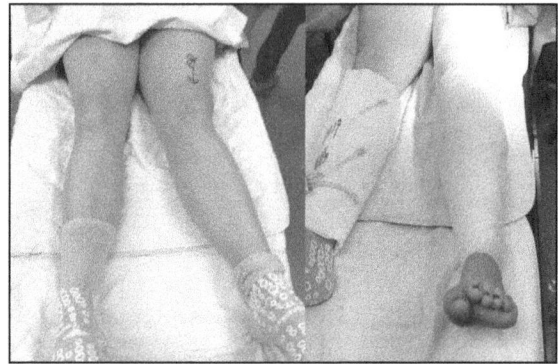

36 Pre-op and post-op comparisons.

37 Operative corrections: (a) making the bone cut, (b) making the correction angle with metal wedges, (c) final correction.

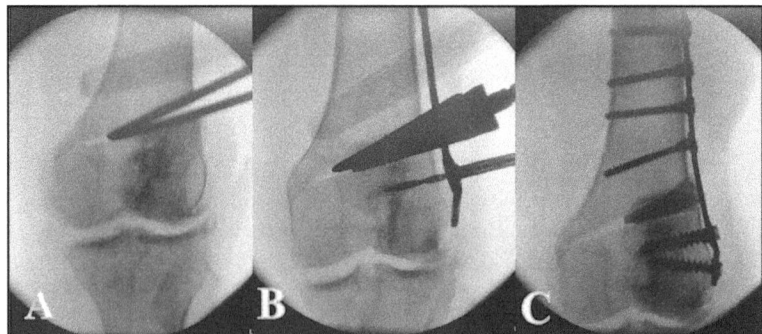

9 MENISCUS TEARS: TORN "CARTILAGE" IN THE KNEE

Torn cartilage is an old term and can be confusing to patients. The truth is the knee has two types of cartilage. One is the special cartilage that covers the bones. It is called the articular cartilage. It is specialized to be the most slippery surface (lowest friction) to make the knee motion smooth and use the least energy possible.

The other is the meniscus cartilage. This is a special "C" shaped piece of a different type of cartilage that is designed to transfer load from one side of the knee joint to the other. This is the type of cartilage that tears, so when we say torn cartilage, we often mean a torn meniscus and not damage to the articular surface on the bone. When the cartilage on the bone is damaged, that is called articular cartilage damage; when it is soft or thin, it's called chondromalaci; and when severe, it is called osteoarthritis. In general, using the term torn meniscus is more specific and clearer than torn cartilage since there are two types of cartilage in the knee.

What Is a Meniscus?

The menisci are two gasket-like cartilages that are inside the knee and sit on top of the tibia; they help its flat surface better match the curved surface of the femur. Together, the two menisci fit snugly around the rim of the knee (see Image 38). They act as a cushion for the femur as it sits on top of the tibia. The menisci work to absorb shock, and with the articular cartilage, they help the leg bones move smoothly.

It was once thought that the menisci were of no use. But it is now well-known that they can carry up to 50% of the weight (force) across the knee, and if they are completely removed, arthritis will develop in short order. The lateral (on the outer side of the knee) meniscus is smaller than the medial side and almost "O" shaped (semicircular). The medial (on the inner side) meniscus is "C" shaped and is more likely to be injured. Once a meniscus is injured, the patient may experience locking, buckling, and giving way (see Part Two, Chapter 5, "The Unreliable Knee").

When a meniscus is torn, the torn edge can catch between the two bones and cause pain. The knee may lock or give way. This frequently causes swelling in the knee, loss of motion, and the sense that the knee is unstable. Pain can be worse when the leg is bent fully, twisted, or with an impact load of any type. Recurring swelling is a concern for ongoing damage to the knee as the knee is trying its best to lubricate itself without being able to fix the problem of the torn fragment getting caught between the bones. Over time, this causes arthritis and chronic pain. Doctors cannot reverse the damage that a locking or catching fragment causes if it is left untreated for too long. Left alone, over time the constant rubbing of the torn meniscus on the articular cartilage will cause more damage and degeneration of the knee joint. As a result, the knee may also become swollen, stiff, and tight. Therefore, to help protect the knee, many orthopaedic surgeons think that correcting the problem is best done sooner rather than later.

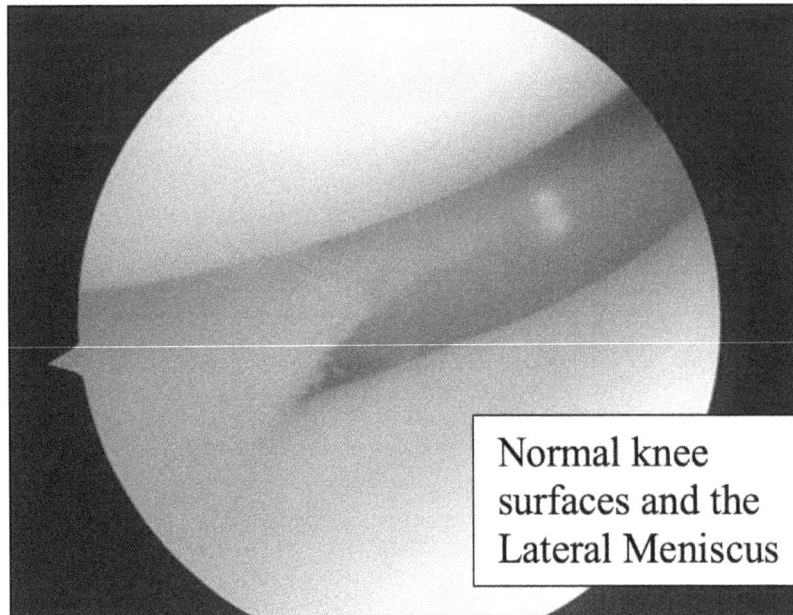

38 Normal meniscus.

Tearing the Meniscus

A tearing of the meniscus can occur in any age group. The meniscus does soften with age, and it is more common to see tears with less trauma as people get older. A tear usually results from forceful twisting of the knee with the knee loaded (the weight is on the knee) or planted on the ground. It can also occur when squatting or when the knee is hyper-flexed (bent back too far). It can happen after jumping and landing with the knee flexed or from twisting as the foot hits an obstacle, like a hole, a rock, a heavy object, or uneven ground. In addition, sometimes a very minor activity can cause a tear when there is a previous injury or a predisposing factor present. Tears can also come with a trauma that causes damage to the other ligaments. An injury to both a ligament and the meniscus makes the knee very unreliable, causes swelling, and usually prompts a visit to an orthopaedic surgeon.

Meniscus changes occur as we age, so be aware that getting an MRI after 65 frequently shows meniscus tears and arthritis; these are very common and may not be the cause of the pain (see Image 39c). More and more studies show that "cleaning up" meniscus tears in the older population gives short-term relief, but the long-term prognosis does not change. In my practice, I am careful not to order an MRI on older patients with arthritis since it almost always shows "tears," but these findings are most often a result of degenerative "wear and tear" and not caused by injury. It is important to remember these arthritic changes on an MRI are typically not a good enough reason, by themselves, for surgery. In general, "cleaning up" wear and tear changes in the knee often gives only short-term improvement that fades and sometimes worsens the knee symptoms. An MRI is helpful only after an older patient fails nonoperative treatments and/or we are concerned about a painful stress fracture, loose bodies, loss of circulation in the bone, a bone tumor, or knee issues other than just a degenerative meniscus tear.

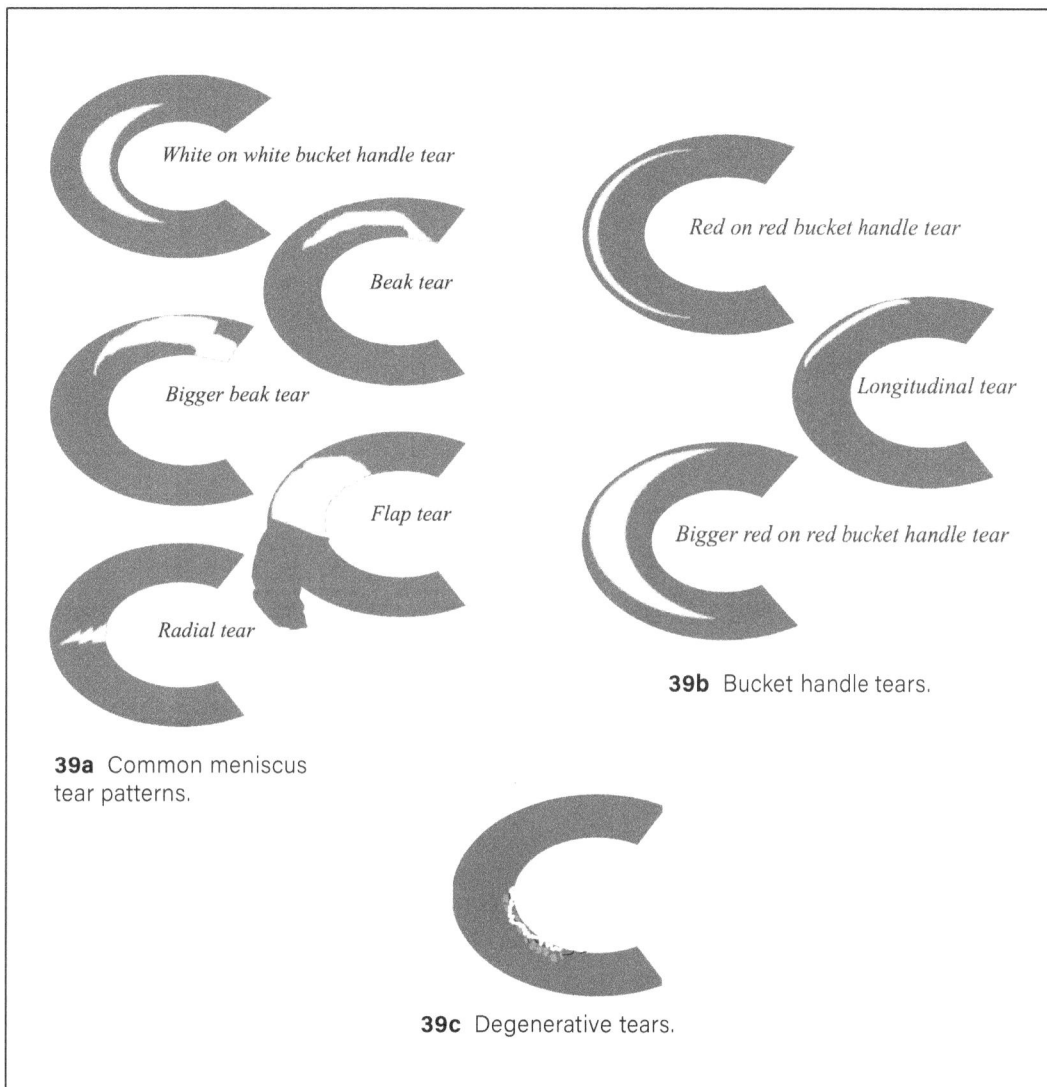

White on white bucket handle tear

Beak tear

Bigger beak tear

Flap tear

Radial tear

Red on red bucket handle tear

Longitudinal tear

Bigger red on red bucket handle tear

39b Bucket handle tears.

39a Common meniscus tear patterns.

39c Degenerative tears.

Why Do They Tear?

Tears in the meniscus usually occur because of a forceful twisting injury, squatting fully or with rapid, sharp, full bending (hyperflexion) of the knee. Playing sports, falling, twisting the knee while moving on uneven ground, work injuries, and trauma to the knee are all causes of a torn meniscus. In younger people, the meniscus is a tough and rubbery structure, and meniscal tears are more likely to be caused by a sports injury or trauma to the knee. In more mature individuals, the meniscus can be weaker and easier to tear, and it can occur because of a minor injury, even from the up-and-down motion of simple squatting.

Degenerative tears of the meniscus can also be seen as a part of osteoarthritis of the knee, gout, and other arthritic conditions. In those patients, the damage is more gradual, and the symptoms will appear over time. Repetitive compressive or rotational stress on the knee can cause the bones to strain the cartilage, causing further wear and tear. Finally, pieces of the meniscus can detach and go into the joint; these are called loose bodies, and they can cause pain and swelling (see Chapter 13).

How Will I Know If My Meniscus Is Torn?

In many cases, no one injury leads to a meniscal tear. Knee pain is the most common complaint, and sometimes it is accompanied by locking, buckling, swelling, or giving way. The pain may be felt along the joint line where the meniscus is located. Sometimes the symptoms are vague and occasionally involve the whole knee.

After the initial swelling goes away, a patient with a meniscus tear will usually complain of recurrent swelling without warning, the inability to squat or kneel, locking, or giving way. In other words, the knee gets stuck, requiring some twisting to unlock it and restore motion. There may be locking or catching while walking or twisting the knee, causing the knee to stop supporting the body's weight and give out. Less commonly, the knee becomes locked in a bent position and cannot be straightened at the time of the initial injury. This happens when the torn part of the meniscus is large enough to get stuck between the bones, which stops the hinge mechanism of the knee, causing a true block to knee motion. Walking is difficult with a locked knee, and running is almost impossible. Surgery is required to reduce and repair or remove the trapped, torn meniscus.

In general, even in knees that only lock intermittently, if meniscus tears are left untreated they can cause rubbing of the torn section against the tibial or the femoral surface. The knee may become swollen, stiff, and tight. In time, this will cause damage to or degeneration of the knee joint.

Special Case: Discoid Meniscus

The meniscus begins as a disc-shaped structure in utero. As the knee develops, the thick middle part becomes thinner, and it changes to the more common "C" shape or semi-lunar partial "O" shape. On occasion, the lateral meniscus does not change and will retain its "discoid" shape. Unlike the normal "C" or partial "O" shape, it looks like a filled in letter "D." People with this condition may never become aware of it until it becomes unstable or tears. When the damaged discoid meniscus causes locking, swelling, or pain, surgery is required to treat the problem. If the patient has surgery to repair this, the surgeon may remove the torn portion of the meniscus and reshape the meniscus into the natural "C" shape. A discoid meniscus may be one of the few tears we see in young children. Some people have a discoid that does not cause any symptoms until it tears, and some have an unstable discoid meniscus that slides around more than normal menisci do and can even lock inside the knee without a tear.

LATERAL MENISCUS

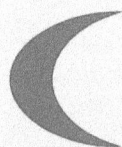

The More Normal "C" Shape   The Abnormal "D" Shape

Diagnosis

To make the diagnosis of any meniscus tear, a physician will ask for the history of the injury and examine your knee (see Image 40). We will test your knee when it is bent and straight, check for swelling (an effusion), check your ligaments, and check for joint line tenderness (pain over the tear when touched).

Also, there are some special tests we can perform. A McMurray's test is done by twisting your knee while bent in a direction that may catch the tear and seeing if straightening it causes a pop or pain, which would be positive for a tear. An Apley's compression test is done by twisting the knee when loaded to see if there is pain, and a flick test causes pain when flicking the knee in short, quick rotation to either side. Of course, other causes of knee swelling need to be excluded, as discussed in Chapters 5 and 6.

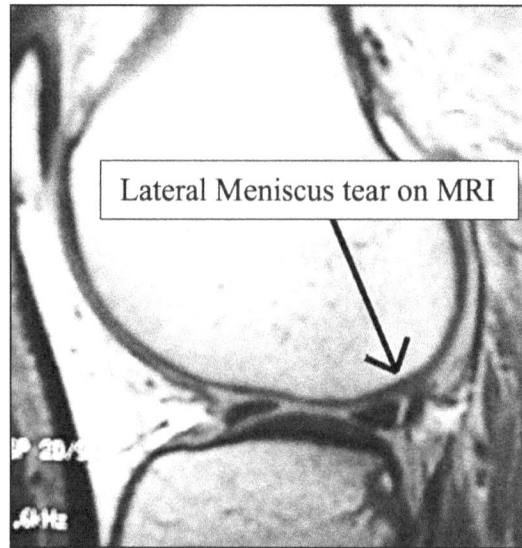

40 MRI of lateral meniscus tear.

Healing of the Tear

Some tears are small and with poor blood supply; these will be trimmed using the arthroscope and small instruments. This is called a partial meniscectomy. Other tears are on the outer edge (peripheral) with a good blood supply and can be repaired by sewing the edges together using special stitches. This is called a meniscus repair. People commonly mix these two procedures up. They are not the same, and they have very different postoperative care. Repairs require a modified physical therapy protocol, postoperative knee protection with a brace, and more time to heal.

For all types of meniscus repairs, how long it takes the body to heal after surgery is inversely proportional to the tear length, the patient's age, and the location of the tear.

The shorter the tear is, the younger the patient is, and the more blood flow there is, the faster the tear will heal. More details on repairs verses removal are discussed later in this chapter.

Meniscal and Baker's Cysts (Popliteal Cysts)

Occasionally, a meniscal cyst may accompany a tear. The tear irritates the knee, and the knee will react by trying to increase its lubrication by making more joint fluid. The fluid can be trapped by the tear and cause a local cyst that is connected to the tear. In practice, medial cysts occur more often than lateral cysts. Lateral meniscal cysts are harder to treat than medial meniscal cysts, and they have a higher risk of recurrence.

The joint fluid also can pump into the back of the knee through a tear into the popliteal space. This fluid collection is then called a popliteal, or "Baker's" cyst. The name implies that bakers get them; however, they are named after Dr. William Morrant Baker, who first described them in 1877. Just the same, the idea that bakers stand on their legs all day, and this causes swelling, rings true with my patients. The mental image of a baker standing on their feet helps them understand the problem. In either case, a sack of fluid forms that feels like a hard lump on the joint line, or a sense of fullness is felt in the back of the knee. The swelling causes pain when the knee is bent and often blocks the ability to squat.

When a Baker's cyst becomes large enough, it can rupture, causing pain and swelling down the calf. A rupture may feel like a pop and/or warm water running down the back of your leg followed by calf soreness and then days later maybe some bruising. Large Baker's cysts can also disturb the circulation to the foot and cause foot and ankle swelling. A cyst won't usually completely resolve unless the problem inside the knee, like a tear, is removed or repaired. Once the knee problem is treated, the cyst should go away on its own. If it doesn't, draining it may help. If it still does not go away, the cyst may need to be surgically removed.

What Are My Treatment Options?

If the knee is locked and cannot fully straighten, trying to force it straight will damage the knee more. In these cases, physical therapy is not a good idea, and a locked knee requires surgical (arthroscopic) treatment. Similarly, a mechanically unstable knee with frequent locking and giving way can put you at risk for a fall down the stairs or even while just walking down the street; fixing the knee is key. A repaired knee helps prevent falls. In many cases, an MRI is helpful for a doctor to fully understand if other structures are damaged. In a locked knee, the MRI helps us plan to fix everything torn or damaged at the same time, if that is what is best for the patient.

If there is an ACL or other ligament tear, the torn meniscus or cartilage damage should be treated arthroscopically at the same time. The results are far better when these procedures are done together than separately, since stabilizing the ligaments is important when the meniscus is repaired. Fixing the ligament or ligaments helps the healing of the repaired meniscal cartilage and prevents reinjury once it is repaired.

NOTE: Many insurers now have minimal requirements to preapprove surgical treatment in knees with a torn cartilage. They may include no advanced arthritis (see treatment in the next paragraph), at least six weeks of nonsurgical treatments such as anti-inflammatory medications (Advil, Aleve, Motrin, ibuprofen, etc.), and doctor-directed therapeutic exercises or physical therapy by a professional. An injection of cortisone or draining the knee may also be helpful in some cases for a swollen knee before considering surgery. That is a clinical decision made by the orthopaedic surgeon depending on your history, physical exam, and X-rays.

When a patient already has advanced arthritis and a torn meniscus, the treatment options for the torn meniscus may be limited since the damage to the bone surface may be the primary cause of the pain. In those cases, injections, a lubricant, platelet-rich plasma (PRP), therapy, glucosamine/chondroitin, and braces have all been used. In many cases, symptoms can be controlled without surgery or knee replacement. Cortisone may last six months or more and a lubricant from nine to 12 months, and sometimes much longer. PRP is a product that is made from your own blood. It can be drawn in the office setting, spun down, and the platelets separated from the red and white cells. The yellow liquid that remains contains plasma that is now enriched, or "rich" in platelets (hence the name platelet-rich plasma). Many star athletes have turned to PRP for treatment with some regularity, but the data is mixed. Some patients report great results individually but larger studies on the benefits of these treatments have been limited to subsets of patients with less severe arthritis. The PRP treatment is, in general, not covered by insurance, yet it has gained popularity due to its theoretical benefits.

In a knee with arthritis, arthroscopic treatment can clear the debris in the joint. This makes half of patients' knees feel better and makes the other half feel worse. If there are mechanical signs and symptoms from loose bodies, removing those fragments can reduce swelling. The mechanical symptoms can be related to a loosened fragment of cartilage or a torn meniscus that is caught between the two bones or locked. If there is already no cartilage left on the two bones and an X-ray shows the bones rubbing on each other ("bone on bone") and you have chronic pain, a replacement can be a better option over arthroscopy, depending on your age.

If you have no other options, there is a lot of recurring swelling, and the lining is inflamed (so-called synovitis), an arthroscopic "washout" may give six months or more of relief. If you are younger and have an inflammatory disease like rheumatoid or psoriatic arthritis, a synovectomy (arthroscopic removal of the inflamed lining) often gives ample relief for six months or more and may reduce your need for high-powered arthritic medications, at least temporarily.

One caution: recently there has been a lot of discussion about arthroscopic surgery in patients with advanced osteoarthritis in the knee and X-rays that show both bone and cartilage loss with bowing or knocked knees. In this type of advanced wear-and-tear osteoarthritis when there is not a lot of inflammatory lining to remove, arthroscopic "cleaning out" of the knee does not yield great outcomes. If you elect to do this, expectations are limited and results are guarded. While arthroscopic "cleaning out" for osteoarthritis may help some patients in the relative short term, it does not give true long-term relief for many.

Some patients may even feel worse a few months after arthroscopic treatment for osteoarthritis only. For advanced arthritis, depending on the patient's age and health, the knee may be best treated by performing a total knee replacement.

Exceptions

In patients considered too young for knee replacement, if there is deformity with only very localized arthritis on one side of the knee, surgical correction of the deformity may be the best option. There are also very promising new technologies for very localized loss of cartilage, which I will address in Chapter 13. Sometimes grafting the defect while you correct the deformity is the best option. This may include the local transfer of cartilage (sort of like hair plugs for areas of balding, or autograft), donated cartilage (allograft), or your own cartilage that is grown in the lab and reimplanted into your knee (the MACI procedure). More details are in Chapter 10, "Other Cartilage Defects."

Meniscus Cartilage Repair or Removal?

Since meniscal cartilage has the function of supporting the knee, adding stability and spreading the loads more evenly inside the joint, when it is torn it causes a problem. The question arises, what can we do about it? In some cases, we will see that removal of the torn fragment is best. In other cases, we will see that repairing the torn segment preserves more long-term function, may decrease the risk of arthritis, can improve stability, and is worth considering.

Meniscal Repair vs. Partial Meniscectomy

Once a meniscus is torn, it won't heal on its own. The torn fragment will intermittently trap between the bones, causing unpredictable locking, giving way, and swelling. Continued swelling is often a sign that further damage is being done to the knee. Arthroscopic surgery may be required to either remove the torn portion of the meniscus (partial meniscectomy) or repair the tear (meniscal repair).

If a repair is needed, its success depends on the overall condition of the cartilage. Very small tears have no blood supply and cannot be repaired. Old cartilage does not always heal well. The location of the tear is also important. A location with a better blood supply improves the chance of healing.

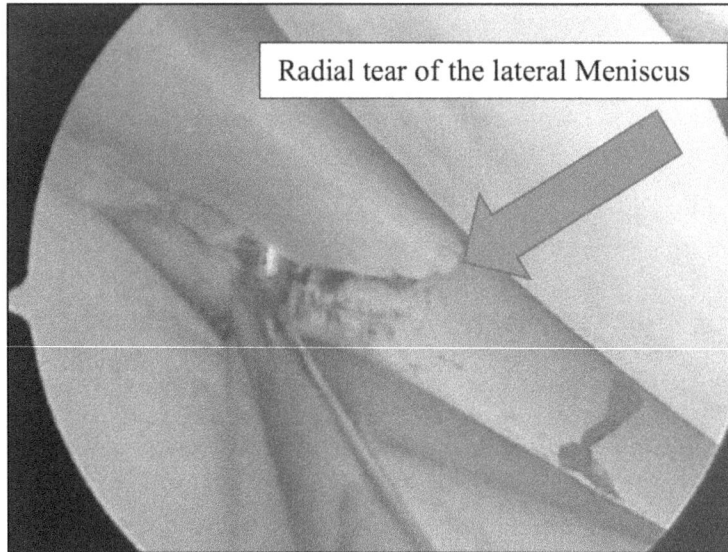

41 Radial tear of the meniscus.

The best conditions for repair are seen more frequently in patients under age 40 and when tears are in areas referred to as the "red on red zone" or the "red on white zone." The red zone of the cartilage is usually the outer third on the medial side of the knee and the same in the posterior lateral meniscus. The inner third is the white zone; there is no blood flow in this zone, and as a result, little to no healing will occur. The zone in between is the red on white zone. There is an intermediate chance of healing in this zone. If the cartilage can be repaired, I use the arthroscope to place tiny sutures or stitches to fix the tear. Sometimes I can supplement the repair (particularly in the red on white zone) with a clot made from the patient's own blood, which contains the patient's own platelet-rich factors and aids in the healing of the cartilage tear.

When the tear is in an area of poor blood supply (the white zone), chronic in nature, or a degenerative tear, a suture repair of the meniscus is not possible. In this case, arthroscopic surgery is required to remove the torn, impinging fragments of the meniscus. Removing the loose, irreparable fragments frequently resolves the mechanical problems caused by the tear. This is necessary to return the knee to good function. Radial tears can be repaired on rare occasions.

Uncommon Case: Meniscus Root Tear

Some patients have torn their meniscus where it attaches to the bone. When this happens, the support for the entire meniscus is lost. It slips out from between the two bones enough to lose its ability to share the weight and evenly spread out the load of the femur on the tibia. It is like a suspension bridge with its cable cut. The bridge would not hold the weight of the cars on it. In the same way, since the meniscus cannot bear the loads it was designed to hold, the knee will see too much force. It would be the same as if we took the entire meniscus out. With the load not being evenly shared across the knee, the knee will wear faster than normal and, we now know, it will lead to early osteoarthritis in that part of the knee. To prevent this from happening, a root repair is required to save the meniscus, which can restore its load-sharing function and protect the knee

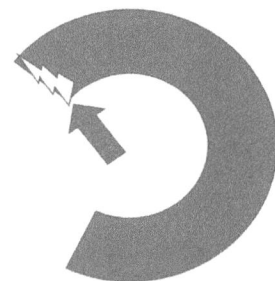

42 Root tear.

from overloading and wear. The big "C" in Image 42 is a graphic representation of a root tear. An MRI of a root tear and surgical repair photos are shown in Images 43 and 44.

A root tear also requires a special type of more complicated repair, as we are trying to get the root to heal back to the bone. That means patients must avoid weight-bearing activities for at least six weeks and wear a protective brace for four months after surgery. Since a root tear is the same as cutting out the entire meniscus, the good news is that, when the repair works well, it is very helpful in protecting the knee from the long-term effects of losing the entire meniscus. When I do this type of repair, I also order a special unloader brace to help protect the meniscus and allow the patient to move the knee while helping it to heal correctly.

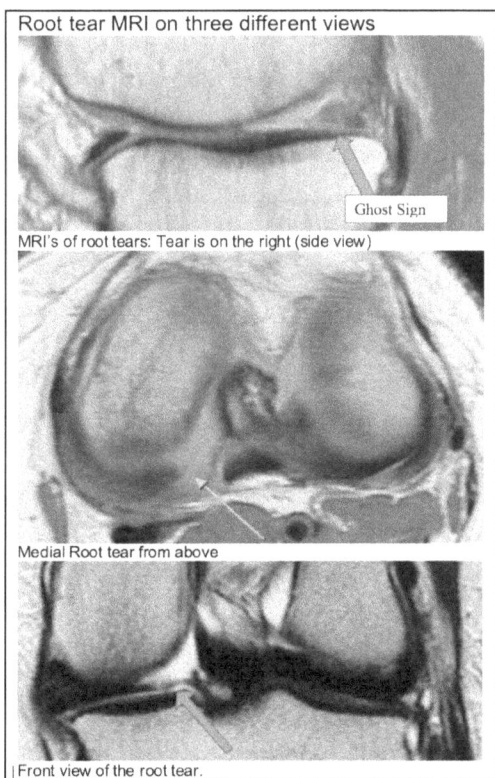

Root tear MRI on three different views

Ghost Sign

MRI's of root tears: Tear is on the right (side view)

Medial Root tear from above

Front view of the root tear.

43 MRI of root tears from three different image directions: top–sagittal plane (perpendicular to the plane of the body), middle–axial plane (parallel to the floor when standing upright), and bottom–coronal plane (in the plane of the body or parallel to the plane of your face).

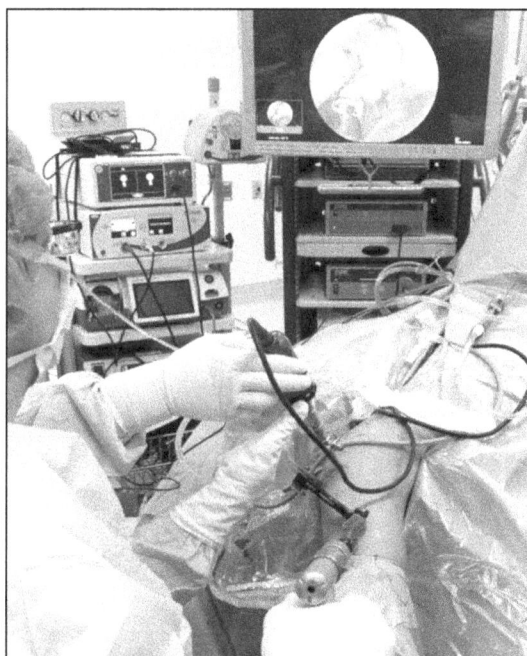

44 Intraoperative photo of a standard setup for a root repair procedure.

10. OTHER CARTILAGE DEFECTS

THERE ARE TWO TYPES OF CARTILAGE IN THE KNEE: MENISCAL AND ARTICULAR. We have already talked about the meniscus (Chapter 9) and deformity-causing arthritis (Chapter 8) in detail. In this chapter, we are going to explore issues concerning the less discussed, but still very important, articular cartilage, which can be found on the surface of every joint in the body. It is the specialized cartilage surface in the knee that covers the ends of the femur, patella, and tibia, and is a smooth covering that makes the surfaces glide freely. It also serves as protection for the bone and as a shock absorber. As smooth as it is, it can still wear or become damaged. It can be worn by the repetitive stress that's put on the knee by heavy activity. It can also be damaged during trauma or ligament injuries.

Once the area is damaged, the surface is prone to degeneration since it will not heal on its own. Sometimes the cartilage is softened, and occasionally the bone underneath the cartilage is damaged, removing its natural support. Sometimes the cartilage defects are shallow, and sometimes they are deep. All these conditions can cause knee pain and swelling. This ongoing damage or roughening of the smooth surface can lead to arthritis. When these defects are symptomatic and they cause pain, locking, or recurrent swelling, surgery is often needed to improve knee function.

Shallow Cartilage Defects

Shallow cartilage defects are different from osteochondritis dissecans, or OCD (find more information about osteochondritis dissecans in Chapter 4, "Knee Pain in Young Children and Teenagers") and are more common in adults. They may be caused by trauma, wear and tear, or arthritis. These defects can be treated nonoperatively or with anti-inflammatory medications, cartilage food supplements (glucosamine and chondroitin sulfate), cortisone, or synthetic lubricant injections (hyaluronic acid). They can also be treated surgically with simple debridement (removing the loose fragments), the microfracture technique, replacement with a synthetic scaffold, transfer of cartilage from another part of the knee (autograft), or frozen cartilage grafts (allografts). Finally, your doctor can harvest your own cells, growing more of them and replanting them back into your knee, a process called an ACI (autologous chondrocyte implantation).

Nonsurgical Treatment

NSAIDs are the mainstay of nonsurgical treatment for inflammation anywhere in the body. In a knee with surface defects, NSAIDs decrease the swelling and reduce the pain associated with wear. In theory, some anti-inflammatory medicines can reduce the swelling in the cartilage itself and "toughen" the cartilage. Gastrointestinal upset is the most common side effect, and these drugs also can increase bleeding times (that is, the time it takes your blood to clot is longer than normal). In this sense, many of the drugs can protect against a clot, like aspirin does. At the same time, they, as a class of drugs, can reduce the stomach's natural protection against acid and cause ulcers. Selective NSAIDs that block only part of the inflammatory pathway can have fewer side effects, but many individuals react differently to different drugs. Therefore, one drug may work well for you, with few side effects, but not be tolerated well by your neighbor. When matched with a patient's specific needs, these drugs can be both safe and effective for most people.

Glucosamine and Chondroitin

Glucosamine and chondroitin (G+C) sulfate are food supplements that are touted to have a wide range of benefits, including regrowing cartilage and restoring the joint space. These benefits are somewhat overstated, to say the least. The advertisements that show knee X-rays with improvement in joint space after treatment have been proven false. However, it does seem that there are patients that benefit from taking these supplements. A few studies have shown that up to 50% of patients experience some reduction in pain, as well as improvement in function. One blind study in Europe showed similar benefits to Celebrex, an NSAID, after six months of use. Keep in mind that the placebo effect alone helps 30% of all patients.

The chemical mechanism of how G+C may work is not clear, and there is no direct proof it "fortifies" the cartilage.

Other supplements like methyl-sulfonyl-methane, turmeric, and garlic are also thought to help the joints and preserve cartilage. These are all food supplements and not FDA-approved as medications. Still, some patients report that they have experienced an improvement in their symptoms. In others, it seems to make no difference. If a supplement does not help your symptoms within a month, it is unlikely it will make a difference with longer use. Therefore, I recommend that my patients try these for only one month, stop using it for a week, and only go back to using it if they see a difference (increased symptoms after stopping). If there is no difference, then the supplement is not helping them.

Just the same, there may be patients who lack the building blocks of cartilage in their diet, and a food supplement may replace that deficit. G+C may be like chicken soup for the knee. In my practice, patients looking for alternatives can try G+C, which is available over the counter and is usually taken twice a day. There are many brands, and generics are made by some of the major companies. G+C sulfate is available at Walgreens, CVS, and other popular stores. Wholesale outlets, like Sam's Club, Costco, and BJ's, may also have their own brands. Your local pharmacist may be most helpful in finding a brand you like. The pills are relatively large. Remember, many of these products are prepared from shellfish, so don't take this if you are allergic to shellfish (there are vegetarian versions available).

Note: As with all foods and medications, if you develop a reaction, stop taking the supplement immediately and notify your primary care physician.

Cortisone Injections

In an inflamed knee, when oral agents fail and there are no true mechanical symptoms from an injured structure, a cortisone injection may be of great help (see section on cortisone injections on page 38). Injections may also be an alternative treatment to consider before any surgical treatment for arthritis, the inflamed lining of the knee (synovitis), gout, pseudogout (false gout), and even some degenerative meniscus tears.

One note on cortisone injections: Most doctors mix a local anesthetic with the injection so even if the patient has only a few hours of relief, we can be reassured that the knee is the cause of the patient's pain. When the knee injection contains a local anesthetic, if the numbing medication in the knee gets rid of the pain, the knee is the most likely source of the problem. Conversely, if the knee does not improve at all and the local has no benefit, other sources of the referred pain to the knee (like a herniated disc or hip arthritis) must be investigated.

In many cases, patients get significant relief from pain and can return to activities within a week to 10 days. In some cases, the relief is short-lived in terms of weeks, and in others, it lasts only a few hours. Patients with short-term relief may benefit from hyaluronate (hyaluronic acid, hyaluranon) lubricant injections as they may last longer. There is some new data just released at the very end of 2022 that correlated increasing the number of injections over time with developing worsening arthritis and needing a total knee replacement.

Synthetic Lubricant

Every joint makes its own lubrication. The lubricant is mostly hyaluronic acid, a large molecule that forms a thin oily substance that, in combination with the microstructure of the articular surface, creates an extremely low-friction surface that can last a lifetime. Many companies make synthetic lubricants in higher and lower molecular weights, using differing synthesis and purification methods. The original FDA approvals ranged from three to five injections one week apart, depending on which product you used. The FDA approved a single injection form (naturally a larger volume of lubricant) that is being used in some settings. In my experience some patients don't tolerate the larger volume as well as the three smaller injections over the single injection (see Image 45).

In 2023 many insurance companies have stopped paying for the lubricant shots on the basis that, on average, they are not that great. I believe it is because the data is a mixed bag. There are those patients that respond and those that don't respond. In general, very advanced arthritis with bone on bone on an X-ray usually doesn't respond well. Those with less arthritis do better. The patients who get good pain relief swear by these injections. I have some happy patients getting shots every 9 to 12 months for five years or more with good relief. So, my approach is they are not for

45 The author's set up for a knee injection in the sitting position. This position mimics how we approach the knee for knee arthroscopy. Some orthopaedic surgeons prefer lying down injection positioning.

everyone. They don't work well on patients with advanced arthritis (bone on bone), but they seem to be good for many patients with early arthritis. Lubricant may be the only good option for those patients that are not good surgical candidates. It is very low risk when compared to knee replacement surgery.

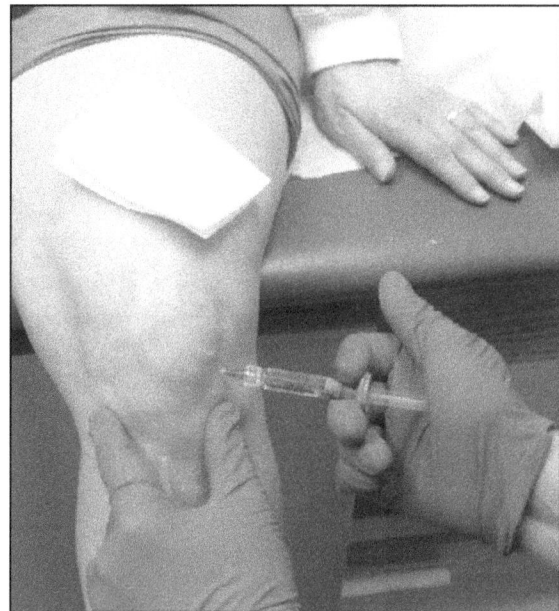

Surgical Treatment

For patients who have mechanical symptoms (locking, buckling, giving way), an arthroscopic debridement may help with limited cartilage damage and loose fragments in the joint. At the same time, one must be aware that some experts have criticized debridement alone as a treatment for advanced arthritis as not that helpful over time. In one large study, arthroscopic debridement for an already arthritic knee was shown to be no better than a "sham" operation. Many physicians have taken issue with this study because it was not clear if there was significant bone loss preoperatively, and there was no clear discussion of true mechanical symptoms.

Since that study, there have been other studies noting that short-term results may yield some initial improvement, yet the overall results are often the same with or without surgery two years later. **Still, even in that study some patients who were placed randomly in the nonoperative treatment group dropped out of the study to have surgery because of continued knee pain.** The patients and the physical therapist believed that therapy alone would not "fix" the knee. So, even in these studies, the researchers are not exactly saying knee surgery makes no difference. Remember, this is for patients with only known arthritis and cartilage loss. In patients without advanced arthritis and who have known mechanical problems like an ACL tear, a torn meniscus, a loose body, a cartilage defect, a fracture, and persistent swelling that has failed other treatments surgery may be their best option.

In a younger population with higher demands (sports or work), patients usually benefit from surgery in many ways. So, again, these studies do not mean that all knee surgeries are not helpful. That is not the case. Many studies show that ligaments, cartilage defects, and meniscus tears should be repaired and loose bodies should be removed, especially when leaving them alone causes recurrent knee instability and decreases the quality of the patient's life or risks further damage to the knee. Sometimes doing nothing is not the same as doing no harm.

Nonetheless, when all else fails, if the knee is the clear source of the pain, an MRI or a diagnostic arthroscopy may show the cause of the problem. If there is minimal or no arthritis, and there is a mechanical problem, as noted already, arthroscopic surgery will help correct the current mechanical problem.

Defects in the Cartilage Surface

For many patients, if the symptoms of a cartilage defect are ignored and spontaneous healing does not occur, the cartilage and its base will separate from the diseased bone, and fragments will break loose into the knee joint. If the fragments are loose, your surgeon may clear the cavity to reach fresh bone. Fragments that cannot be mended will be removed, which will leave a defect hole that needs to be repaired. When there are measurable defects in the bone and cartilage is loose, other options should be considered.

For example, a microfracture technique is used for smaller lesions (less than 2 square centimeters in size) (see Image 46). The involved surface is cleared of the damaged cartilage, and tiny holes are made in the bone to allow the marrow to "leak" out and cover the boney bed. To accomplish this, the cartilage surface is drilled, or "cracked," with a microscopic drill or awl to help blood and marrow get to the surface, just like you might aerate soil when you want grass to grow. The new cartilage will cover the surface with fresh tissue, and the surface defect will fill in with fibrocartilage over time. Unfortunately, although it helps, this repair does not make the same hyaline cartilage that we normally have in our knees, and it is not as effective as hyaline cartilage.

In larger defects (between 2 and 4 square centimeters in size), local transfer of cartilage plugs from one location in the knee to another work well (see Image 47). The only downside is that the area that the cartilage comes from in your knee, and the remaining cartilage near the donor

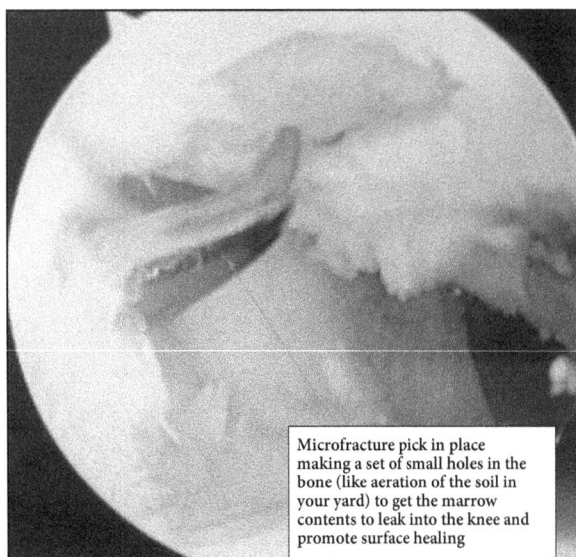

Microfracture pick in place making a set of small holes in the bone (like aeration of the soil in your yard) to get the marrow contents to leak into the knee and promote surface healing

46 Microfracture technique for marrow stimulation.

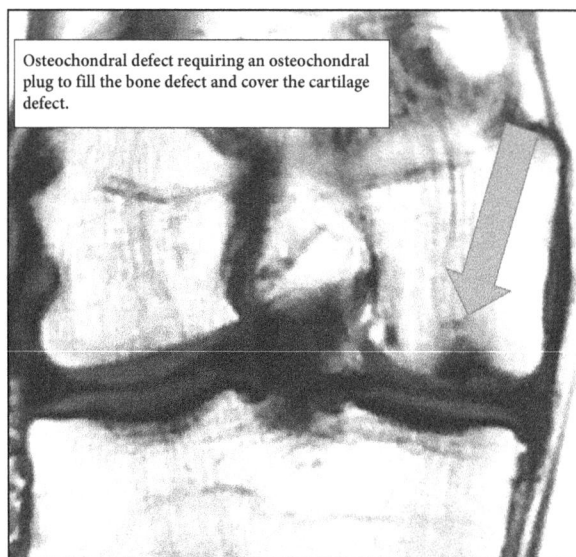

Osteochondral defect requiring an osteochondral plug to fill the bone defect and cover the cartilage defect.

47 Deeper defect in the bone under the surface of the knee (OCD - osteochondritis dissecans).

site, may have to stand up to higher loads. Therefore, that area's surface will be compromised after the plugs are taken, which can cause its own issues in the future.

With even larger defects (greater than 4 square centimeters in size) or where there is bone loss along with the cartilage defect, frozen allograft (human donor tissue) has been used to cover the surface. Freezing preserves the cells in this donor cartilage. However, the cells can live only a limited time once harvested, so timing the donation well and implanting the graft is important. Some patients can wait "on call," for lack of a better term, for the correct size donor bone to be available. It is also known that so-called kissing lesions (defects on both the tibia and femur that touch) cannot be treated with two allografts. Still, large defects on the femur can be replaced with frozen grafts, often yielding good results.

Lastly, tissue can be harvested at the time of a diagnostic arthroscopy; the cartilage cells are grown in a lab and later reinjected under a flap of the periosteum (the thin membrane that covers bone). This procedure, ACI, is the preferred technique for larger defects. It requires at least two surgeries, waiting at least six weeks between them while the lab grows the cells and prepares them in a liquid. There is a long rehabilitation period. MACI (matrix-induced autologous chondrocyte implantation) is a similar procedure where the cells are placed in a matrix before implantation. This makes locating and placing the cells much less difficult at the time of surgery and eliminates the need to harvest and sew the periosteum in place. The MACI technique is a clear improvement over ACI. The good news is that MACI is now available in the US. It promises to make this technology more predictable and easier to use (see Image 48).

Other technologies are being developed all the time. Allograft cultured "neo" (juvenile) cartilage cells have been tested as a possible cartilage surface replacement. This technology has the advantage of using young cells. I had a patient take advantage of this treatment when it was just developed, and he has done very well over the long term (more than 10 years). He recently told me, "It has given me back my knee." Interestingly, at the time of this writing, he has developed the same problem of cartilage loss in the other knee, and, after discussing the options, we are planning to use his own cells—that is the MACI procedure—for that knee.

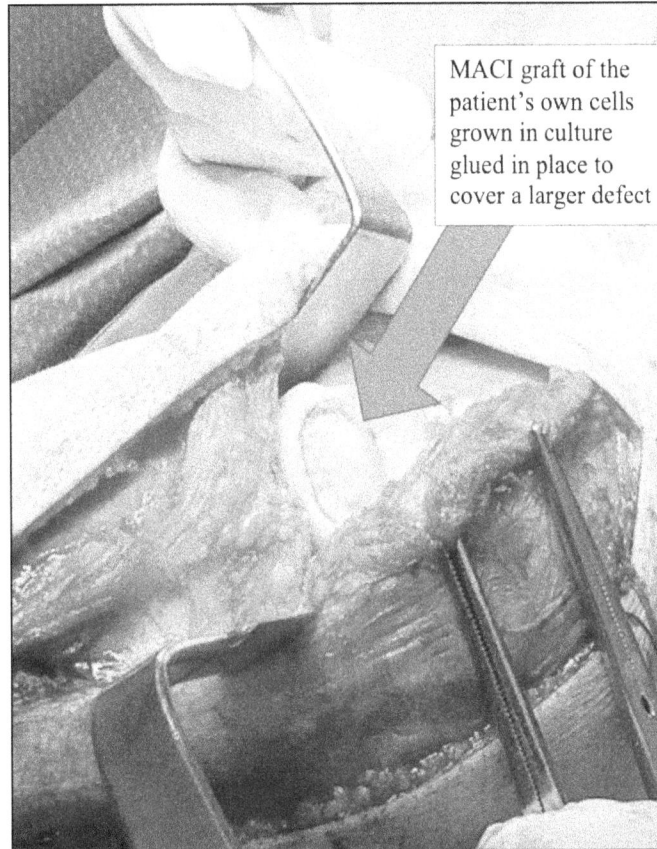

MACI graft of the patient's own cells grown in culture glued in place to cover a larger defect

48 Matrix cartilage cells grafting. Here, the cartilage cells are embedded in the membrane and glued in place.

Summary

In summary, small defects can be treated with the microfracture technique, but larger defects require grafting of some type (autograft, allograft, or cultured cartilage). The full healing process takes time regardless of which technique is used. If you have one of these repairs, you will use crutches and a brace to protect your knee while it heals. Since impact loading or trauma is usu-ally the original cause of the defect, patients need to stop all impact loading on the knee for an extended period after repair to allow the body to heal properly.

To protect these repairs, many surgeons will first use a knee immobilizer while the patient is on crutches that allows for a little weight-bearing. After the initial healing phase of four to six weeks, a knee-hinged brace is often used to continue protecting the cartilage as it heals during the first three to four months after surgery. A brace is needed for heavier activities for up to one year after surgery. Some patients with large defects and bowed legs may need a special unloader brace to allow a return to activity while the graft incorporates and the new cartilage grows. Other patients with bigger deformities (bowing or knocked knee) who are too young for knee replacements will also need a corrective osteotomy (as discussed in Chapter 8, "Deformities of the Knee and Osteoarthritis").

11 KNEECAP PAIN AND DISLOCATIONS

THE KNEECAP (PATELLA) HAS MANY IMPORTANT FUNCTIONS IN THE KNEE:

- It protects the front of the knee, carries the forces from the thigh muscles to the tibia, and moves the patella tendon away from the center of the knee, improving the knee's mechanics.

- In addition, the kneecap's position makes the muscles supporting the leg more efficient.

- As a result of this efficiency, the kneecap allows us to run, kick, jump, squat, and balance our body weight on one leg while going downstairs.

- When working perfectly, it even makes it possible to get out of a chair or a squatting position without using our hands.

Because of its importance in all these functions, we notice when the kneecap is damaged, dislocated, or tracking abnormally. When the kneecap is not doing its job, many people will feel anterior knee pain; pain while climbing stairs, squatting, or kneeling; or a sense of the knee giving way.

So, What Ails the Mighty Kneecap?

The most common problem is simple wear, cracking, and softening of the undersurface. The underside of the kneecap is covered with cartilage that helps it glide in the groove on the end of the femur (trochlear). The patella and the trochlear together are called the patellofemoral mechanism. The "wear and tear" is known as chondromalacia patella, which is the loss of the articular cartilage's structural integrity (see Image 49). Problems begin to occur with wear and tear, and the underlying cartilage begins to degenerate.

The degeneration can occur from normal aging. It can also happen because of the way the patella moves in the trochlear groove. If there is abnormal tracking of the kneecap in its groove, weight applied to the kneecap is uneven. This causes one side to wear faster than the other. Therefore, excessive loading of the kneecap, like deep squats with heavy weights, running downhill, or playing sports with fast starts and stops, make this worse and can accelerate the arthritic process.

Patients typically complain of pain walking up and down stairs, squatting, kneeling, and running downhill. There may be swelling, maltracking of the kneecap, or a crackling sensation upon bending. Sometimes the sounds are so loud they can remind people of a creaky door hinge. The problem is most often aggravated by overuse, being overweight, inappropriate weight training exercises, trauma, or sports, and the root cause is the malalignment or maltracking of the kneecap.

When the cartilage under the kneecap starts to fail, changes are seen on its surface. In patients with chondromalacia patella, an exam using an arthroscope can reveal everything from a soft surface instead of its normal firm plastic-like consistency (Grade 1 changes) to patches of advanced worn spots or cartilage loss down to the bone (Grade 4 changes). If the underlying issues are not addressed early on, arthritis and loss of knee function almost always follow. Interestingly, this is an area of AI (artificial intelligence) research that I was involved in with a company called ImageBiopsy Lab that uses AI to look at the X-ray and determine an arthritis Kellgren and Lawrence grade (the Kellgren and Lawrence classification was developed and reported first in the 1950s in England for the evaluation of arthritis stages on X-rays).

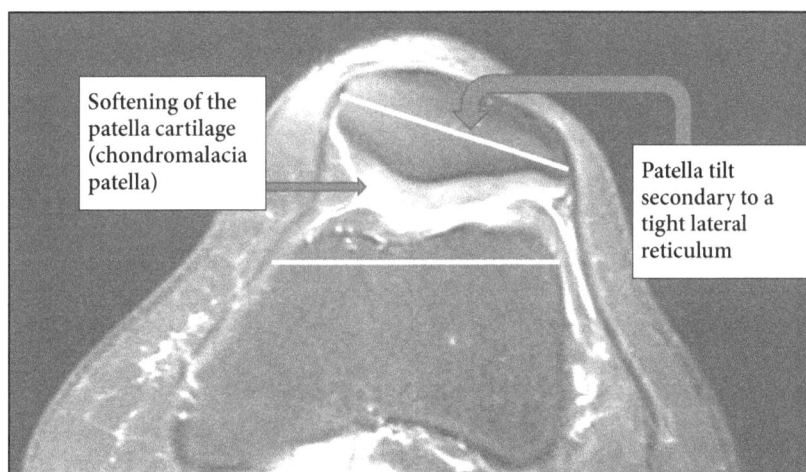

Softening of the patella cartilage (chondromalacia patella)

Patella tilt secondary to a tight lateral reticulum

49 CMP chondromalacia patella (arrow: defect in the kneecap surface) and patella tilt from a tight lateral retinaculum.

Nonsurgical Treatment

When the patella is painful, tracks poorly, or is softening, the initial treatment includes rest, ice, and NSAIDs. Therapy for maltracking, including patella taping and vastus medialis obliquus (VMO) strengthening, can help (see exercises in Appendix II). Patella braces can also be used, which benefit some people, but there can be mixed results. Orthotics can help decrease foot pronation and help unload the kneecap. Weight loss is also important when indicated and modifying activity can be a helpful part of the treatment as well. Another treatment is glucosamine and chondroitin, oral cartilage food supplements believed to reduce inflammation and support cartilage growth (see sidebar in Chapter 10 page 71).

Patella Subluxation or Dislocation

Tracking of the kneecap is another cause of chondromalacia patella and a source of pain. As the knee bends, the patella is supposed to slide up and down the center of its groove. A normal patella should move relatively straight up and down the trochlea (its groove). However, the patella can slip out of place due to injury or congenital abnormalities affecting the shape of the knee (see Image 50). Sometimes the groove can be steep, and sometimes very shallow. In addition, bands of tissue holding your patella in place can become too tight on one side, causing the patella tendon to align with the inner or outer side of the knee.

First-time dislocations of the kneecap occur more often between the ages of 14 and 18. However, the average age of first-time dislocations of the kneecap is slightly higher at 21, meaning the range of age is wide, and it can occur at almost any age with trauma to the knee. It is slightly more common in females than males (54% verses 46%).

When the trochlea is shallow or the tendon is misaligned, the kneecap can jump over the edge of its groove. This problem is commonly known as patella subluxation or dislocation. In subluxation, the patella tracks to one side more than the other and slips partway out and then back again. In dislocation, the kneecap comes out of its groove completely, and can either pop back in by itself or get stuck out of place.

When kneecap subluxation occurs, the shift can weaken the soft tissue support for the patella. If it only partially slips out as in patella

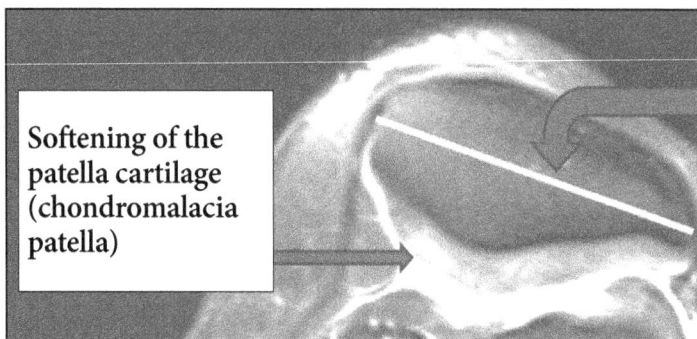

Softening of the patella cartilage (chondromalacia patella)

50 Closeup of patella cartilage defect.

subluxation, it could be minor and hard to see. It can also be more serious, and you may be able to see that it's in the wrong position at first glance. If subluxation happens frequently, it will cause damage to the kneecap cartilage, pain, and a physical disability because the knee will be unreliable.

Recurring patella subluxation or dislocation gives rise to the sensation of the knee giving way. Sometimes it's hard to describe the feeling since other knee problems (like ligament or cartilage tears) cause a similar sensation. Patella instability is also associated with pain along the outside or underneath the kneecap when patients squat, bend, or go up and down the stairs (like symptoms in patients with chondromalacia of the patella). The location of the pain, along with a good physical examination, can help a doctor make the correct diagnosis. Image 51 shows a knee with abnormal mechanical alignment of the patella tendon attachment to the tibia and the center of the groove the kneecap rides in.

When the kneecap is dislocated, it completely slips out of its groove, a problem that can be caused by trauma or a sports injury. The supporting ligaments tear, and there can be a chip or fracture of the kneecap or the groove. If there is blood in the knee, a tear is likely. If there is blood with fat droplets in the knee, a fracture is likely. Drawing the fluid out of the swollen knee will take tension off the knee after a dislocation and reduce the pain. The fluid may help a doctor diagnose a torn ligament or a fracture that may not be apparent on an X-ray. If your orthopaedic surgeon finds that the knee fluid shows signs of blood and fat droplets, further tests, including an X-ray and possibly an MRI, are required to rule out a fracture or loose fragment of cartilage in the knee joint.

After a dislocation, the bone on the patella and the edge of the femur may be bruised from the patella slipping over (see Image 53a). In cases of more significant trauma, as in some collision-related dislocations in sports, a piece of the bone and cartilage can be sheared off as the patella dislocates or comes back into place. If an X-ray shows a loose chip of bone after a dislocation, it will need to be either removed or fixed, depending on the size of the piece. Sometimes only a piece of cartilage is broken off. In those cases, an X-ray may be normal since the loose piece can only be seen on an MRI. If an MRI shows a loose fragment, the treatment is the same as when an X-ray shows a loose fragment of bone.

Other patients have an anatomic divergence between the tibial tubercle and the center of the groove in which the kneecap sits. In other words, the attachment of the patella tendon is not aligned with the groove, increasing the likelihood of patella subluxation or dislocation. Measuring this distance, called the tibial tubercle–trochlear groove or TT-TG distance, helps the doctor to select the best treatment. When it is high (greater than 1.4 centimeters in females and 1.0 centimeter in males), there is increased mal-tracking, and the poor alignment should be addressed if the mechanical problem is the root cause of the patella instability or pain.

Treatment

Physical therapy is often the first line of treatment to correct patella alignment. Patellafemoral pain associated with chondromalacia can also occur if the quadriceps muscles are weak, which causes an imbalance in the joint. Since the quadriceps dictate the movement of the patella, the weakness can cause the patella to pull to one side more than the other. This puts more pressure on one side and can damage the cartilage over time. Physical therapy, patella taping (a technique invented by an Australian physiotherapist named Jenny McConnell), orthotics, and bracing all aim to correct the quadriceps muscles' pull on the patella.

If these conservative measures fail, surgery may be required. Two types of surgical procedures can help fix these problems. The first is a lateral release. If the outer side of the knee is tight, painful, and reproduces the patient's pain on palpation, this type of surgery may be helpful. This procedure releases the tight tissue near the outer kneecap and helps to shift it to the medial side. It can be done arthroscopically, and a video of this procedure can be seen on my YouTube channel (www.youtube.com/DrAReznik). In many cases, this removes enough pressure to solve the problem.

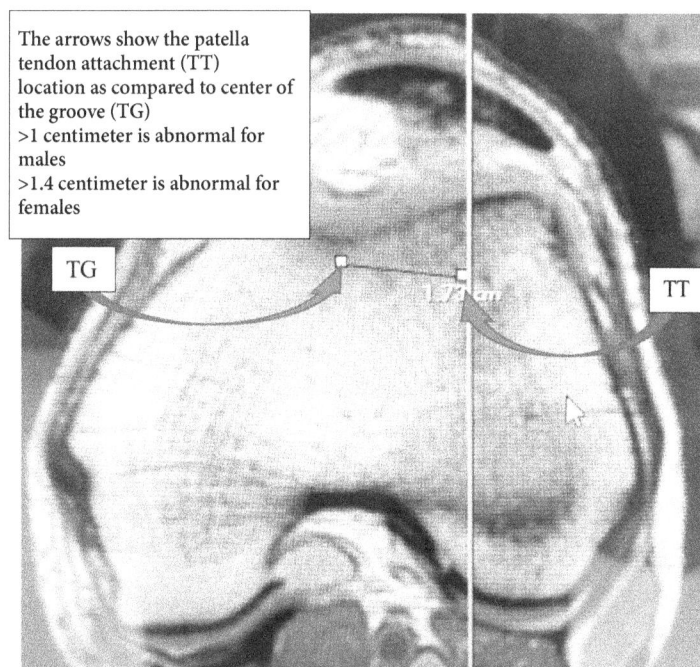

The arrows show the patella tendon attachment (TT) location as compared to center of the groove (TG)
>1 centimeter is abnormal for males
>1.4 centimeter is abnormal for females

TG

TT

51 The TT-TG (Tibial Tubercle–Trochlear Groove) distance as a measure on MRI.

Some people have both tightness of the lateral side of the knee and malpositioning of the tibial insertion of the patella tendon (an increased or abnormal TT-TG distance). The best way to control the patella's position is with the tibial tubercle transfer (TTT, or patella realignment procedure; see Image 51). The tibial tubercle is the bony prominence below the patella. In this operation, the location where the tendon attaches to the tibial tubercle is moved forward and toward the inner side, and it is then held in place by two screws while the bone heals. Once it heals, the screws are not needed, and if the patient can feel them or is bothered by them, they can be removed with a minor procedure, which has a fast recovery (days, not weeks). A video of this more complex reconstruction for a failed prior soft tissue correction of a dislocating kneecap is also on my YouTube channel.

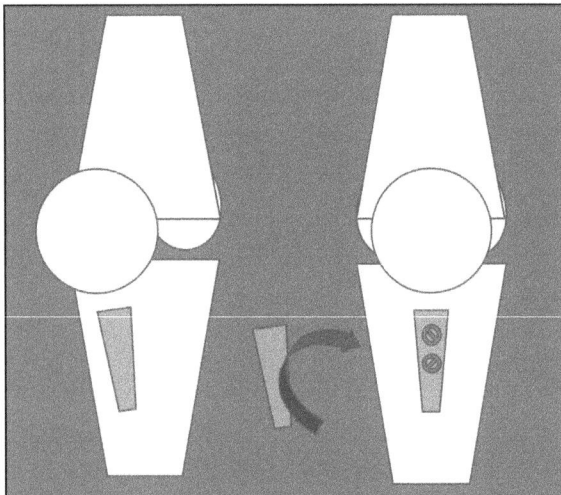

52 Diagram of a TT-TG surgical correction, note the rotation of the tubercle to center the kneecap.

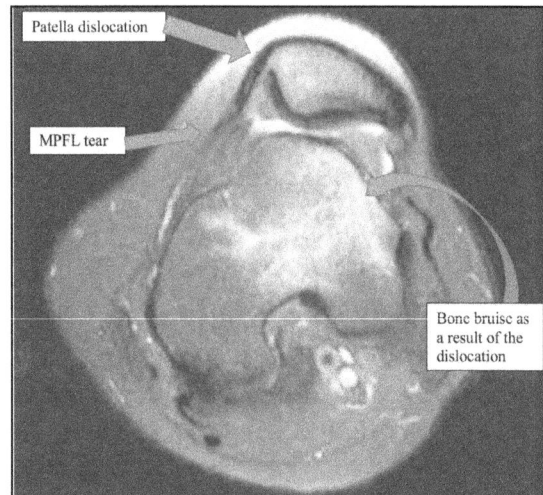

53a MRI image of a knee after dislocation. The patella is still out of place, tilted and mal-positioned, and the MPFL (medical patella femoral ligament) is torn. The bone on the side of the femur is bruised from the trauma of the knee cap popping out of place and hitting the side of the femur.

Loose Medial Patella (Torn Medial Patellafemoral Ligament)

Lastly, when the kneecap dislocates the ligament that connects the inside of the kneecap to the inner side of the knee is frequently torn at the time of dislocation. This ligament is called the medial patellafemoral ligament (MPFL). It attaches to the upper third of the kneecap, and when it is torn, the kneecap can dislocate with less force. Luckily, after a first-time dislocation, the MPFL usually heals with simple treatment. It heals provided there are no other significant bone alignment issues. Therefore, testing for instability or having an MRI show a tear is important in people with recurring dislocations. For many years its importance in holding the kneecap in place was not fully appreciated.

More recently, repairing or reconstructing this ligament has been found to be important to prevent future dislocations. There are many procedures that have been developed in recent years to fix or reconstruct this ligament.

There is some disagreement on what is more important, medial structure's looseness or lateral tightness. At the same time, abnormal kneecap shape, groove shape, limb alignment, or/and location of the attachment of the patella tendon are also major causes of patella dislocations. In reality, all of these factors play a role in the risk for recurring dislocations of the kneecap depending on the patient's own anatomy.

The Role of the Medial Side of the Knee

The surgery for medial looseness tightens the natural structures on the medial side of the knee. Over the years, many authors have described moving the VMO muscle to help solve this problem. More recently, arthroscopic versions of tightening the medial side have also had good results. Now, more surgeons believe that tears of the MPFL are a source of patella subluxation. The main reason this issue is more recognized now than in the past is that many of the injuries to the MPFL healed with simple treatment (a knee immobilizer) and typically are self-healing. Knowing that 80%–90% of these heal with initial immobilization and then therapy without surgical treatment is reassuring to most patients after a first-time dislocation. The other 10%–20% require more discussion.

When MPFL tears cause medial side instability, it can be tested by pushing the patella laterally with the knee relaxed. If the patella glides over the lateral edge of the femur without resistance, the medial side may be a problem. When this happens, the MPFL can be repaired or reconstructed with suture anchors, part of a local tendon or frozen tendon graft. In my practice, after careful study of the MRIs I have found that many of these are torn from the kneecap or off the medial femur. In these cases, I prefer to repair the ligament directly instead of reconstructing it because the procedure is less invasive and very effective.

Note: When the MPFL is reconstructed with a strong ligament graft there is a risk of overtightening the graft. This can cause other issues for the patella down the road and tensioning the graft correctly with the knee slightly bent in the operating room is an important part of the repair.

Complex Patella Instability

In rare cases of chronic recurrent patella dislocations, all three problems can be present at the same time. Namely, the lateral side is too tight, the medial side is too loose (MPFL tear), and the bone is not well aligned (abnormal TT-TG distance) The patient has failed after trying options like NSAIDs, physical therapy, patella taping, and orthotics. At the first writing of this book, I had seen this only a few times in my practice. Now I see a good number of these patients and offer them a more comprehensive approach to this problem. Some patients are referred to me after failing to heal from more simple procedures that did not fully address all the issues at the same time.

In these cases, a tibial tubercle transfer, lateral release, and MPFL reconstruction may all be required at the same time to solve patella instability. Patella alta is a congenitally high-riding kneecap. Some of these patients dislocate the patella because, in patella alta, the kneecap starts so far above the groove when the knee is straight it cannot find its way to the center of the groove as the knee bends. This can also be corrected at the time of surgery. I had one such case recently. The patient needed an MPFL repair, removal of a loose body, lateral release, a correction for an abnormal angle (TT-TG distance that was larger than normal), and a correction for a kneecap that was also too high (patella alta—interestingly, a fourth reason for patella instability). It was a bit more complicated than the average case. When the patella tendon is longer than the groove (as in patella alta), the kneecap has trouble finding the groove as the knee bends because it starts above it. To correct this, we must remember to also move the tendon lower down to get that issue corrected at the same time we correct the location of the tendon.

Another reason for patella instability is knocked knees (a valgus deformity as shown in Image

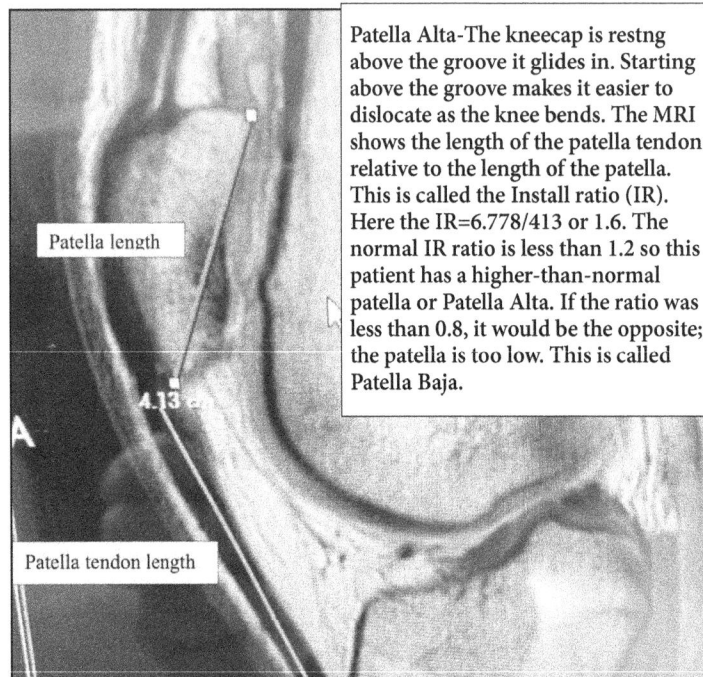

Patella Alta-The kneecap is restng above the groove it glides in. Starting above the groove makes it easier to dislocate as the knee bends. The MRI shows the length of the patella tendon relative to the length of the patella. This is called the Install ratio (IR). Here the IR=6.778/413 or 1.6. The normal IR ratio is less than 1.2 so this patient has a higher-than-normal patella or Patella Alta. If the ratio was less than 0.8, it would be the opposite; the patella is too low. This is called Patella Baja.

Patella length

Patella tendon length

53b Patella Alta measurements explained.

36). If the knee is very knocked, as the tibia is angled away from the midline, the tibia tubercle is significantly pushed to the outside. That creates an outward force on the kneecap, which can pull the kneecap out of place when loading the knee in a semi-bent position. In minor cases, the tibial tubercle realignment works nicely. In more severe cases, correcting the knocked knee is required by doing an opening wedge osteotomy (cutting the bone and correcting the alignment of the leg) in the femur just above the knee joint.

In summary, the options for correcting kneecap problems increase a fair amount when we factor in the malposition or misalignment associated with the tibial tubercle, the possibility of MPFL tears, a patella that rides too high, tilting of the kneecap, VMO laxity or weakness, valgus or knocked knees, and tight lateral retinaculum. Surgery can correct lateral tightness, medical looseness, bone misalignment, or any combination of these issues.

12 INJURY TO THE KNEE EXTENSOR MECHANISM

FOR THE KNEE TO MOVE OUR BODY, THE KNEE MUST BE CONNECTED TO POWERFUL muscles. For most movements and standing there is no doubt the quadriceps are extremely important in powering the knee. The four muscles of the quadriceps with their common tendon (the quadriceps tendon), the kneecap (the patella), and the patella tendon together make the "extensor mechanism." If any of its components are injured, the knee will become unstable. In this section we will examine how the knee extensor mechanism can be injured and what we can do about it.

Fracture of the Kneecap, Patella Tendon Rupture, or Quads Tendon Rupture

Most people understand that the kneecap protects the knee, helps the quadriceps work more efficiently, and enables us to go up and down stairs, get out of a chair, kick a ball, run, and even jump. Many people also understand what happens when the kneecap slips out of place or dislocates. However, very few people understand what happens if the quads mechanism is broken by an injury. Imagine, for a moment, a pulley and a rope. The pulley can break (the kneecap fractures), and the rope can break on either side of the pulley. On one side, the quadriceps attachment to the kneecap can tear (a quads rupture). On the other side, the patella tendon, the strong ligament that attaches the kneecap to the tibia, can tear. All these injuries remove your ability to balance on one leg and make it almost impossible to walk. For all practical purposes, these injuries need to be repaired surgically unless there are overwhelming medical reasons not to do so.

Treatment for Extensor Mechanism Injuries

Once the extensor mechanism is damaged, we can no longer apply the force through the knee from the thigh muscles. This makes walking very difficult without bracing the leg in a straight position. If braced in extension, the quads are not needed. If not braced and the knee flexes during normal walking, it will give way since the quads cannot stop the knee from bending too far without giving way. These injuries almost always require repair or immobilization to heal. In this section we will discuss these injuries from patella fractures to the tendon ruptures.

Patella Fractures

Patella fractures are failures of the bone, which can occur by direct trauma, as in a direct fall onto the knee, a car accident, or a forced hyperflexion injury (the knee is bent back very quickly, and the quads muscle tries its best to stop it). This applies a lot of tension force to the kneecap. The bone is more like cement than steel. It does well when force is applied in compression (a direct load placed on it), but not as well when it's stressed in tension (a pulling or bending force). As a result, a rapid load to the bending knee can cause high-tension loads in the kneecap and the patella can split in two. When we add the trauma of hitting the ground or a hard surface, the fracture can split into multiple fragments or become comminuted (splintered or crushed). The treatments for kneecap fractures range from wiring the pieces together to complete excision of the kneecap.

When there are very small pieces near the tip, they can be removed, and the patella tendon can be repaired directly to the bone. When there are two pieces, aligning the cartilage surface and tension band wiring are the treatments of choice. Tension band wiring is the method that converts the tension forces on the healing fracture to compression forces (as previously stated, the bone likes compression more than tension). This repair method helps the bone press together as the muscles contract, allowing for earlier rehabilitation. When the patella is so crushed that it cannot be repaired, it can be removed, and the tendon can be reconnected to itself. This is effective, but there is a loss of approximately 50% of the strength.

Patella Tendon Ruptures

The patella tendon can tear with an acute trauma, chronic inflammation, and in some cases with recurring tendonitis for conditions like jumper's knee. One of my patients tore his by attempting a deadlift of over 600 pounds. Patella tendon tears can be repaired by reattaching the torn tendon directly to the patella (to the bone) when it is torn off the bone. This works reasonably well in many cases; however, the repair applies all the stress to the healing ligament. Therefore, it has the potential of failing to heal due to that stress in a reasonable amount of time. My personal preference is placing some type of tension-relieving suture or wire through (or around) the patella and attaching it to the tibial tubercle. In this way, the tendon repair can be protected as it heals, and early movement or motion of the knee can be accomplished safely as the tendon heals.

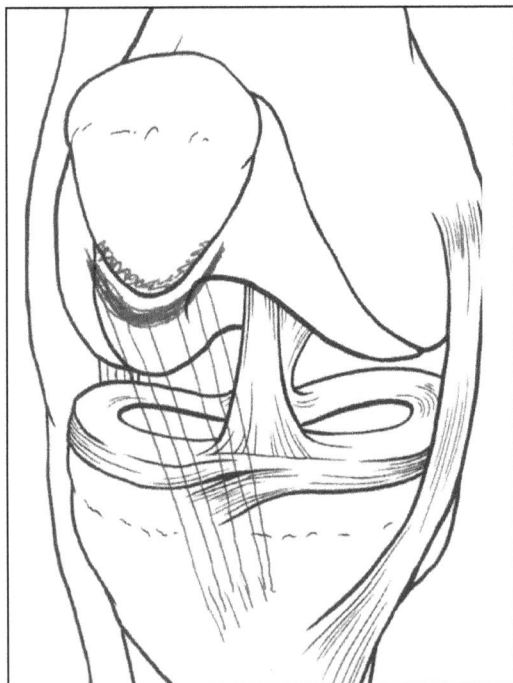

54 Jumper's knee: microscopic tearing at the bottom edge of the kneecap.

Quadriceps Rupture

Lastly, the quads tendon can rupture with a flexion injury or a fall. However, the tendon is very broad and strong, so rupture is not common. Some patients have a history of prior tendonitis, gout, or inflammatory arthritis as predisposing conditions prior to this injury. These can be repaired directly to the bone using strong sutures and drilling holes through the bone.

After all these injuries and treatments, patients should expect to experience stiffness and quadriceps weakness, and they will need to wear a long, straight brace to protect the site. In time, the tendon or the patella will heal, range will return, and strength will follow slowly. Care must be taken not to overtighten the repair during the procedure and to protect it in the early phases of healing. To accomplish this, your surgeon may use any one of the tension-relieving techniques I have described. Your doctor may combine this with strict bracing, with the brace to be worn when you are not participating in closely supervised therapy with a licensed physical therapist. Patients should follow

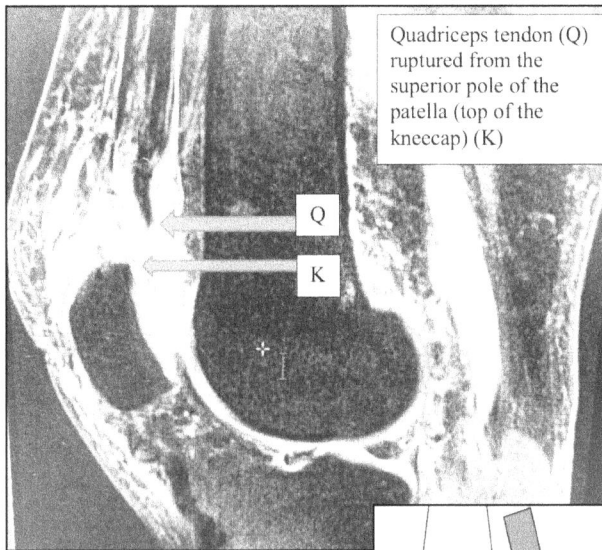

Quadriceps tendon (Q) ruptured from the superior pole of the patella (top of the kneecap) (K)

55 Quads tendon rupture. When the quadriceps tendon is torn, the kneecap is no longer connected to the muscle, and walking is next to impossible.

56 All three types of injury to the patella-quads mechanism.

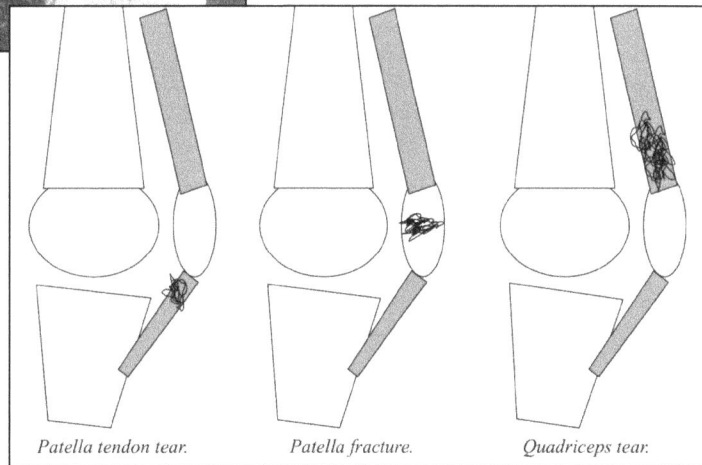

Patella tendon tear.   *Patella fracture.*   *Quadriceps tear.*

the rehab protocol and not pretend to know better than their surgeon or their therapist. As I like to tell my patients, Mother Nature has her own plans, and you cannot fool her.

Tibial Plateau Fractures

The knee has several weight-bearing surfaces. The primary loads (weight) in the knee pass from the femur to the tibia, with the curved surface of the femur resting on the relatively flat surface of the tibia. Like a mountain with a flat top, this flat surface is called the tibial plateau. It's a very sturdy surface, yet it is vulnerable to trauma and can break. The most common injuries result from a side blow to the knee. This can occur in sports, like skiing and football, or from trauma, like a fall or a car accident. The fractures shown in Image 57 occurred when a skier fell, injuring both legs at the same time. The stress applied to the outer side of the knee can cause one of two injuries: rupture of the medial ligaments (medial collateral ligament sprain or tear) or collapse of the lateral plateau as shown in Image 57. You can imagine how the femur acts as a hammer as it hits the plateau in this type of injury.

There are many types of plateau fractures involving the outer (lateral) side, inner (medial) side, or both (bicondylar) sides of the plateau. If the surface is depressed or the sides of the bone are cracked, the plateau can no longer support the femur. This is exacerbated if there is a ligament injury associated with the fracture. The unstable knee will be painful, swollen, and often grossly deformed after the injury. The fracture can be detected by checking the medial and lateral stability of the knee, getting X-rays, and performing CT scans (as in the CT-generated 2D and 3D images in Images 57 and 58). When instability is found during the exam or the fracture is significantly depressed (pushed down into the bone), it should be surgically repaired to preserve knee function. A high percentage of patients with a depressed lateral tibial plateau fracture also have a meniscus tear.

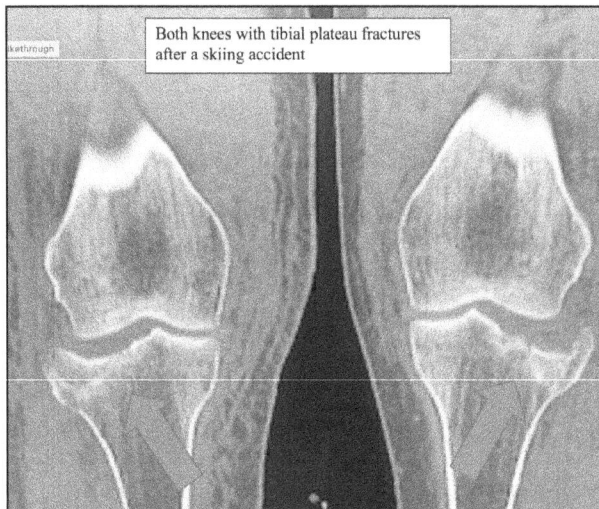

Both knees with tibial plateau fractures after a skiing accident

57 Tibial plateau fractures in both knees after a skiing injury.

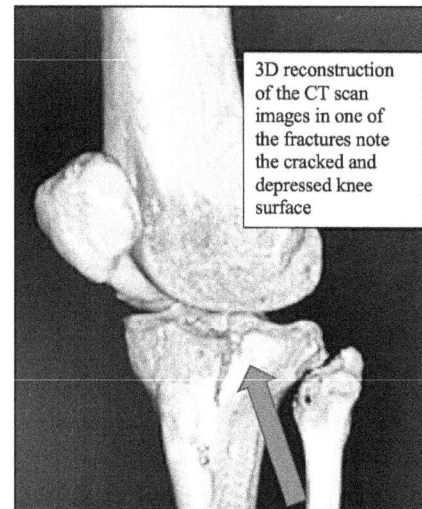

3D reconstruction of the CT scan images in one of the fractures note the cracked and depressed knee surface

58 "3D" computer image made from a CT scan for operative planning of a split compression tibial plateau fracture (arrow).

Treatment

Surgery is indicated when the surface is depressed or displaced significantly. Many years ago, up to 1 centimeter of displacement was the prerequisite for surgery. Now, with CT scans and arthroscopic-assisted techniques, the cutoff is no more than 0.5 centimeters. If the plateau is injured and the fracture is depressed, the femur will "fall" into the defect, and the knee will be unstable in the direction of the fracture. Walking on the fracture will worsen the condition. Once the plateau is fractured, the patient should be braced or splinted and placed on crutches. A CT scan is used to view the displacement, the number of fractures, and the location of the pieces. It can also aid in surgical planning if surgery is necessary.

At the time of the surgery, an open or arthroscopically assisted method may be used to reduce the fracture and realign the joint. A bone graft, screws, and a plate with screws may also be used to support the surface. Newer plates with "locking" screws have improved the strength of these repairs, and precontoured "anatomic" plates have also improved our ability to reduce the fracture and restore the normal anatomy. Images 59 and 60 show the use of a precontoured locking plate. Remember that even with a perfect reduction, ideal plate fixation, and bone grafting, we cannot undo the crushing injury to the cartilage surface at the time of the fracture. Many of the cartilage cells are killed in the initial blow to the knee, and that cannot be reversed.

Once the fracture is reduced and fixed in place with the plate and screws, the wound is closed, and the patient is placed in a straight knee brace to protect the knee. He or she may not do weight-bearing activities for at least six to 12 weeks postoperatively, depending on the nature

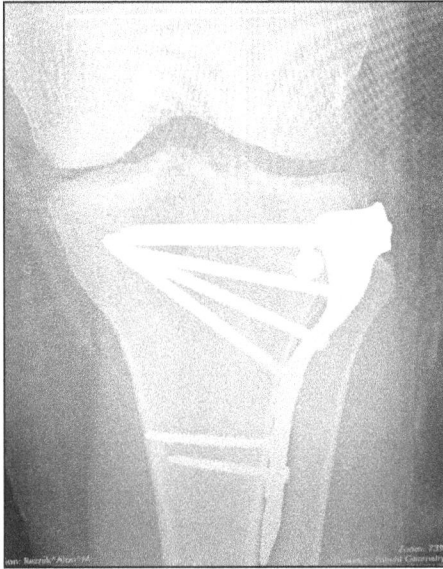

59 Frontal view (AP view): X-ray of plate in place after operative repair of the fracture.

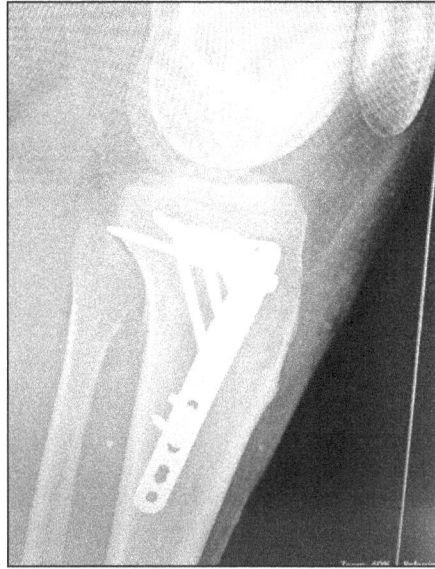

60 Side view (lateral view): X-ray of plate in place after operative repair of the fracture.

of the fracture, the depth of the defect, the amount of bone graft used, and the surgeon's assessment of the quality of the bone fixation. These are generally accepted guidelines to help patients understand the naturally slow healing times. In each case, follow-up X-rays are required to see if new bone is forming before the patient returns to weight-bearing activities.

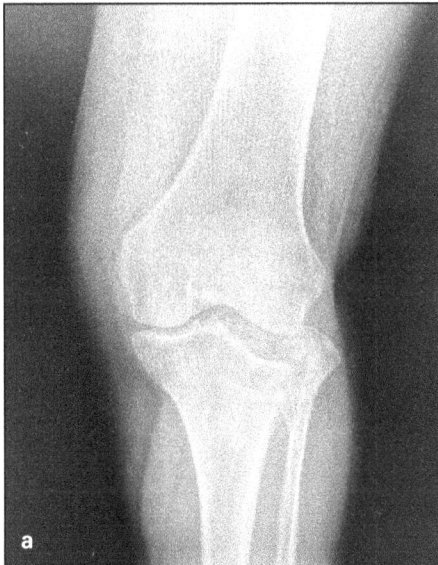

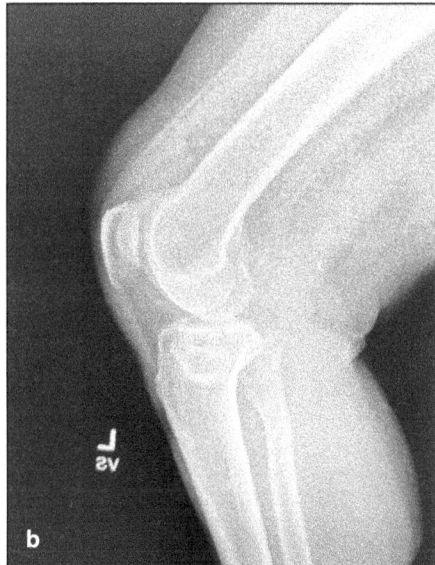

61 a and b Severe tibial plateau fracture in osteoporotic bone (thin, soft bone from lifetime calcium deficiency) (a) AP X-ray of fracture, (b) lateral view of fracture.

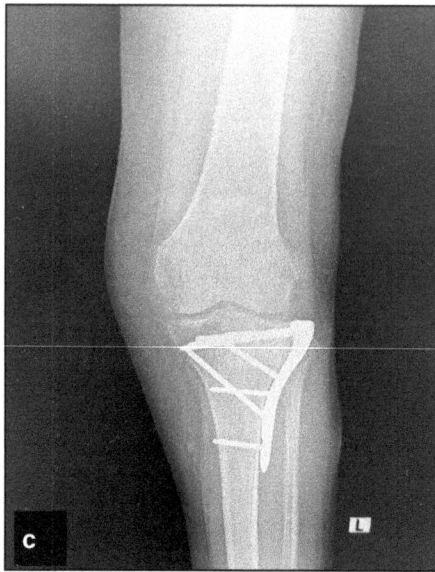

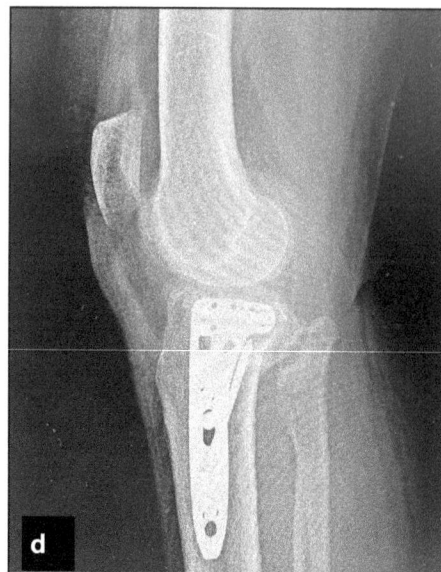

61 c and d Severe tibial plateau fracture in osteoporotic bone (thin, soft bone from lifetime calcium deficiency) (c) AP view of fracture reduction with bone grafting, and (d) lateral view of reduction and plating.

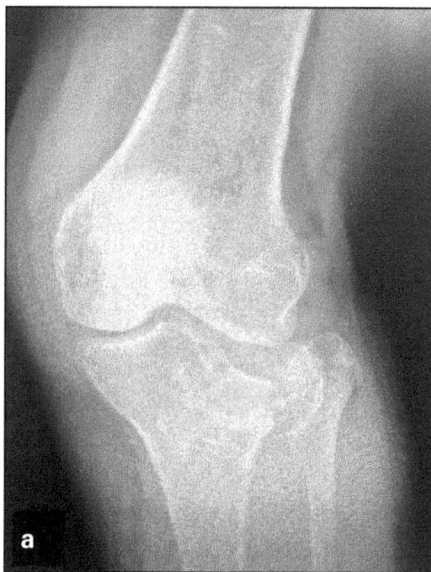

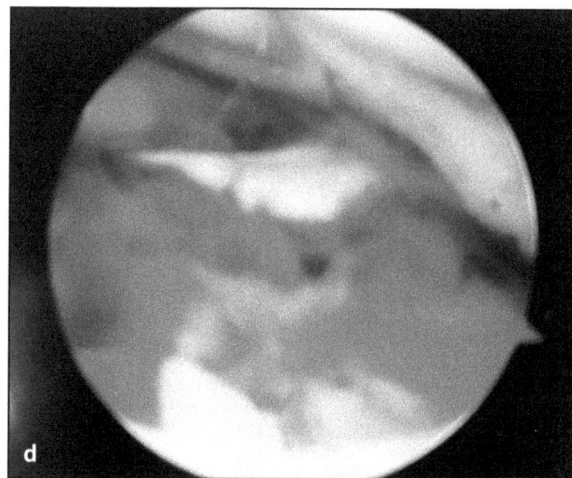

62 a and b Arthroscopic assisted open reduction internal fixation of severe tibial plateau fracture in osteoporotic bone: (a) AP X-ray of fracture, (b) arthroscopic (fiber optic) view of fracture.

No two fractures are exactly alike, and treatment varies based on the type of fracture, type of hardware used, and bone quality. Keep in mind that diabetics are at increased risk of infection and wound problems. Smokers also heal slower and are at increased risk of developing wound complications compared to the general population. The combination of smoking, alcohol abuse, and poorly controlled diabetes is a serious problem and can put the lower leg at risk of amputation after significant trauma. If you are having this surgery, stop smoking.

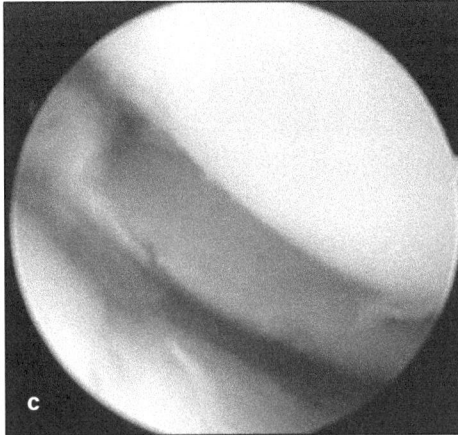

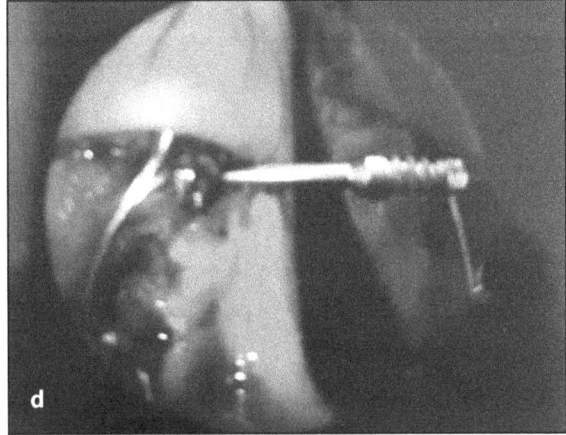

62 c and d Arthroscopic assisted open reduction internal fixation of severe tibial plateau fracture in osteoporotic bone: (c) arthroscopic view of fracture reduction to an anatomic position, and (d) view of applying the plate through a minimal incision because of the arthroscopic assist reduction of the fracture.

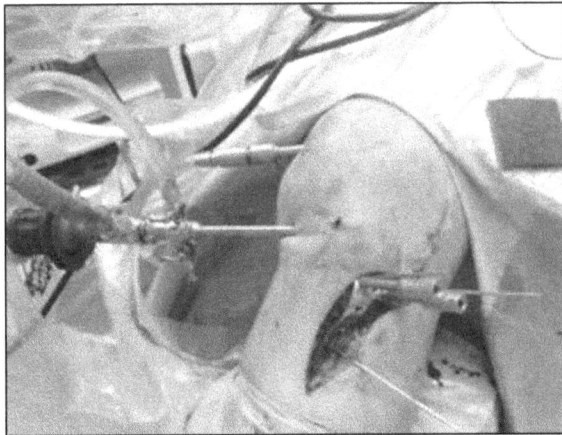

63a Arthroscopic set up for reduction and plating with minimal plate incision.

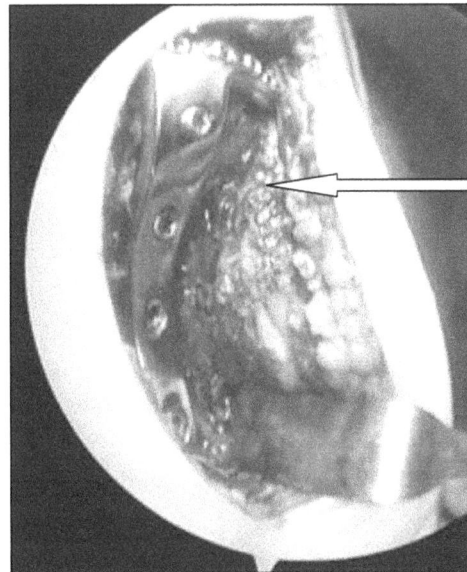

63b Plate in place holding the final reduction (fracture repair).

13 LOOSE BODIES, CARTILAGE DEFECTS, BONE BRUISES, STRESS FRACTURES, AND CARTILAGE LOSS

WHEN THERE IS DAMAGE TO THE INTERNAL STRUCTURES OF THE KNEE CARTILAGE fragments may become loose within the knee or become partly attached. It can be the articular cartilage or the meniscal cartilage or even a piece of a ligament that can get stuck as the knee moves. It is these mobile segments of loose tissue that can cause intermittent locking of the knee, swelling, pain, and/or instability with activity. This section is devoted to making this diagnosis and sorting out the best treatments.

The Knee in Motion

As you know from previous chapters, three parts of the knee make it move very smoothly: the femur and its smooth surface cartilage; the tibia and its smooth surface cartilage; and the meniscus, or the bushing like a gasket (or an "O" ring) in between the two surfaces to make them match more completely as the knee bends. These special surfaces contain water and a lubricant that make the knee the smoothest moving joints with the lowest friction possible. The low-friction surfaces of the knee are among the lowest friction surfaces ever created.

These special surfaces are some of the many reasons our bodies are such amazing machines and why we can walk a mile and only use, or burn, 100 calories. In comparison, a gallon of gas for your car carries 31,000 calories of energy, and if we could use the energy of one gallon of gas, we could walk 310 miles, or get 310 "mpg" on those calories. In other words, on the 100 calories of energy we use to walk a mile, an SUV could not even drive one football field. Our bodies are truly amazing in this way, and your super-smooth knee joints are a big part of that efficiency.

What Can Go Wrong?

Given how important the smooth surfaces are, when something happens to them we often notice that something is just not right. We may feel pain, the knee may swell, or we may find ourselves unable to do certain things. For example, walking longer distances or running may be a problem. The damage and swelling are often a result of an injury or wear and tear. If there is an injury, the knee's special surfaces can get scratched, dinged, dented, and chipped—just like the metal on your car. If dented or dinged, there may be a hole in the surface. The surface can also wear down like a car's tire, and if the knee is injured or misaligned, just like a tire, its surface can wear unevenly. All of these can cause pain and swelling. Once the cartilage is damaged and arthritis begins, the joint no longer works as smoothly, it wears much faster—and your magical 310 mpg drops!

What If I Have None of Those Problems and Still Have Swelling?

Infections (like Lyme disease), swelling and inflammation caused by problems like crystals in the joint from gout or the similar crystal deposits of pseudogout, inflammation, and arthritic diseases can all irritate the joint and damage the surfaces. The body may respond by trying to lubricate the surfaces and make more joint fluid, which results in joint swelling.

Lastly, the bone under the cartilage can be bruised, stressed, or cracked. These are all different injuries from torn ligaments, kneecap dislocations, meniscus tears, and fractures (discussed in Chapters 9-12). Keep in mind that all the problems described here can cause arthritis down the road and may eventually create the need for a knee replacement. It is my goal, as an orthopaedic specialist, to identify these issues early and, when possible, offer ways to repair or help the body heal the damaged area. The issues that we can treat include:

Loose Bodies

Simple loose bodies can occur when a small piece of cartilage is chipped off the surface and then floats around inside the knee. In time, the knee fluid nourishes the cartilage cells and they grow, just like a grain of sand in an oyster. Once it gets bigger, a large, loose body can get trapped between the bones and cause locking as it gets stuck and unstuck. Sometimes patients can feel it moving around and experience swelling. Patients often know when the loose body is in a "good" place and not a problem and when it moves to a "bad" place and causes locking. In any case, the loose piece will continue to cause trouble and will need to be removed using an arthroscope to prevent more locking and more damage to the knee. In general, with simple loose bodies, there is little else to do after they are removed, and the recovery is relatively easy.

Loose bodies with deeper surface and bone damage can occur with trauma to the knee or when fragments of bone below the joint surface lose their local blood supply, crack, and separate from the rest of the bone. The condition is called osteochondritis dissecans (OCD), and it is frequently due to repeated stress or trauma to the area, which can cause microscopic fractures to appear (see Image 64). They cannot heal because of the repetitive use of the leg. Imagine if you bend a plastic fork thousands of times; eventually, the pieces break off and become loose. The knee hurts and may swell, but you keep pushing it and hoping it will get better, but it does not. The loose fragment can move out of the hole it is in and move around in the knee. Even if it moves only a small amount, it can hurt. Sometimes the piece becomes completely loose like the loose body mentioned above, which causes swelling, pain, and locking (see Image 65). Other times it is not completely loose and can be repaired.

The most common site for OCD is the outer (lateral) side of the inner half of the knee (the medial femoral condyle). Although no one knows why a segment of bone loses its blood supply, most doctors believe that it is due to repetitive microtrauma. Classic OCD occurs commonly in older children and adolescents who actively participate in sports. The theory is that the repetitive impact during a sport like soccer or basketball causes a small segment of the bone to crack or fracture under the surface. The continued microtrauma on the already injured knee prevents the defect from healing and loosens the bone fragment. The younger the patient is, the more likely that OCD will heal if treated correctly.

Shallow cartilage defects in adults are different from OCD in growing children and teens. In

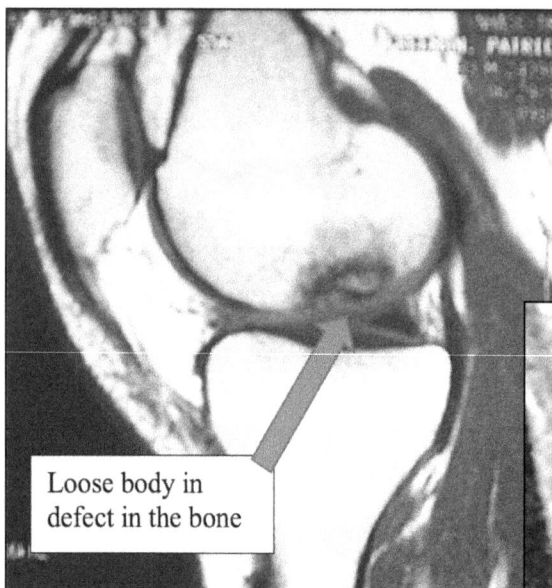

64 OCD (osteochondritis dissecans) with a loose body in the defect.

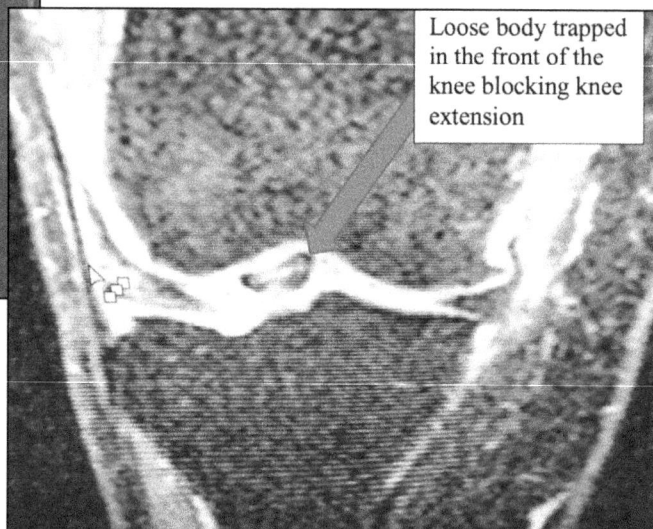

Loose body in defect in the bone

Loose body trapped in the front of the knee blocking knee extension

65 Loose body blocking knee motion.

adults they can be caused by local trauma, wear and tear, or arthritis, and the defect or damage can be treated by a technique called microfracture, in which the surface is drilled or "cracked" with a very tiny (microscopic) drill or awl to help blood and marrow (along with the patient's own stem cells) get to the surface. The idea is to promote the formation of new fibrocartilage and gain access to the stem cell–rich bone marrow just below the surface, similar to aerating the soil before seeding the lawn. Microfracture makes small channels in the bone surface, and the channels allow the stem cells into the knee, after which new cartilage grows and covers the surface with fresh tissue.

It's important to note that there are size and shape criteria for all these treatments, and clinical judgment is needed for each treatment option in each age group. After a microfracture, you may be asked to decrease weight-bearing activities for four to six weeks or use an unloader brace to unload the surface to help it heal. Healing may take three to four months and impact loading of the knee like running, jumping, climbing hills, or hiking down steep inclines should be completely avoided during that time.

Complex Loose Bodies

If the symptoms from a cartilage defect are ignored and healing does not occur, the cartilage and its base eventually separate and a fragment or fragments break loose into the knee joint, as is the case with OCD. They can then cause locking, sharp pain, and leg weakness. If the fragments are loose, the surgeon may scrape the cavity to reach fresh bone, add a bone graft, and fix the fragments in place. If the fragments cannot be mended, they are removed. This leaves a defect or hole that needs repair.

Stress fractures in older patients may occur after a more traumatic injury. They can also occur after significant repetitive stress like a sudden increase in walking for very long distances on concrete floors, or increased running when you have not been running for some time. In this setting, we are more likely to see a stress fracture that does not break off completely. The outer bone is intact, which is why a plain X-ray will not show much. But when pain persists and simple treatments like rest, crutches, and NSAIDs fail to help, an MRI may be needed to make the diagnosis.

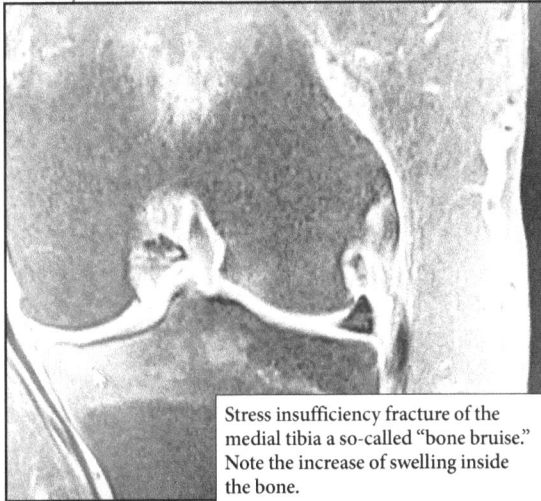

Stress insufficiency fracture of the medial tibia a so-called "bone bruise." Note the increase of swelling inside the bone.

66 Stress fracture of the bones—these are not seen on plain X-rays—MRI shows water or "bruising" inside the bone, and this is diagnostic of a stress insufficiency fracture if not traumatic or, if traumatic, a "bone bruise."

When we see a stress fracture on an MRI that is not healing, it can be treated with drilling, pinning, or if a larger area is involved (a so-called stress insufficiency fracture), calcium grafting may support the bone and reduce the pain. This is most useful in patients over 55 who don't need their knee replaced or are hoping to avoid a replacement with an alternative treatment for bone pain after a stress injury.

The graft material can be injected into the fracture with arthroscopic instruments and X-ray imaging. The calcium graft is made of calcium pyrophosphate, the same calcium crystals in your healthy bone. Once placed, the graft hardens and supports the bone like an internal cast. Once it hardens, the calcium grafting seems to treat the pain of the fracture very well as the fracture heals.

Classic OCD is usually diagnosed with specific X-ray images. If OCD is suspected or seen on an X-ray, an MRI is often necessary to grade the lesion and determine the best treatment. In a growing child, an early lesion may heal with use of a brace or cast and resting the leg by using crutches, avoiding weight-bearing activities, and absolutely avoiding all sports while healing! If the defect is displaced or loose, or an MRI shows fluid under it, surgery is necessary to restore the blood flow and stabilize the loose piece.

When surgical repair is necessary, I have fixed many of these defects using dissolving pins or screws that are sunk into the cartilage after drilling the base to stimulate a new blood supply, a procedure that is successful if the cartilage fragments have not broken loose. The dissolving pins or screws are bioabsorbable and slowly dissolve in the bone, so they do not need to be taken out once the bone heals. If fragments are loose, your doctor may need to clean the cavity to reach fresh, healthy bone and then attach a bone graft in position with dissolving pins or screws. Fragments that cannot be mended are cleaned and drilled to stimulate new cartilage growth. For smaller lesions, a graft can be taken from another part of your own knee and transferred into the defect. We are robbing Peter to pay Paul by doing this, but if an area is less important for normal activities it may be worth it. For very large defects, there are many treatment options. Sometimes a live cartilage graft from a donor is best; however, other cases, depending on the depth of the defect, may be treated with cartilage grown from the patient's own cells. MACI grafting with bone grafting is also an option in larger defects (see pages 26 and 74-75).

As noted above, small defects can be treated with the microfracture technique, but larger ones require grafting. Grafts can be obtained through autograft (transplanting cartilage from one part of the knee to another, osteochondral autograft transplantation, or OATS); allograft OATS (using frozen grafts from a donor, a technique used for very large defects with bone loss); the patient's own cultured cartilage cells (see the discussion on MACI in the next section); or a newer, synthetic bone substitute that fills in over time with the patient's cells. If the graft is a culture using the patient's own cartilage cells, this requires two procedures. In the first procedure the doctor removes the loose pieces and cleans the knee of fragments. Then for the second procedure the doctor harvests cells to use to grow new cartilage cells for later implantation.

Growing Your Own Cells

The newer version of grafting defects with your cells is called the MACI technique (matrix-induced autologous chondrocyte implantation), which was discussed in Chapter 10. It has been used in Australia and Europe with great success for many years. It has taken a long time for the market to be big enough in the US to justify going through the FDA, but it is now FDA-approved and is used in the US. Once your cells are grown in a lab, a second procedure is needed to implant your newly grown cells and have the defect fill with new cartilage. It is truly made up of your cells and your own DNA so there is no chance of rejection. There are strict age and defect size criteria for MACI's use, and these criteria may vary slightly depending on a patient's medical insurance.

In general, depending on the patient's age and the location of the defects, we can make good choices on the treatment plan using the following guidelines:

- **Microfracture** technique for defects 1–2 square centimeters in size.

- **OATS** (transfer from one part of the knee to another—borrowing from Peter to pay Paul idea) for defects 1–2 square centimeters or more with deeper loss of bone below the surface. It is used because both bone and cartilage are lost.

- **MACI** for defects more than 1.5c-d centimeters or multiple defects with good sidewalls, or "shoulders."

- **Allograft OATS** (from a donor body within a short time of donation to preserve the transplanted cells) for defects greater than 2–4 square centimeters with a bone defect below the surface that needs replacement.

Older patients (over 55) with larger defects may need partial or total knee replacements. Those with deformity (bowed or knocked knees) may need that corrected at the same time or an earlier date. Those with recurrent patella dislocations with patella cartilage surface loss will need the dislocation problem fixed first or at the time of the cartilage repair.

Regardless of which type of repair is done, the healing process takes time. You will be asked to use crutches and wear a brace and will need to protect the knee from impact loading (often the original cause of the problem). This is meant to let the body do the hard work of healing these defects. At first, you may be in a knee immobilizer, which is a straight brace with Velcro straps. This allows you to protect the repair and still place your toes down with very little weight on the leg for balance while using crutches. Then you will need to wear a custom knee unloader brace for at least four months after the procedure.

14 KNEE REPLACEMENTS

MILLIONS OF KNEE REPLACEMENTS ARE DONE WORLDWIDE EACH YEAR. IT'S HARD to believe that the first attempts were described in the early 1860s, when hinges made of iron were tested by German surgeon T. Gluck. However, it was not until 1968 that the first successful modern replacement was performed. The materials were better than iron, but still not the best for the long-term test of human motion. The overall benefits were limited by the lifetime of the materials used. In time, advances included special polyethylene and metal made of cobalt-chrome alloys. These days, knee replacements can last 20 years and beyond.

Knee replacements can eliminate the pain from bone rubbing on bone when there is no cartilage left in the knee. Partial replacements are also possible. For example, some patients have much more wear on one side of the knee and that can be replaced. Other patients have a damaged kneecap, but the rest of the knee is in good shape; for them, a kneecap or patella replacement can be helpful. A knee replacement can be used to correct a knee deformity.

The choice to replace the entire knee or just part of it is not as straightforward as it would seem. The extent of any deformity, bone loss from wear and tear, age, and body weight are all factors to consider with your surgeon.

Knee replacements are used to restore quality of life, and as such, they are one of the top surgical procedures—along with hip replacements and rotator cuff repairs—in improvement made in quality of life after the surgery. They can also be used in bone tumors around the knee with larger metal extensions to replace the bone removed with a metal bone replacement and a hinged knee joint.

One word on knee replacement risks and results: It has been found that those patients with recurring infections in other parts of the body have a high risk of getting a knee replacement infection. Recurring infections, poor health, poor nutrition, high body mass index (over 40), low body mass index (less than 18.5), diabetes, and extreme osteoporosis (soft bones) all increase the risk of complications when having a knee replacement.

Results as measured by range of knee motion are related to the range with which the patient starts. In other words, if your knee is in pain and you continue to wait until you lose motion, the ability to restore motion decreases as the preoperative motion worsens. There is a value in not waiting too long if you need a knee replaced. Also, results worsen with increasing deformity. Again, if there is an angular deformity of the knee and it is getting worse, waiting does worsen the possible replacement results and increases the risk of complications.

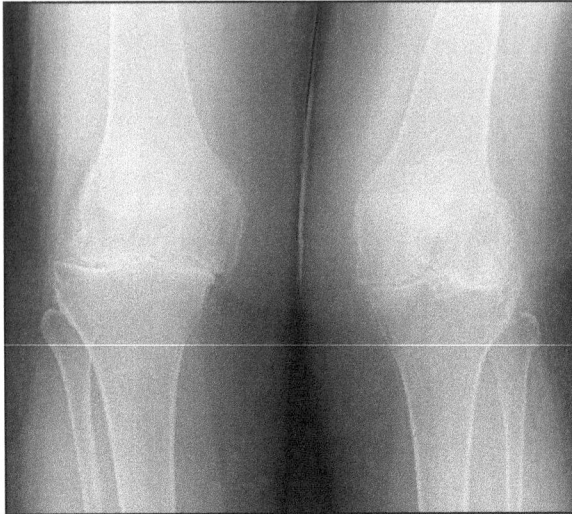

67 X-ray of advanced osteoarthritis in both knees with both being "bone on bone."

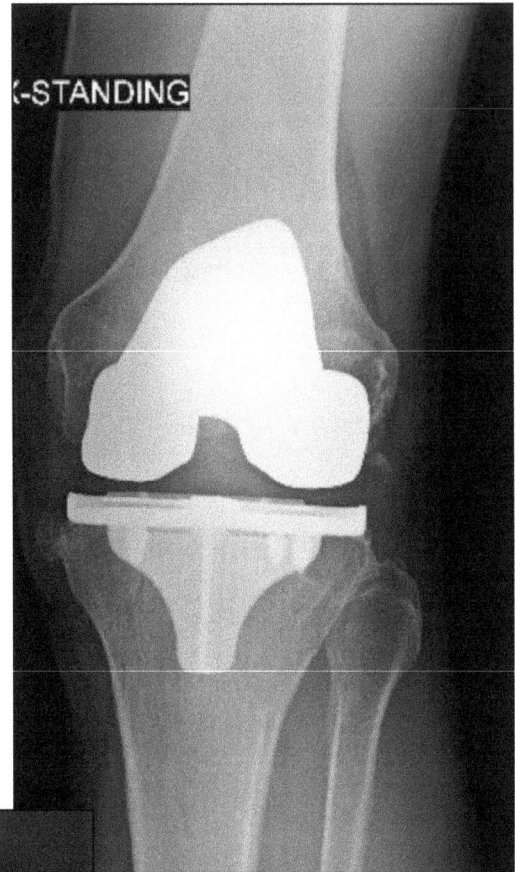

68 X-ray of standard knee replacement with femoral and tibial components in place.

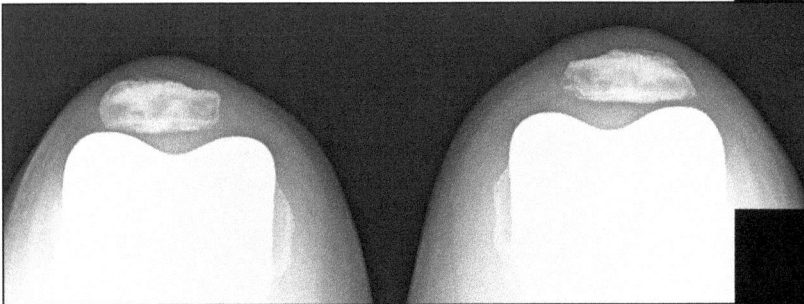

69 X-ray of knee cap replacements in both knees.

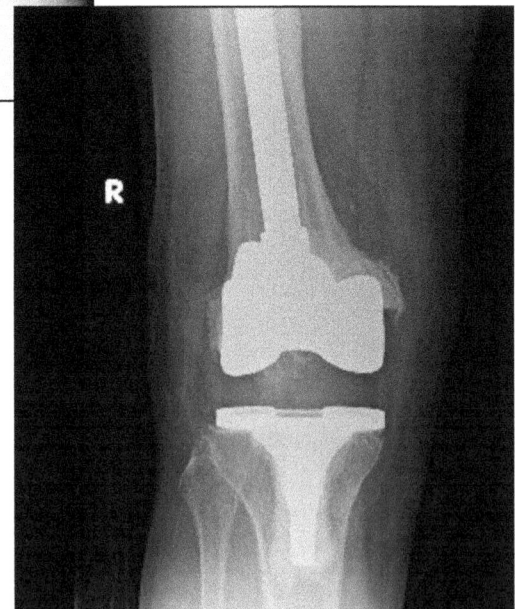

70 X-ray of a special long stem knee replacement for patients with very soft bone, large pre-surgery bone deformity, or revision of a prior knee replacement.

PART THREE

THE SHOULDER

The shoulder is the most complex joint in the human body (see Image 71). It has the greatest range of motion, and it plays an important role as the base that supports your arm and hand through all their movements. This makes the shoulder extremely important for most activities of daily living, work, and self-care. Of course, it also has a primary role in all overhead sports. When the shoulder is hurt, its function decreases, and as a result, the person's quality of life is diminished. Whether the injury is a result of trauma, overuse, or arthritis, shoulder problems can make it difficult to dress, work, reach a high shelf, throw a ball, or even lift a small child.

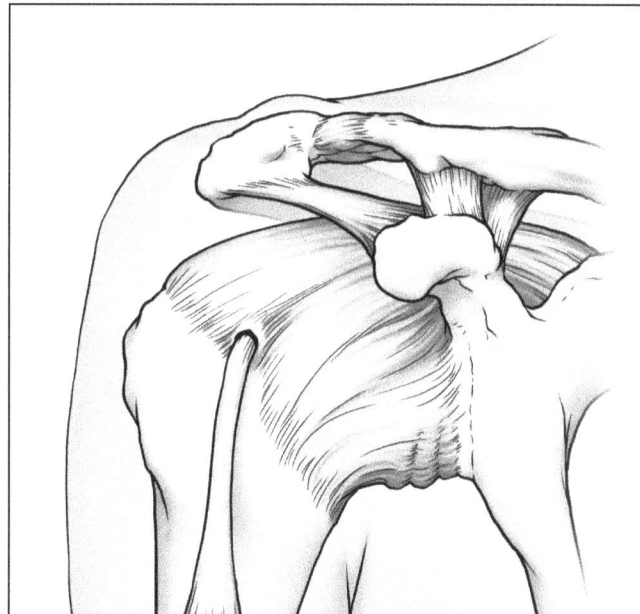

71 Line drawing of the shoulder bones, ligaments, joint lining, and biceps tendon without the muscles covering them.

What Could Go Wrong?

Below are several things that can go wrong with your shoulders:

Tendinitis and Bursitis
Inflammation of the tendons and bursae (small, paper-thin, fluid-filled sacs that lubricate the spaces around a joint). Tendonitis and bursitis cause pain when your arm is lifted; it may result from an inflammatory disease such as rheumatoid arthritis or from tendons being pinched by local bone spurs or surrounding structures.

Rotator Cuff Tear
A tear in the tendons or muscles that stabilize the shoulder, causing pain, weakness, or interference with daily activities; it's often due to uncontrolled inflammation, repetitive use, traumatic injury, or age-related degeneration.

Separation
A condition that occurs when torn ligaments in the shoulder cause the clavicle (collarbone) to slip out of place where it meets the scapula (shoulder blade). This may be caused by a fall or other trauma, weak shoulder muscles, or a shallow joint socket.

Subluxation
A condition in which the ball of the humerus (upper arm) slips partly out of the shoulder socket but does not dislocate, causing some pain, fear of dislocation (apprehension), muscle spasms, and weakness in certain motions.

Dislocation
A condition in which the ball of the humerus (upper arm) pops out of the shoulder socket, causing acute pain, muscle spasms, swelling, and deformity until the shoulder is put back in place (reduced). It is often caused by a fall or other trauma. If the humerus does not go back in place by itself, see your doctor as soon as possible.

Multidirectional Instability
In some patients, the ball and socket are loose in more than one direction, meaning the ball can slip partly out of place in more than one direction. Multidirectional Instability (MDI) can occur in any combination of slipping toward the front, the back, or downward. Some patients have had more than one traumatic dislocation and have torn more than one structure. Most concerning are patients with some laxity who continue to dislocate and have symptoms that affect their normal activities.

Other patients with MDI were born with general ligamentous laxity. In other words, their normal collagen has more give, or stretch, than the average person's. Some people are said to be "double-jointed" when they have this condition, while others have a known disease or syndrome. One example is Ehlers-Danlos syndrome, a group of genetic connective tissue abnormalities. One of the issues in most of its forms is very loose joints, and these patients have MDI when tested but often don't have symptoms. Regardless of whether it is named, it is the level of symptoms related to the instability that becomes our main concern. If the MDI (looseness of the joint) is mild and does not cause pain or functional limitations, we are not as concerned about the laxity.

Frozen Shoulder

Shoulder stiffness or immobility due to abnormal tissue formation between the joint surfaces (also called adhesive capsulitis). This may be caused by an injury, a genetic tendency to develop thick scars after trauma (keloids), or occur in patients with diabetes (who are predisposed to frozen shoulder). On rare occasions, a frozen shoulder may be the first sign of diabetes. Patients with inflammatory conditions like rheumatoid arthritis can also lose motion and are predisposed to frozen shoulder.

Osteoarthritis

Degeneration of the shoulder joint, particularly the acromioclavicular (where the upper part of the scapula meets the clavicle), causing pain and stiffness.

Rheumatoid Arthritis

Inflammation of the shoulder joint that is a result of antibodies and an inflammatory response that causes advancing, painful arthritis.

Inflammation, Arthritis, or Injury of the AC Joint

The acromioclavicular, or AC, joint attaches the shoulder blade and the ball and socket to the collarbone. The shoulder's only boney connection to the rest of the body is through the collarbone, hence the importance of a properly functioning AC joint. Like other joints, there can be sprains, subluxations, dislocations, inflammation, arthritis, spurs, or fractures at or around the AC joint, which can cause pain, loss of motion, stiffness, and swelling of the entire shoulder.

In this section of the book, we are going to discuss all the conditions listed above, as well as treatment options—and more—to help you to understand what can go wrong with your shoulder and what can be done about it.

15 FROZEN SHOULDER (ADHESIVE CAPSULITIS)

ALTHOUGH THIS IS NOT THE MOST COMMON OF ALL SHOULDER PROBLEMS, patients with adhesive capsulitis, or frozen shoulder, experiencing severe loss of motion often make an appointment to see me when they cannot easily get dressed and lose normal daily function. It is less common than bursitis and tendonitis from overuse, and it can occur for many more reasons. Most often, there is a smaller underlying shoulder injury or problem that causes the patient to have difficulty moving their arm. In time, the patient barely notices that their range of motion is slowly decreasing. As the frozen shoulder worsens, the lining of the joint is, in fact, shrinking in size without the patient realizing it. At some point, the tight lining causes motion to be limited and activities of daily living become more difficult. Pain often increases with lost motion, and eventually, the patient notices that they have trouble reaching for the back seat of the car or putting a shirt or sweater on. Many people don't seek an orthopaedic consultation until sleeping becomes a problem. The number one complaint I see in shoulder patients that force them to come into the office is that they cannot sleep at night.

A frozen shoulder can be a response to local pain and inflammation. It is often related to a seemingly small trauma and can also occur after more significant trauma, surgery, or fracture. I also see frozen shoulders when patients delay moving the arm after a treatment for an injury because of residual pain; any prolonged period of immobilization can set it off. Therefore, when a sling is necessary to treat a shoulder problem, a watchful eye is required to see the warning signs of a frozen shoulder before it becomes a larger problem. In some severe cases, almost all motion is lost over time.

Frozen shoulder is more common in women than men, in people 40 to 60 years old, and in people with diabetes. Loss of internal rotation (the ability to reach behind your back) is an early sign of a frozen shoulder. Most women tend to notice the loss of internal rotation much earlier than men because many need to reach behind the back to put a bra on every day. It makes sense that women are often seen by a doctor earlier in the process than men.

Patients who have skin hypersensitivity or have a history of forming keloids may also have an increased risk of developing a frozen shoulder (see sidebar on keloids on page 101). Sometimes a frozen shoulder seems to be related to a genetic predisposition, especially if a patient also has a history of keloids. A few patients in my practice have had a frozen shoulder on one side, only to have another one on the other side years later. Even though the initial cause may be clear, it is important to note that there is a strong association with diabetes in some populations. Diabetes itself seems to affect cells in the lining of the shoulder, causing it to become stiff and shrink after even the most minor insult or injury. Once the lining thickens with scar tissue, it becomes less flexible.

Interestingly, on rare occasions, a frozen shoulder can be the first sign of underlying diabetes and may be the only presenting symptom. If a patient develops a frozen shoulder after a minor injury and they are very thirsty, drinking a lot of liquids, or tired or weak, getting blood tests like a fasting blood sugar level and a hemoglobin A1c (glycated hemoglobin) level may be worthwhile to rule out diabetes as a cause. Moreover, when a person with diabetes develops a frozen shoulder, it tends to be harder to resolve than in a nondiabetic person.

Keloid Treatment

What is a keloid? A keloid is a scar that doesn't know when to stop making scar tissue after a wound heals. It starts as a thin scar and then begins to thicken with time. It may become itchy, stiff, and even a little sore. It may start in one spot or a number of small spots and then involve the entire length of the scar. Worse yet, when the body forms a keloid, it makes the scar thicker and denser well after the wound has already healed.

In a healthy person, when the skin is cut or open, cells grow back to fill in the gap. Somehow, the skin knows when the scar tissue is even with the contour of the skin, and the wound is sealed over. At that point, the scar tissue cells normally stop multiplying. When the cells keep producing scar tissue after the wound should have healed, the result is a thickened, overgrown (hypertrophic) scar—a keloid. It can be raised, thick, discolored, ugly, itchy, and stiff, and it tends to run in families. If you are genetically predisposed to getting these thickened scars, early treatment is best.

RECOMMENDED TREATMENTS

✓ Apply hydrocortisone cream every day to reduce inflammation, itching, and the scar-forming activity of the inflammatory response.

✓ If the itch persists, taking an antihistamine (such as Benadryl) or using a silicone bandage overnight, such as Curad Scar Therapy, ScarAway Band-Aids, or NewGel silicone pads, may be helpful.

✓ The combination of the cortisone cream, silicone pad, and Benadryl (when the scar is itchy) are all helpful.

✓ Continue these treatments for at least two months.

WHAT TO AVOID

✓ Sun exposure (cover the scar when in the sun with a bandage or zinc oxide cream. Sunscreen or sunblock does not give enough protection for surgical scars).

✓ Scratching, rubbing, or irritating the area.

✓ Creams and other products that promote scar healing as they can make the keloid get thicker. The idea is to stop any extra healing since the wound is already healed and the problem is too much scar tissue as opposed to not enough.

A person with a frozen shoulder may also develop persistent swelling (lymphedema) in the arm on the same side. The lack of shoulder motion decreases the body's ability to move fluid back to the heart. This can be worse after shoulder surgery or other surgeries near the shoulder joint. This is a special concern after surgery for breast cancer. If the lymph nodes have been removed as a part of removing the tumor, fluid will stay in the arm and the hand may swell. Radiation to the area may worsen the condition. If the surgery is long and the arm is still for hours, a postsurgery frozen shoulder is also possible. Therefore, movement after the surgical wounds heal in these cases can help reduce the risk of a postoperative frozen shoulder (see the section on postoperative frozen shoulder later in this chapter).

Treatment

General treatment for a frozen shoulder includes reducing the inflammation, stretching the tight tissues, regaining the normal motion, and preventing recurrence. The nature of the frozen shoulder, the presence of diabetes, the severity and how long the patient has been frozen all alter the treatment cost and the difficulty in curing the problem.

Initial Treatment for Frozen Shoulder

The initial treatment for a frozen shoulder is anti-inflammatory medications and physical therapy. If the shoulder has been frozen for a long time or suddenly becomes much more painful, a cortisone injection will loosen things up and help the therapist get things moving again. A Medrol Dosepak (a tapered dose of oral steroids) can also be helpful. You can reduce the risk of recurrence by keeping up with the recommended home exercise program and taking anti-inflammatory medications as prescribed. Fortunately, a high percentage of patients improve with nonsurgical methods.

Manipulation and Lysis of Adhesions

If a patient's capsulitis does not resolve or recurs, he or she may need surgical treatment. This includes moving the arm under general anesthesia (a manipulation), removing the scar tissue (arthroscopic lysis of the adhesions), or cutting the tight lining tissue to regain the motion that has been lost (a surgical capsular release). If there are other underlying shoulder problems, they can be treated at the same time.

For example, if large spurs, wear, or a stress injury or degeneration at the end of the collarbone (osteolysis of the distal clavicle) are the primary causes of shoulder pain, these problems should be treated. A simple manipulation and removing the adhesions without removal of the spurs may give the frozen shoulder a "reason" to return. Still, before surgery, the initial treatment should almost always consist of NSAIDs, physical therapy, an injection of cortisone (when not contraindicated), and oral cortisone if those treatments fail. (Remember, cortisone can increase blood sugars, especially in people with poorly controlled diabetes, so additional caution is required in those patients.) If a patient fails to see any improvement after three or more months of nonoperative treatment, surgery may be necessary.

Whether surgery is successful depends on several factors. Once the manipulation is carried out, the most important goals are to maintain the gains in motion made during surgery and to prevent the scar or adhesions from reforming. Anti-inflammatory medications, steroids, and even muscle relaxers to control pain are very important after surgery. The risk of scar recurrence can be further reduced by a very early and aggressive therapy program. To accomplish this, I ask my patients to start their exercises in the recovery room and begin formal physical therapy within a few days after surgery. Provided there are no specific contraindications, post-op anti-inflammatory medications are absolutely required in all patients to keep the inflammation in check.

In difficult cases, an oral steroid (like a Medrol Dosepak) may also be useful in the early post-op period.

Since many frozen shoulders develop very slowly without a clear cause, the muscles have often been tight or contracted for some time. Many patients can feel this tightness and require both time and physical therapy to prevent more muscle shortening after treatment has begun. Even after the adhesions and the tight lining are fully released, it is still possible that motion may not be fully restored. This is because the muscle memory tends to want to shorten the muscles back to their frozen length. Also, your body's defenses remember the pain with motion and want you to avoid the painful movement, even though that is what created your problems. Therefore, once a manipulation and release are done, early motion is very important to avoid refreezing. Home exercise programs, following the instructions on stretching, and the watchful eye of a talented physical therapist can make all the difference. Good outcomes don't occur without hard work.

If a patient is doing well at first, but the motion seems to be deteriorating each week, medical management of the recurring inflammation is urgently required. Nonsteroidal medication can help, but steroids may be needed in complicated cases. Please tell your doctor if you feel like you are regressing at any time during the treatment. (Be careful around three months post-op—some frozen shoulders can recur in that time frame.) If this happens, new medications may be tried, such as muscle relaxers (like Skelaxin or Flexeril), drugs to settle the nerve endings (like Elavil, gabapentin, Lyrica, or trazodone), and others, up to and including oral or injected steroids. In some cases, there will be an improvement to a point, and the shoulder will be more functional, but still not fully recovered. In those rare cases, a second manipulation may be beneficial.

Posttraumatic and Postoperative Frozen Shoulder

One cannot forget that the underlying case of a frozen shoulder is tightening of the lining or capsule of the shoulder joint. This can happen after major trauma to the area. This includes motor vehicle accidents, falls, fractures of the arm, and the normal postoperative inflammatory process of healing. In the process of any surgery there is a healing response, and this can cause a frozen shoulder. This happens more often with patients who are diabetic.

Any shoulder surgery that is an open procedure carries some risk of a postoperative frozen shoulder (postoperative fibrosis), including shoulder repairs of the rotator cuff, repairs for instability, plating of fractures, and shoulder replacements. Some patients who have undergone these procedures have had pain and difficulty moving their shoulders before surgery. In these cases, many patients have a frozen shoulder before the surgery and, naturally, movement after surgery is much more difficult. This combined problem of preoperative frozen shoulder and the trauma of surgery itself requires more attention early after surgery and most often physical therapy for a long time after that.

In addition, cancer patients who undergo long surgeries are also at risk. During a long, complex surgery the arm may be positioned so it is out of the way and then become inflamed. If the operative side is near the shoulder, the shoulder may be immobilized after surgery to protect the surgical area. This is most common with breast cancer surgeries and partial or complete mastectomies. If the surgery is combined with reconstruction after the tumor is removed the operation will be longer and increases the risk. Radiation and/or chemotherapy can also increase stiffness and scar formation. The combination of all three—surgery, chemo, and radiation—are a setup for postoperative stiffness. These patients should be aware that maintaining shoulder motion may require physical therapy as soon as their cancer surgeon will allow it. Lastly men more often than women after open heart surgery are also prone to frozen shoulders and can be treated the same way.

Early Treatment Is Best

Remember, a frozen shoulder is best treated nonoperatively first, using NSAIDs, plus or minus injections, and a physical therapy program that includes both stretching and strengthening exercises for the rotator cuff. Only those individuals with a frozen shoulder who have failed to improve with good medical treatment and physical therapy should consider surgery—and only if they are prepared to work hard in therapy afterward. Please don't wait too long to start the nonsurgical treatments! Many patients have had symptoms for more than a year by the time I see them; they are fed up and tired of having a limited range of motion and pain with activity. They are usually happy to comply with the therapy program but don't have their full stamina left after having pain and stiffness for so long. Most of them would have been better served if seen by an orthopaedic surgeon sooner.

When successfully treated, patients with a frozen shoulder regain most of their range of motion with forward flexion and elevation first, external rotation second, and internal rotation last. Men notice this when they can reach overhead but still cannot get their wallet out of their back pocket. Women notice this when they can move their arms in front of their bodies without pain but still cannot hook a bra behind their back. These patients' symptoms have improved, but they need to continue a daily stretching program for a year after a successful manipulation, especially if they have diabetes or form keloids, which means they face a higher risk of recurrence.

16 SHOULDER INSTABILITY AND DISLOCATIONS

A SHOULDER POPPING OUT CAN BE A DRAMATIC EVENT AND IS FREQUENTLY portrayed as happening at the worst time in the middle of an action movie. You may have a vivid memory of a well-known actor popping his shoulder out and then putting it back in by slamming it against a locker, or a captured hero dislocating their shoulder to escape being tied up. You may have also seen contortionists put their arms in seemingly unreal positions or escape artists get out of tight chains by popping their shoulders out and then putting them back. You may even have friends who voluntarily shift their shoulders in and out of the socket to make a popping sound. Just gross, right?!

These images have lasting visual effects because they are all abnormal motions of the shoulder and represent fundamental problems with normal shoulder structure and function. In fact, these party tricks are really a medical condition. These people either have had a traumatic dislocation that weakens the ligaments and makes it easier and easier to dislocate each time, or have a general ligament looseness that leads to easy dislocations (see "Multidirectional Instability"on page 98 for information on double-jointed shoulders) because the lining of the shoulder is like an overstretched rubber band and does not hold the ball in the socket well. This occurs in very flexible people who are "loose" or "double-jointed." In general, these are the two main types of shoulder dislocations. Some dislocations can go back in place with ease, while others require emergency treatment with an anesthetic or sedation to get it back in place. Here, we are going to look at these broad groups of patients in more detail, so you can better understand the wide range of issues and treatments for these problems.

As I mentioned at the beginning of Part Three, the shoulder joint has the widest range of motion of any joint in the body. This is because the joint itself is positioned on the end of a very mobile stick (the collarbone, as discussed in other chapters), and the shoulder blade sits loosely over the ribs with no bone attachment to them. Because the socket that the ball moves on is part of the shoulder blade, the socket itself is free to move widely with the motion of the blade. This means that the ball and socket starting point varies greatly with the shoulder blade motion, which already makes the shoulder's range of motion greater than that of any other joint. In addition, the ball (humeral head) that sits in the socket is round, and the socket is very small and flat. Imagine a smooth golf ball on a slightly larger than normal tee; this adds even more flexibility to the shoulder joint. Unlike the hip, where the ball and socket are well-mated and stable, the shoulder's ball and socket are not. There is a big trade-off for the flexibility and motion of the joint, in that it is less stable than all the other joints in the body. It makes us wonder: How does the shoulder stay in place? This is a big part of our next topic, shoulder instability—the opposite of frozen shoulder.

Dislocations, Instability, and Shoulder Structure

Shoulder dislocations make up at least half of all major joint dislocations (see Images 72-74). They can occur with trauma at almost any age but are much more common in a younger population. The peak age is between 20 and 30, with males nine times more likely than females to dislocate. The incidence is highest in athletes between the ages of 18 and 25 and people over age 60 who dislocate their shoulders because of a fall or trauma. Younger patients have higher recurrence rates after a first-time dislocation. It is well known that high-demand athletes and military cadets are at high risk for recurrent dislocations after their first traumatic dislocation. Data has shown that high-risk patients should have torn ligaments or labrum repaired after a first-time dislocation to reduce the risk of recurrent dislocations.

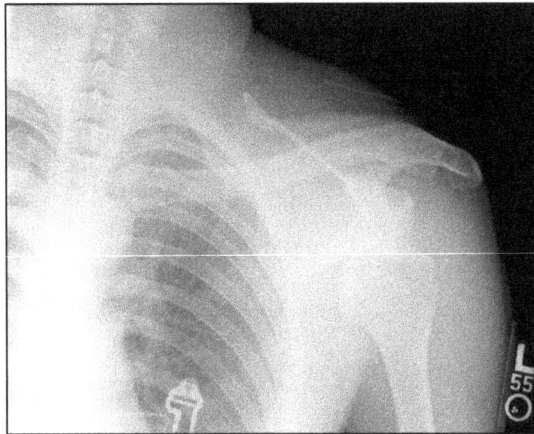

72 Dislocated shoulder.

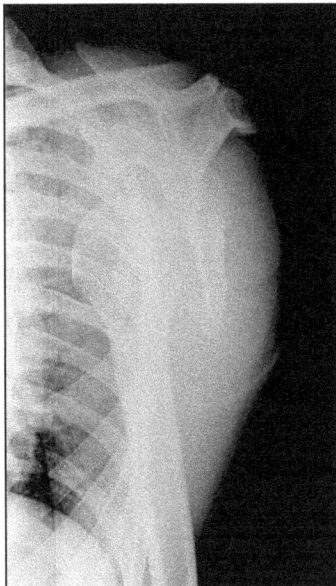

73 Scapular "Y" view on X-ray shoulder at the direction of dislocation. In this case, an anterior dislocation.

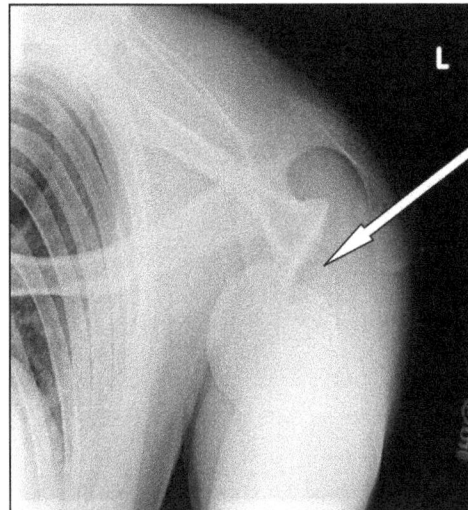

74 Axillary or trauma view of the shoulder. Here we can see the glenoid (socket) causing a dent in the humeral head, forming a Hill-Sachs lesion.

The Shoulder Is Designed for Function

The shoulder is designed for placing the arm and hand almost anywhere around the body. By design, and for its full function, it is also the easiest joint to slip out of place. Primarily this is because the shoulder socket is flatter than those of any of the other larger joints to allow its wide range of motion.

The socket (glenoid cavity) of the shoulder joint is reinforced with ligaments and a rim of tissue that surrounds the glenoid cavity called the glenoid labrum. That soft tissue rim deepens the socket, making the bone lip of the socket wider and adding stability; the ligaments add additional stability. The rotator cuff (the muscles and tendons surrounding the shoulder) adds even more stability by pulling the shoulder into the socket. This is particularly true when the rotator cuff muscles contract in a coordinated way with shoulder motion. The body of the scapula also moves to line up the forces on the shoulder. The shoulder blade motion puts the ball squarely in the center of the socket, making it more stable and reducing the risk of dislocation during heavy lifting, pushing, or pulling. It is a true marvel of anatomy to look at the shoulder as it functions in each patient every day.

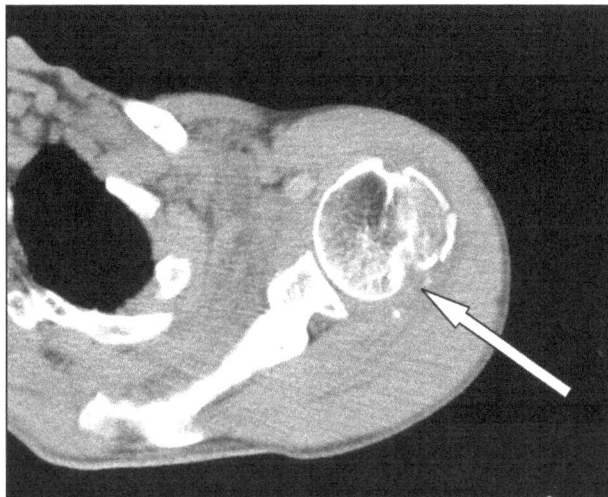

75 CT scan showing a shoulder that was dislocated that has been reduced (put back in) showing a Hill-Sachs lesion (arrow: dent in the humeral head).

Even though it's a masterpiece of protective engineering, the shoulder can be dislocated more easily than any other joint. If any excessive force is applied to the arm parallel to the flat glenoid surface, like a golf ball being hit off a tee, the shoulder may dislocate. When this occurs, the supporting ligaments and the labrum may be torn, displaced, or stretched out of shape. The labrum itself can be torn off the bone (called a Bankart lesion). Furthermore, when the smooth cartilage surface of the head of the humerus slides over the labrum, it can become impinged against the sharp rim. This can fracture the lip of the socket or dent the back of the ball. When this happens, it is called a "boney" Bankart lesion, a small fracture on the lip of the socket that is still attached to the ligaments that tear away with the broken fragment. When the defect is in the ball, it's called a Hill-Sachs lesion (see Images 75 and

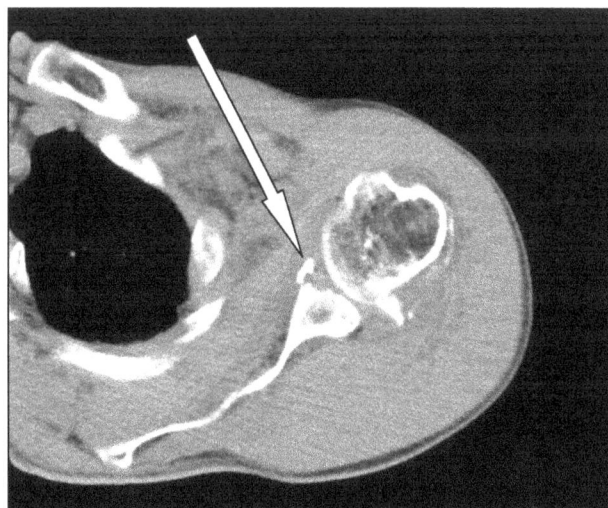

76 CT scan showing a shoulder that was dislocated that has been reduced (put back in), showing a fracture of the glenoid (arrow: a chip off the front of the socket).

76). The defects in the socket or the ball change the normal anatomy and further destabilize the shoulder; each of them can lead to recurrent dislocations.

The combination of the dent size and the amount of ligament damage dictates the future instability of the shoulder. The same is true for a glenoid lip fracture; the ligaments come off with the lip piece, and the larger the fracture, the more unstable the shoulder will be. In time, and with recurrent dislocations, more damage will be done to the joint. Naturally, with larger dents in the ball or the larger the chips off the socket, the easier it is for the shoulder to dislocate again and again. The larger defects combined with a very unstable shoulder cause these patients to give up many physical activities. This is with good reason since these defects, loss of stability, and repeat dislocations can eventually lead to arthritis of the shoulder.

What Does It Mean If Someone Is "Double-Jointed"?

What about the contortionist and those people who are double-jointed? They seem to be able to dislocate their shoulders at will, even without a traumatic event, torn cartilage, torn ligaments, or damage to the bone. This natural looseness is an interesting finding and occurs to varying degrees in 10%–25% of the general population.

Sometimes it is related to abnormal genes like Ehlers-Danlos syndrome, Marfan syndrome, or osteogenesis imperfecta (these terms are all defined in the glossary). Other times there are some minor abnormalities in the chemical structure of the natural connective tissues (collagen) that have no exact description. These patients, in general, have naturally loose joints because the collagen that lines their joints and makes up all their ligaments is more flexible or elastic in nature.

Many of these patients can bend their fingers back more than most people; have loose wrists, knees, and elbows (they can be over straightened or hyperextended); and can touch their toes or the floor easily without bending their knees. This ability often runs in families and is something to which a person is genetically predisposed. Although it is natural for double-jointed people to be able to subluxate their joints, once they do it on a regular basis, it may worsen, limit activity, increase the instability, or cause pain.

The treatment for these problems is not straightforward and can pose a dilemma because some of these patients have "learned" to dislocate their shoulders. This means they have learned how to use their muscles to make the shoulder come out at will or, worse, repeat it by habit, sometimes subconsciously. These party tricks cannot be unlearned easily, although some patients can be taught to retrain their muscles and correct the problem. The goal for most of these patients is to treat this problem with therapy and home exercises, but others cannot fix the overstretched ligaments, and stability cannot be restored without surgery. One caution: if the learned party trick is not altered by corrective behavior modification and therapy, even the best surgical treatment can be undone by the patient's own muscle actions over time.

Other Considerations

Be aware that some patients have secondary gain from continued shoulder pain and instability. This can occur in the teenage years when life transitions are stressful or competitive sports are being driven by parents and coaches. Athletes may need a way out of the pressure that they can no longer handle. It may be that they have loose joints, and a dislocation gets them the out they need.

Since the injury and its recurrence is the only way out of a bad situation, they have no desire to stop the ability to dislocate their shoulders. This is very rare but important to recognize when it happens because the root physiologic issues become an underlying reason not to truly resolve the dislocation problem. Only extracting the child from the high-pressure situation will ultimately help the physical problems at hand. It is difficult for the surgeon to be an expert here.

If the problem is recognized, and the child needs help, a discussion with the child's pediatrician may shed light on the issues. When asking questions along these lines, sometimes my hunch is right and there is even more going on at school or home, while other times it is just a coincidence. That's why I tread lightly when approaching the possibility that the problem is more than the orthopaedic issue. Again, it's a hard thing to think about, discuss, and correct, and yet it's very important to address when recognized.

Treatment

The Bankart repair, labral repair, and glenohumeral ligament repair are all surgical techniques to repair the damage from either a single joint dislocation or recurrent joint dislocations. In these procedures, the torn labrum and ligaments are reattached to the correct place to prevent further dislocations (see Image 77). For those with capsular looseness, shifting or tightening the lining is equally important. The areas of looseness need to be identified clinically and arthroscopically and then corrected at the time of surgery.

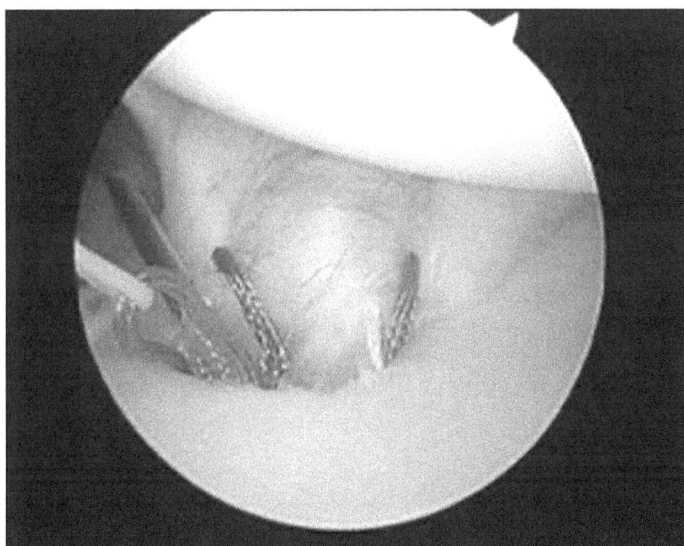

77 Repair of the torn labrum with sutures in place with anchors in the bone (not visible).

In some patients, the ball gets dented as it comes out of place or as it is put back in place, creating a Hill-Sachs lesion. In patients with small Hill-Sachs lesions, if you correct the ligaments, the small lesion will not hit the rim with routine motion. The shoulder is thus more stable, and the chance of reinjury is greatly reduced by avoiding dent-to-rim contact. On rare occasions, the dent is so large that other methods are required to prevent a recurrence. Medium-sized defects can be treated by covering the dent with local tissue (called a remplissage). Very large defects must be grafted in young patients, and these may be best treated with a shoulder replacement in older patients.

More than 30 years ago, when I was starting my career as an orthopaedic resident, these repairs, as well as all other shoulder surgeries, were done as open procedures. These require removing a muscle from its attachment points and putting it back, and the recovery was longer and more painful. When I was a fellow in San Diego a few years later, shoulder arthroscopy was in its infancy, so we made a real effort to convert the simplest of these procedures to an arthroscopic procedure. There were many theories on how best to do this, and one by one, we added more procedures. Almost 30 years later, arthroscopic repair using state-of-the-art techniques are the standard of care for most patients. I was lucky enough to participate in the early stages of these advances, and I have developed some of the techniques I use today, inventing new instruments and equipment. I currently hold six patents (including five for surgical equipment), some of which are used all over the world.

When the glenoid is fractured, the lip fracture needs to be addressed at the same time the ligaments are repaired. Tiny fragments (less than 15% of the socket) can be safely removed, and the labrum will be repaired over the defect. Slightly larger fragments can be put back with arthroscopy and are often repaired with the ligaments. Lip fractures involving more than 25% of the surface should be put back; some of these may even require screw fixation. The cases in between with a defect in the ball (humeral head) require a repair for the tear in the front and filling the defect in the back by covering it with part of the rotator cuff to prevent dislocations.

In rare cases, the bone edge of the socket is badly damaged and a bone graft or transferring the bone and tendon into the defect is required. The first procedure can be done with a donor piece of bone. The second procedure is a bone transfer to cover up the defect in the socket. This requires moving the coracoid process over and screwing it down into the defect with the short head of the biceps still attached; the attached tendon acts like an internal sling to help hold the ball in place and prevent future dislocations. Similarly, when the ball is badly damaged the defect can be filled with a graft of bone from a cadaver, or in an older patient, the shoulder may need replacement.

Loose Joints and Shoulder Subluxation

When the ligaments and capsule lining are stretched out of shape, they can cause instability and subluxation or recurrent dislocations. This can also occur traumatically or as a result of general ligament laxity (like the double-jointed people noted previously). Many patients with this problem cannot do work requiring overhead movements, which causes difficulties for patients like electricians, pipe workers, carpenters, and painters. These patients have equal difficulty with overhead sports like volleyball, basketball, gymnastics, baseball (when overhand pitching), and water polo. In swimmers, the backstroke and the breaststroke can also be an issue for patients with very loose joints. The throwing motion can cause pain, as can overhead weight lifting movements like the pec dec, pull-ups, the bench press, or the TRX program.

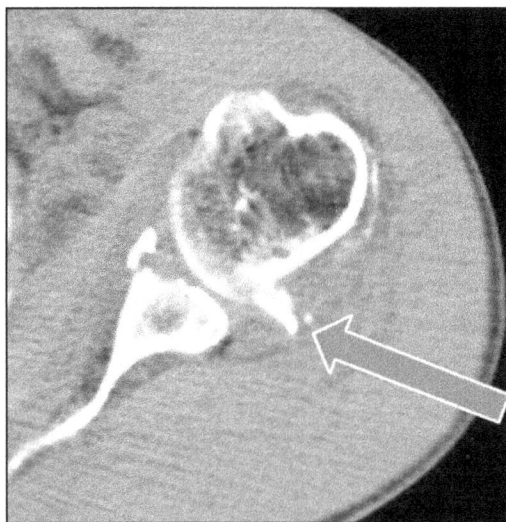

78 A loose body in the shoulder after dislocation. The piece is from the glenoid surface (socket side of the joint) after an anterior dislocation. It was pushed posteriorly when the shoulder was put back in place. The CT scan shown here was taken after reduction.

When this is a concern, an exam including a test for labral tears like Jobe's Relocation test, a reverse Jobe test, an "apprehension" test, and a "sulcus sign" are all helpful in making the diagnosis. In addition to a thorough physical exam, when these clinical signs are positive and the history matches the exam, an MRI arthrogram is helpful in making the exact diagnosis. If the ligaments alone are torn, loose, or stretched and the labrum is still attached, they can be repaired arthroscopically. As previously discussed, some patients with Bankart lesions or a torn labrum also have their ligaments stretched out when the injury occurs. When this is recognized during the corrective procedure, your surgeon can treat this at the same time they repair the labrum.

Special Cases: Posterior Dislocations

Posterior dislocations are less common than anterior dislocations and are therefore often missed. They can occur traumatically, often from a severe trauma like a car accident. or with other more serious or acute injuries—for example, falling on a straight arm from a height, holding on to the steering wheel in a car tightly during a collision, or falling off a bicycle. Occasionally, posterior dislocations are associated with seizures. During a strong seizure, the muscles in the back of the shoulder contract strongly and can pull the ball out of the socket. In those cases, patients have no memory of the event. (It turns out that it is very normal after a seizure to lose the memory of the event itself.) Without a memory of the trauma, many posterior dislocations present with loss of range of motion and pain, but the diagnosis of the actual event and the fact that the shoulder is out of place is not clear at the time of the initial doctor's visit.

When the cause of the posterior dislocation is trauma to the shoulder, the arm is internally rotated and, to the untrained eye, in a seemingly normal position. It is only when someone tries rotating the arm externally that the patient experiences pain and their ability to move is limited. Some of these trauma patients are unconscious and cannot help their doctor make a diagnosis. Moreover, a routine chest X-ray and even routine shoulder X-ray views are not at the correct angle to see the dislocation and are often read as normal. Only an anterior-posterior view of the shoulder joint itself (a view that is perpendicular to the plane of the shoulder blade as opposed to the standard chest view), axillary view (a special view from the top of the shoulder down), CT scan, or MRI will show these dislocations. As a result, many patients are not diagnosed correctly until long after the injury and only when a doctor performs an in-depth exam. Sometimes the dislocation can be seen on a special shoulder X-ray that shows the joint space on one view (the joint space will be absent when the shoulder is dislocated). In other cases, it is first seen on an MRI or a CT scan.

However, if it is diagnosed on the day of the injury, putting the dislocated shoulder back in place with a closed reduction in the emergency room is possible with sedation. Since patients with posterior dislocation are often seen by an orthopaedic surgeon long after the injury occurred, the shoulder can only be put back into place in the operating room under general anesthesia. Many pre-op studies show that if the defect in the front of the ball bone (a reverse of the Hill-Sachs defect seen in anterior dislocations) is large, it requires bone grafting. Even larger defects may require a replacement of the ball.

HAGL Lesions

In very rare cases (even less common than posterior dislocations), the shoulder dislocates anteriorly and the labrum remains intact. This can happen if the ligaments pull off of the humeral head side (ball side) instead of the glenoid lip side. This type of ligament tear is known as a humeral avulsion of the glenohumeral ligaments, or a HAGL lesion. This problem is harder to diagnose than a more common glenoid-labral tear and can be missed—even on an MRI. When instability persists and no tear is seen, the doctor should consider a HAGL lesion as the cause. In these cases, a repair may also be needed, but the arthroscopic repair is a little trickier and an open technique may sometimes have to be used.

Rotator Cuff Tears and Dislocations

Some patients dislocate their shoulders without tearing the labrum or ligaments. Instead, they tear the rotator cuff, which can cause both instability and significant weakness. The use of the arm is often more limited than with a simple dislocation without a rotator cuff tear. These injuries are generally seen in older patients (in patients over age 40, there is a least a 50% chance of a concomitant rotator cuff tear with a posttraumatic dislocation of the shoulder), and the incidence increases with age. Fortunately, repairing the cuff alone usually restores full stability in this population. Rarely, both the cuff and labrum are torn in the same injury. Again, in my practice, these can both be surgically repaired at the same time using fiberoptic, minimally invasive arthroscopic surgery techniques.

17 TORN CARTILAGE IN THE SHOULDER: "SLAP" TEARS

THE SHOULDER COMPRISES A BALL AND, LIKE THE HIP, A SOCKET. HOWEVER, AS stated already, the socket of the shoulder joint (the glenoid) is extremely shallow. The labrum is a lip of cartilage that helps to form a cup (deepening the socket). As discussed in detail in Chapter 16, "Shoulder Instability and Dislocations", this lip (or ring) of cartilage makes the shoulder joint much more stable, but still allows for a very wide range of movements. A superior labral anterior to posterior (SLAP) tear is a specific injury to this part of the shoulder joint and is a common labral injury. More specifically, it is a tear that occurs on the top of the labrum, extending from the front to the back of the cartilage ring. To help you understand this better, in contrast, tears that are associated with dislocations involve the anterior inferior labrum in anterior dislocations or the posterior inferior labrum in posterior dislocations. SLAP tears often involve the attachment of the long head of the biceps brachii tendon (aka the biceps tendon). An injury in this area can be painful, cause a loss of range of motion, and be associated with a partial biceps tendon tear.

SLAP tears of the labrum can be the result of a direct fall, a blow to the arm, a forceful lifting maneuver, or repetitive trauma. In throwing athletes like pitchers and quarterbacks, sometimes a repetitive injury occurs when the normal outer edge of the humerus, the attachment of the rotator cuff (supraspinatus), hits the glenoid lip at the labral attachment and the biceps tendon anchor. This is called internal impingement. This motion and the internal impingement cause the labrum to peel back and come away from the bone, which eventually causes instability or tearing of the biceps tendon attachment.

When this happens, symptoms can include a catching sensation and pain with movement, most typically with overhead activities such as throwing. The labral tear decreases the stability of the joint, which causes the shoulder to drop slightly out of place when the individual is lying in bed; patients often complain of difficulty sleeping. This, in turn, pulls on the muscles and ligaments, causing discomfort. If the biceps tendon is also involved, patients may complain of pain over the front of the shoulder while turning a screwdriver or doorknob. These SLAP lesions are also associated with undersurface tears of the rotator cuff. Anterior SLAPs are associated with the undersurface tears of the anterior cuff, leading to the term SLAC shoulder, or superior labrum and anterior cuff tears.

There are many types of SLAP tears, and the way they are classified helps us understand the best treatment choice for each tear type.

- Type I is a tear of the inner margin and is not associated with any mechanical problem with the biceps attachment to the bone (the so-called biceps anchor). These can be degenerative or traumatic and can be treated by removal of the loose fragments (arthroscopic debridement) alone.

- Type II involves the biceps anchor and treatment ranges from direct repair with sutures and anchors to moving the biceps attachment elsewhere with a repair (see Chapter 16 for information on biceps tenodesis and tendonotomy).

- Type III is a bucket handle tear. The treatment requires removing the tear because the biceps attachment is not involved (just like a torn cartilage in the knee, it causes locking and catching in the shoulder, and removing the torn piece helps dramatically).

- Type IV is a bucket handle tear of the labrum with the involvement of the biceps. This repair can include repairing or relocating the biceps, as well as repairing or resecting the freely trapping labrum. There are other, less common types of tears, including combined lesions. They are SLAP tears that are combined with shoulder instability tears of the anterior, posterior, or inferior labrum. This gets very complicated quickly, but what's most important to know is that all the tears should be treated at the same time; the exact details are beyond the scope of this discussion.

Pitchers and Other Throwing Athletes

Pitchers and other throwing athletes require special attention for several reasons. First and foremost, they require more arm speed than any other athlete. When a baseball is thrown over 90 miles per hour, the shoulder rotation can be over 7,000 degrees per second. Yes, that is 7,000 degrees per second! To put it simply, the arm reaches a speed that would cause it to spin the equivalent of one full rotation in one-twentieth of a second. Luckily, the pitcher releases the ball in a tiny fraction of a second, or we would see some interesting shoulder problems!

Loss of Internal Rotation

Understanding that pitchers are throwing at amazing speeds, it is no wonder we have pitch counts in Little League® and professional pitchers have rotation schedules that allow for long rests between games. The ultra-high stresses seen in the shoulder with overhead pitching causes adaptations in a pitcher's shoulder. These stresses in combination with hitting the limits of natural motion mean pitchers develop problems that we mere mortals don't have.

First, they need extreme external rotation to allow for the coiling or extreme cocking. It is the body turn and the extreme cocking position that starts building energy for the pitching motion. Second, there is a compensatory loss of internal rotation that leads to tightness of the posterior lining or capsule in order to have the extreme motion in external rotation. Unfortunately, this combination of increased external rotation and a tight posterior capsule can lead to a condition called internal shoulder impingement. In these athletes, with internal impingement, the top of the humeral head, undersurface of the rotator cuff, and superior labrum hit each other, causing a superior labral tear often called a SLAP lesion, which is more serious in some pitchers than others.

The initial treatment for internal impingement, as seen in baseball pitchers, is a specific therapy and a stretching program, including the so-called sleeper's stretch. The athlete will lie on the side of the tight shoulder with the shoulder abducted 90 degrees (straight out from the body), and the elbow bent at 90 degrees. Imagine the position a police officer stopping traffic puts their arm in, and then rotate the arm down all the way so the palm faces the table with the elbow still at 90 degrees. Then the athlete will stretch by using the good arm to push the affected arm further down toward the table. The loss of internal rotation is at the root of a lot of the problems caused by internal impingement. The sleeper stretches and a rotator cuff program that increases shoulder internal rotation slowly over time with a physical therapist help often works. About

90% of patients respond to the stretching program with increased internal rotation by gaining 10 degrees of motion within 10 days. Maintained stretching exercises will keep and even increase this improvement in motion and reduce the symptoms. Those who don't respond may need an arthroscopic posterior capsular release.

Core Control in Throwing Athletes

Ask a pitcher, soccer player, tennis player, or even a hockey player, and they will tell you that balance is very important for upper body control, and it creates a stable platform for the sport. It is important to check an athlete's balance in a sports exam, especially if they are a throwing athlete. We test to see if they can balance on one leg and squat without losing their balance; have them stand on one leg and try to throw or catch a heavy workout ball; and see if they can stand on one leg and bend the opposite hip and knee to 90 degrees, then straighten the knee or kick from that position. These are all simple balance tests that many of the "high-level" high school and college athletes frequently fail in my office. **It is often a surprise to them and their parents when the throwing athlete fails the simplest of all balance tests**. It is because, even though they have strong quads and hamstrings, they lack good hip and core control. Moreover, they have not been tested before and don't understand the connection between poor balance and their symptoms.

Remember high school physics? Newton taught us that for every action, there is an equal and opposite reaction. So, if I could throw a ball at 90 miles per hour or hit a serve at 125 miles per hour, where does the "equal and opposite" reaction force come from? The simple answer is the arm. But then where does the force in the arm come from? It must be the rest of the body. And the body's force, where does it come from? The final answer is the ground. At the end of the "force chain" is the ground we stand on, and our legs control how that force is transferred to the ground. Therefore, the next concern we have for a throwing athlete is how well he or she transfers force to the ground. This requires great balance.

What happens to athletes who fail my three balance tests? They develop overuse injuries to the shoulder and elbow. Why? They cannot smoothly transfer force to the ground because their legs are not transferring weight efficiently, so they try to overcompensate by using the arm muscles to force speed into the pitching motion. This shows up as shoulder, arm, and elbow pain; loss of endurance; and slower pitching speeds as the game progresses.

In my practice, I see this mostly at the end of a growth spurt and with an increase in the competitive level of play: for example, when a junior high pitcher has rapid growth, when a high school student moves to the varsity team, or when a high school player goes on to play in college. The treatment for this issue is balance training, core strengthening exercises, and an evaluation by a pitching coach to be sure that the pitcher's form will allow for good weight transfer while they are throwing.

Treatment of SLAP tears

Very few patients with significant SLAP tear injuries return to full capability without surgical intervention. In most cases, surgery is required to repair the tear and reattach the labrum to the glenoid. I do this repair through an arthroscope with sutures and tiny absorbable anchors. The goal is to repair the tear and restore normal function in a minimally invasive way during an outpatient procedure. When a SLAP tear is associated with significant damage to the biceps tendon, a biceps tenodesis (transferring the tendon to a new location and removing its attachment from the superior labrum) may be necessary to correct the shoulder problem.

There are more than four types of SLAP tears now. For our discussion, these four give us the basic concepts. Type I needs a simple removal of the torn edge (see Image 79a). Type II can be repaired with the caution that some Type IIs are really a normal recess in the labrum and should not be repaired. Type III, the bucket handle type, should be removed, but if the biceps anchor is stable, that should be left alone. When unstable, a biceps tenodesis should be performed. Type IV can be repaired or, when very unstable, repaired and then a biceps tenodesis is done to remove the tension on the repair (see Image 79b). In short, more recently there has been a move away from reattaching the biceps anchor since it tends to pull on the repair of the SLAP lesion. For this reason, I will, if needed, repair the SLAP and move the biceps tendon to a location that does not pull on the repair by performing a biceps tenodesis. I have seen better outcomes and less post-op stiffness with this approach.

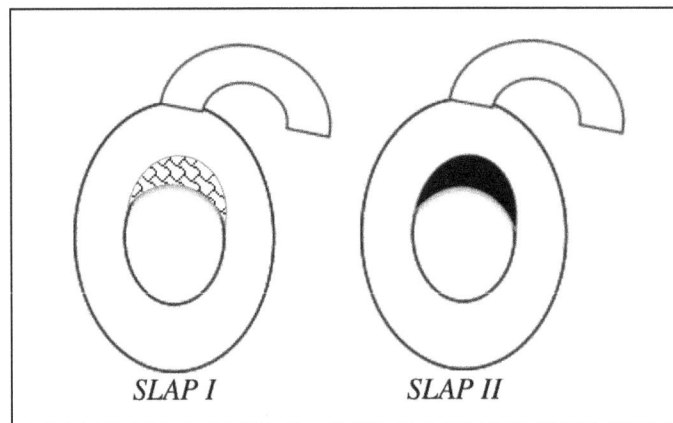

79a Slap Type II: Loose fragments at the edge of the labrum (left) and Type II detached tear but biceps intact (right).

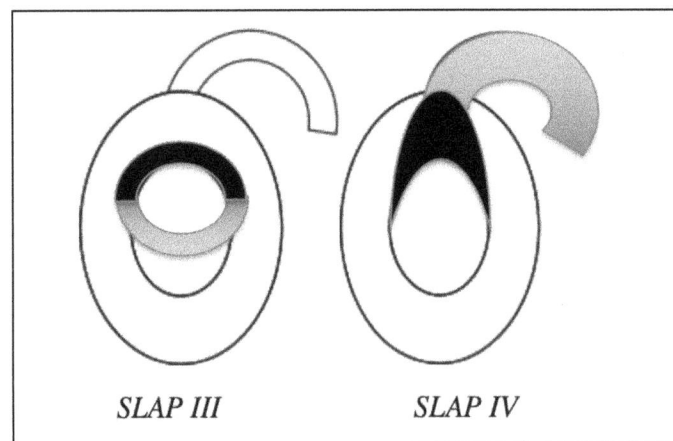

79b Slap Type III: bucket handle tear (left) and Type IV detached labrum and detached biceps anchor (right).

18 ROTATOR CUFF TEARS

PATIENTS ARE OFTEN CONFUSED ABOUT THE SHOULDER AND HOW IT WORKS. THE shoulder has more parts than other joints. Bodybuilders and athletes all know about the big muscles—like the deltoid, trapezius, pectorals, biceps, and triceps—since we can see them. Just the same, under those big muscles are four smaller muscles that are equally important. These four smaller muscles are the subscapularis, infraspinatus, supraspinatus, and teres minor. All these muscles begin on the shoulder blade in separate locations as broad muscle attachments to bone. They then narrow to form tendons that attach at all sides of the humeral head. The four tendons directly control the rotation of the ball in its socket and help keep the ball in place. The tendons grouped together form a strong "cuff" around the head, and they guide and rotate the shoulder joint, hence the name "rotator cuff" (RTC).

The rotator cuff helps to stabilize the ball of the shoulder within the joint, centers the ball when the bigger muscles are working, rotates the humerus, and helps lift the arm. This centering function that helps the shoulder move smoothly does not work when the cuff is injured or torn (see Image 80).

When recapping the history of a rotator cuff tear, most of my patients say that they cannot put plates on a high shelf in the kitchen, take a gallon of milk out of the refrigerator with their arm straight, or reach into the back of the car. Many say they drop things, and most have trouble sleeping because of night pain. The exam almost always demonstrates weakness when the arm is elevated to the side, especially with the hand turned down as if you were emptying a can of soda with your arm out to your side. This is called the empty can sign, and it is one of the signs of RTC impingement. When pressure or downward force is applied to the arm in the "empty can position," we see pain and weakness. Your doctor may also test your cuff with what's known as a drop arm test, by lifting your arm to 90 degrees away from your side and asking you to

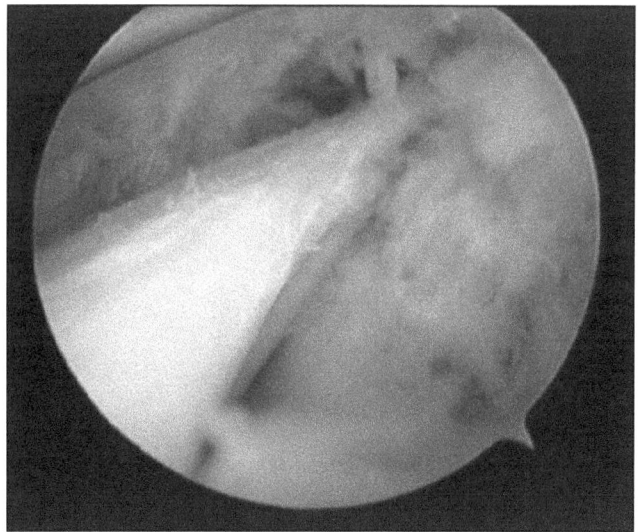

80 Rotator cuff tear.

lower it slowly. If you can't do this, or with the slightest resistance the arm drops to your side, it indicates a possible rotator cuff tear. Some patients with larger tears also have external rotation weakness with their arm at their side.

Patients with rotator cuff tears usually experience loss of motion, weakness, and pain. Night pain and pain with certain arm motions are typically the most difficult for a patient with a rotator cuff tear. Loss of sleep often affects daily life and, along with the inability to lift everyday items (like a container of milk), frequently brings patients to the doctor. In my experience, the most frustrating problem for patients is the loss of sleep. Often it is the chronic sleep issues combined with the loss of use of the arm that are the main reasons people seek treatment for their shoulder ailment.

Rotator cuff tears are most common in people over age 40 who do repetitive overhead work, sports, or weight training. It may also occur in younger patients following acute trauma or athletic activity. Tears can be partial or full thickness. Partial tears can occur within the tendon itself, or on the upper or lower surface. Sometimes partial tears are associated with calcium deposits, a condition called calcific tendonitis. Other times there is chronic tendonitis or a partial tear. A new injury can then complete the tear. In general, partial tears and chronic tendonitis are much more common as we get older. Hence, the rotator is more likely to be torn after trauma or injury as we age.

The centering action of the rotator cuff is more important than it seems. By keeping the ball centered in the socket, the cuff not only prevents dislocation but also keeps the center of rotation of the shoulder in its place, helping the deltoid lift the arm more effectively. When the cuff is not working because it's weak, damaged, or has a torn tendon, the ball does not stay centered in the socket. When the deltoid contracts and the ball is out of place, it will slide on the glenoid surface and the muscle force will pull the ball straight up instead of rotating it in its socket. The upward movement is stopped only when the ball hits the undersurface of the acromion, which causes both pain and further loss of motion. The impingement of its tendons against the bone above it can cause further pain and weakness. The constant rubbing of the RTC tendon on the bone above it is one of the ways the rotator cuff can begin to tear (see Image 81).

Sometimes patients have ongoing shoulder impingement, and then they have an acute event after lifting something or falling. They may have had some chronic changes in the cuff, a thin cuff, or a partial tear, then traumatically ruptured the balance of the tissue. Patients with gout or inflammatory arthritis also have tendons that are weakened by their disease and can tear their rotator cuff after suffering a minor trauma.

Healthy tendons can also be torn at any time with extreme force applied in the wrong direction, like when someone falls down the stairs. Aside from traumatic causes, it makes sense that rotator cuff tears often occur in people who are over 40 years old who do repetitive shoulder motions, overhead work, heavy labor, overhead sports, or regular weight training. Although not too common, tears can also occur in patients under age 40 following acute trauma or a significant sports injury.

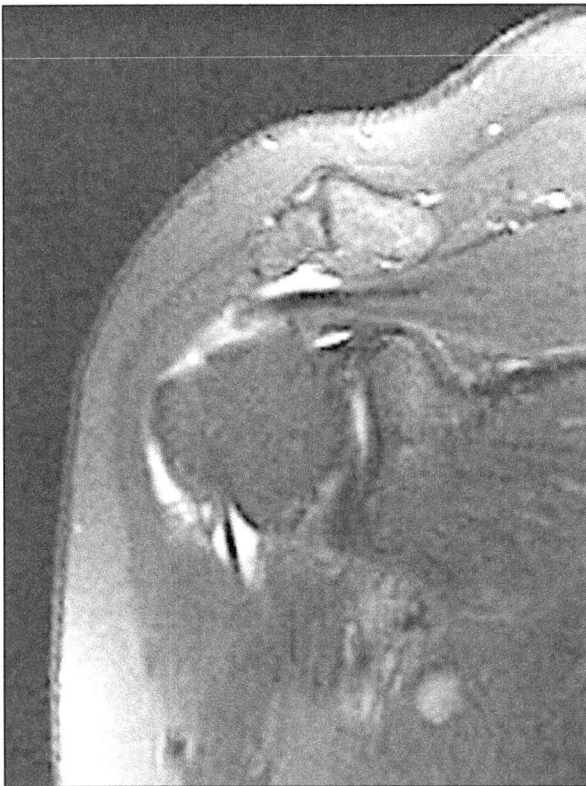

81 MRI of rotator cuff tear.

Calcific Tendonitis

Sometimes partial tears are associated with calcium deposits that can be seen on a plain X-ray of the shoulder. This is called calcified tendonitis (see Image 82). Tears can also be associated with a biceps tendon tear. If the biceps tendon tears spontaneously, up to half of patients will have a rotator cuff tear, too.

Tear Size and Shape

Tears can range from small and slightly open to large and completely retracted. They can be full thickness or partial thickness: full thickness tears can be curved, or "C" shaped, "L" shaped, "V" shaped, or "U" shaped (see Images 83a, 83b, 84a, and 84b). Partial thick-ness tears can occur within the tendon itself, on the upper or lower surface.

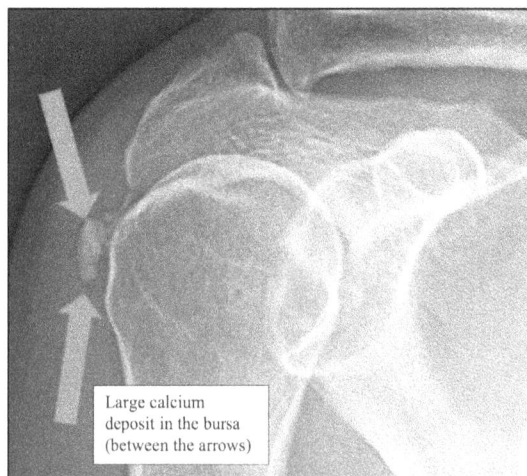

Large calcium deposit in the bursa (between the arrows)

82 Calcific tendonitis of the rotator cuff (arrows).

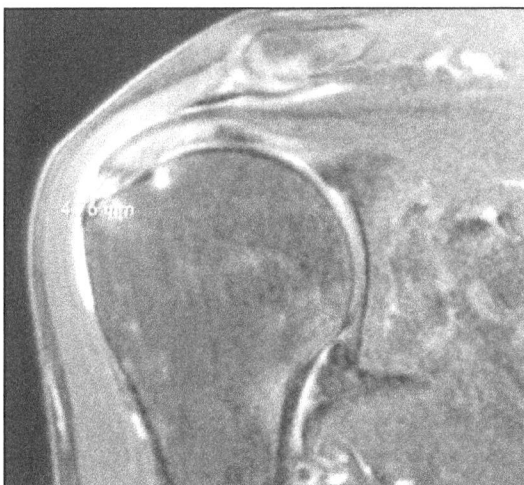

83a MRI small rotator cuff tear.

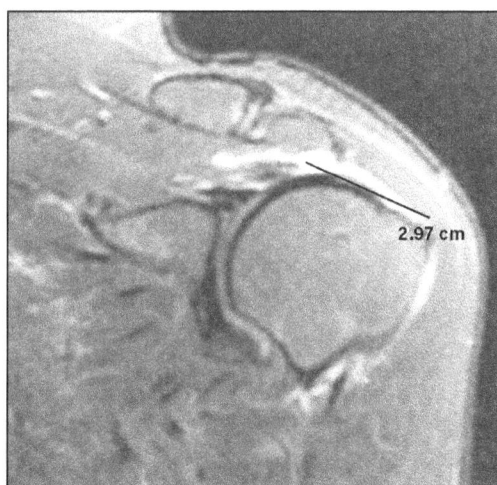

2.97 cm

83b MRI large rotator cuff tear.

Treatment for Rotator Cuff Tears

Very small tears, partial tears, and tendonitis can often be treated with injections, anti-inflamma-tory medications, and physical therapy. If there is a partial tear with spurs rubbing on it, removing the spurs can improve the pain associated with the spur's impingement on the tendon.

Full thickness tears don't heal themselves; instead, the muscles pull on them, and they get bigger over time. The shoulder will weaken, and very large chronic tears are harder to fix. Smaller, more acute tears are easier to fix and are associated with better healing rates. When a rotator

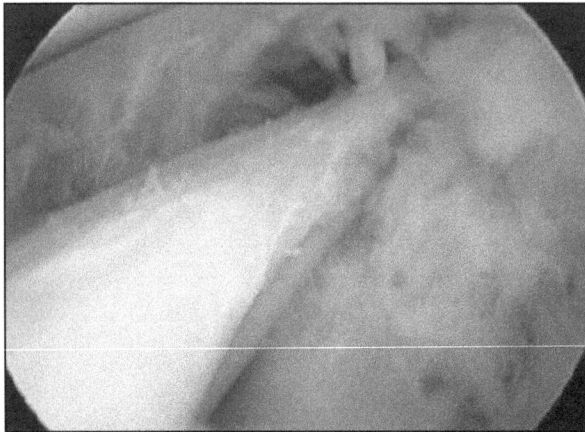

84a Medium-sized rotator cuff tear.

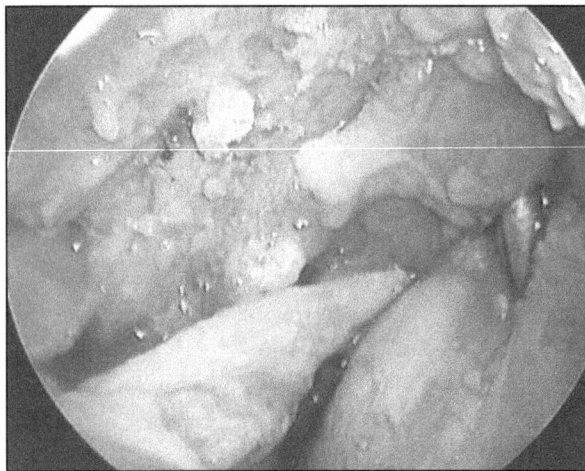

84b Large retracted rotator cuff tear.

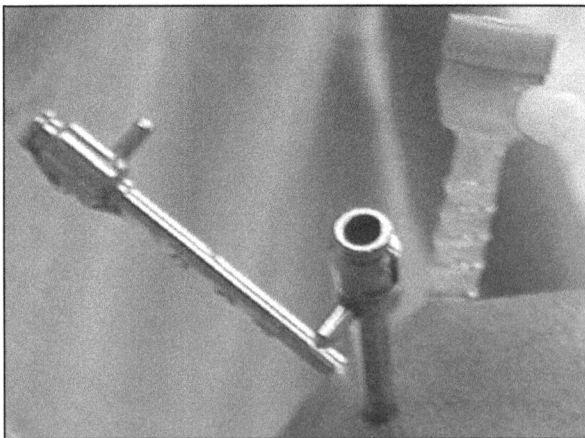

85 Arthroscopic cannulas in place for arthroscopic repair.

cuff tear has failed treatments like anti-inflammatory medications, therapy, ice, and rest, or a patient has lost arm strength, an arthroscopic (minimally invasive) surgical repair is often the best option (see Image 85).

The type of repair and recovery depends on the size, shape, and location of the tear. A partial tear may require only a trimming or smoothing procedure called a "debridement." Removing thickened bursal tissues (bursitis) or calcium deposits may also help.

When bone spurs impinge on the tendon, they can also be a source of pain and should be removed at the same time. Sometimes the small joint at the end of the collarbone is worn out and painful or rubs on the tendons. When this happens, the worn-out bone and spurs should also be removed arthroscopically. This adds more time and effort to the procedure while greatly improving the outcome, reducing pain, and increasing motion (see Images 86a and 86b).

I have been performing minimally invasive arthroscopic treatment repairs of the rotator cuff, damaged bone, and bone spurs for more than 30 years. I perform this surgery using a high-definition fiber-optic scope through small incisions as an outpatient procedure. Newer methods and specialized suture anchors have been developed over time, and this approach has increasingly become the standard treatment for RTC tears.

If the tendon is torn from its bone attachment when done through the scope, as in the prior open procedures, it can be repaired directly to the bone using a very strong suture and special suture anchors. Other tears require suturing the two sides of the tendon together. Some larger tears need both side-to-side sutures and sutures anchored to the bone. Remember, the sutures hold the tendon in place while your body heals the tendon, and the suture is never as strong as the tendon will be when it is fully healed, so your post-op activities and restrictions will depend on the size and type of tear you have. Tears are often classified by size and shape as shown in Image 87.

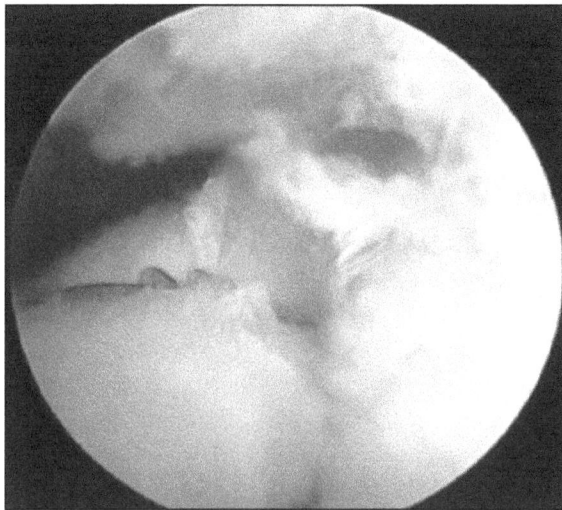

86a Medium tear repaired.

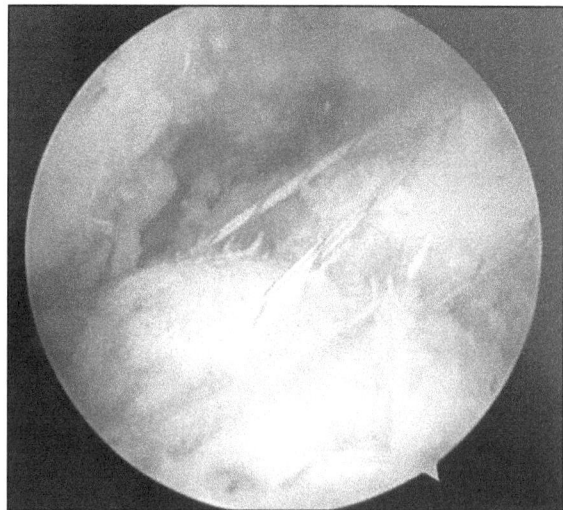

86b Large tear repaired.

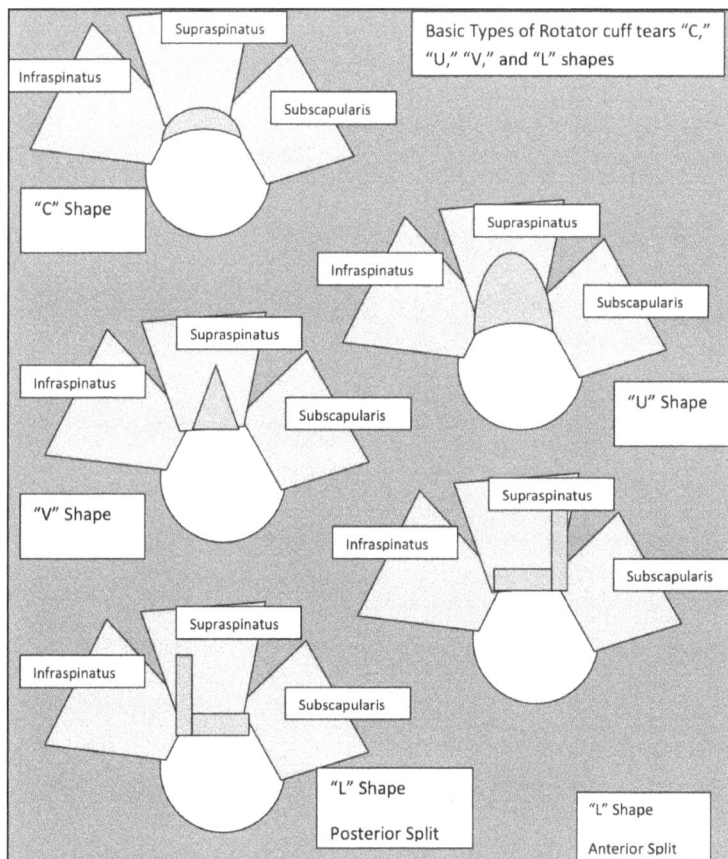

87 Most common rotator cuff tear patterns.

In all cases, the tendon needs six weeks to get "sticky" and start attaching to the bone, and then 80% of the healing will take place over the next three to four months. The larger the tear, the longer it takes. The "healed end" of the tendon takes a year to fully mature, and the natural tissues will continue to become stronger in time. Muscles then regain strength after the tendon heals, and full endurance strength takes a year or more to come back. Remember, most baseball pitchers, even those paid millions of dollars to play, still take a year or more to get full throwing ability back.

Arthroscopic techniques are technically demanding, and patients should rely on their surgeon's judgment as to what the best procedure for their problem will be. In experienced hands, the complication rate for arthroscopic repair is extremely low, yet even the best repairs sometimes don't heal. The risk of infection for open surgery is nearly one in 100, whereas it's less than one in 500 (my personal infection rate is less than one in 3,000) for arthroscopic surgery.

VERY LARGE (MASSIVE) AND CHRONIC ROTATOR CUFF TEARS

A patient may have longstanding rotator cuff weakness and not as much pain—until they have a relatively minor injury, and the loss of function becomes worse than they expected based on the injury itself. These patients may have had a very large tear that was compensated for by other muscles, and the new event or injury has pushed it over the edge. After having an MRI, they are very surprised to learn that, in fact, they have a large tear that has been there for years.

In these cases, the MRI shows a large tear and loss of muscle mass consistent with a chronic problem with the cuff. Some of these large tears are not directly repairable. In those cases, a side-to-side "partial repair" is a good option (a partial "margin convergence repair" involves bringing the sides of the tear together. It is not the same as bringing the ends to the bone but helps improve function in many patients). In others, a repair patch may help bring the edges together. There are newer patches that may also help the cuff "heal."

In even more severe cases, when other partial repairs are not possible, a patch that attaches the ball to the socket (a so-called superior capsular reconstruction) may improve function nicely. These are all "salvage" procedures for less-than-ideal situations, and the results are never as good as repairs of smaller tears. Although not ideal, it is often far better than doing no repair at all. These more complex repairs can all be done arthroscopically, and, when there are massive tears without underlying arthritis, the best option is determined at the time of surgery.

Arthritis in the Shoulder as a Result of a Longstanding RTC Tear ("Rotator Cuff Arthropathy")

Some patients have avoided getting their cuff repaired for years, and they may not recall the original injury, yet they know things are not going well. The ball does not seem to be controlled by the rotator cuff, and it may be rubbing against the bone above the socket. Patients may feel this friction and pain even with simple movements. The shoulder no longer functions well, and the motion is limited, and even simple tasks like getting dressed can be difficult.

The diagnosis of RTC arthropathy can be made and confirmed when the X-ray shows the humeral head riding high and touching the acromion, and when the X-ray also shows signs of loss of cartilage and advancing arthritis in the ball and socket joint (see Image 88). Also, since the

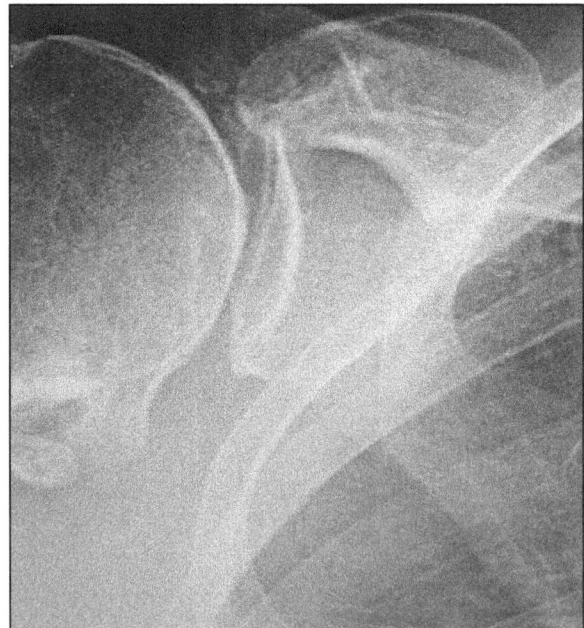

88 Humeral Head arthritis with osteophyte at bottom edge (goats beard deformity and loose body next to the goat's beard on the X-ray).

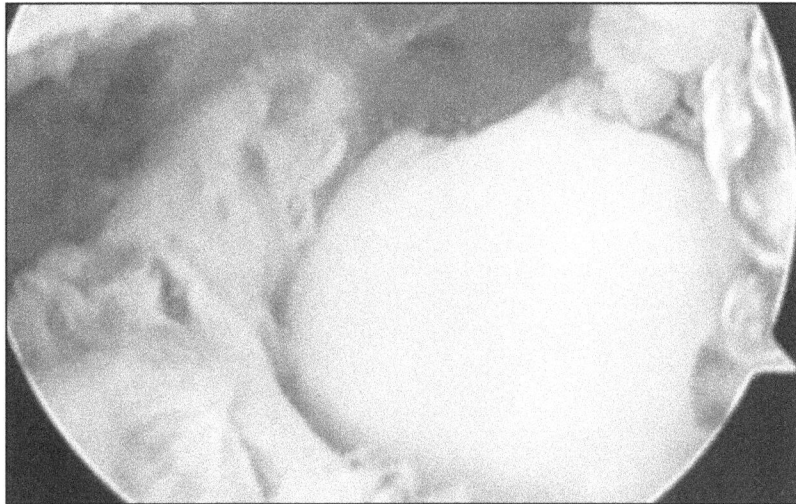

89 Massive tear of the rotator cuff first sutures in place to begin to close the defect.

ball is riding higher than normal and it can be touching the bone above the rotator cuff (the acromion), this may indicate that the cuff is no longer covering the ball of the ball and socket. Rotator-related arthritis and loss of function are exactly what we are hoping to avoid by repairing the cuff tears when they occur.

Repairing small tears before they are big and big tears before they cannot be repaired at all is the best strategy to stop this destructive process from happening. When this does happen, the patient has an unstable shoulder and painful arthritis. A very specialized reverse shoulder replacement may be the only and best option. Like all shoulder replacements, this is not an arthroscopic procedure (see Image 89).

Sometimes a plain X-ray will show a calcium deposit in the tendon or the humeral head riding slightly higher in the socket than normal. These signs may be a tip-off that there is a tear, and the diagnosis can be confirmed with an MRI.

When a plain X-ray shows a complete loss of the space between the humeral head and the bone above it (acromion), the cuff is no longer between the bones holding the head in the socket. This is an indication that there is a large tear of the RTC. If there is no arthritis, the full extent of the tear can be confirmed with an MRI. When there is advanced arthritis on the X-ray and the cuff is torn, then we have a case of RTC arthropathy as explained above, and an MRI is less valuable in making the diagnosis since the shoulder needs to be replaced if it's painful (see Images 90a and 90b on pg. 124). MRIs can be very helpful in surgical planning in many of these cases since the type of replacement depends on the quality of the cuff tendons and tissue at the time of surgery.

Special Conditions of the Rotator Cuff

Sometimes patients have symptoms that appear to be similar to a rotator cuff injury or tear. Their exam will show weakness and yet the cuff may not be torn. These are special cases that require much more thought and often turn out to be different problems than what first meets the eye. Many times, the weakness is a result of a local nerve issue or nerve compression. This can be a pinched nerve in the neck, herniated disc, brachial plexus injury, or other neurologic issue, and these problems need to be treated differently that a classic rotator cuff tear.

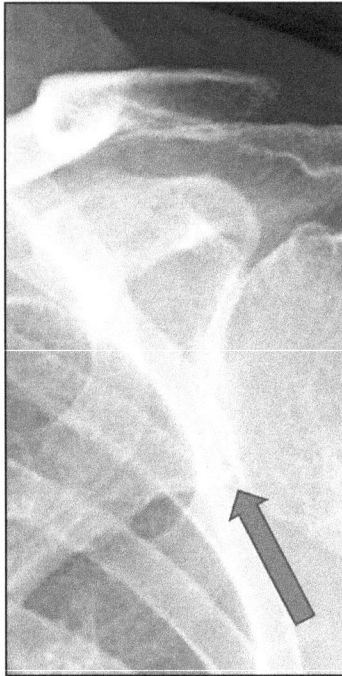

90a Humeral—Glenoid surfaces worn down to bone (common osteoarthritis of the shoulder).

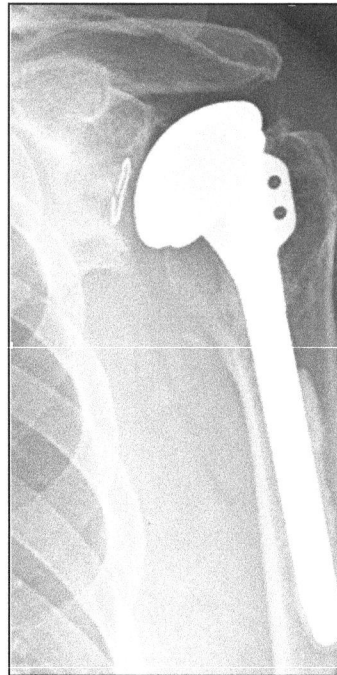

90b Shoulder replacement.

Nerve Issues

Some patients have nerve problems that cause shoulder pain and loss of function. For example, nerves can be pinched at any location along the way as they travel from the neck to the muscle. They can be pinched at the neck, as in a herniated disc and surgery on the shoulder does not improve that issue. Some patients have more than one problem, like a rotator cuff tear and a herniated disc. Most surgeons will try to fix the tear first since the surgery carries fewer operative risks than disc surgery.

Again, if the disc is causing shoulder or arm pain, patients will not improve without decompressing the nerve exactly where it is pinched. This means the disc needs to be removed if there is a cervical spine disc (a herniated disc in the neck) pressing on a nerve root. If there is a narrowing of the spinal cord because bone spurs are pressing on the nerves or the spinal cord, the spurs need to be removed if the patient fails medical treatment, therapy, and injections. See the section "Shoulder Pain, Or Is It?" on page 126.

Ganglion Cysts and Suprascapular Nerve Entrapment

In some glenoid labrum tears (see SLAP tears), cysts form above the socket near the suprascapular nerve. The cyst can press on the nerve, which can cause pain and weakness as if the patient has a tear, but no tear is seen on an MRI. Decompressing the nerve by removing the cyst and repairing the SLAP lesion will often solve this problem. The suprascapular nerve can also be compressed at the sphenoid notch, near a sharp turn it takes before it reaches the muscle. There is a band, or ligament, that crosses the nerve and can get tight; releasing the band and freeing the nerve frequently solves this unique problem. Trying to repair the tendon alone or doing a simple decompression of the space (an acromioplasty, as discussed in the next section) is not helpful in these situations if the nerve is not decompressed at the sight of pressure.

Shoulder Impingement, AC Joint Pain, and Pinched Nerves

The shoulder can be weakened or hurt from several conditions. A few have been discussed already, including rotator cuff tears, subluxations, dislocations, labral tears, SLAP lesions, and arthritic conditions of the ball and socket joint. Tendons can also cause pain as when a patient has impingement syndrome, damage to the AC joint can cause pain and loss of motion, and pinched nerves can cause shoulder pain as well.

Impingement Syndrome

Overhead use, trauma, and repetitive motion can also cause pain when the rotator cuff rubs against the bone above it; in these cases, the tendon can swell or even be partially torn. The tendon can hit the front or side edge of the acromion or the undersurface of the connection between the acromion and the clavicle (the AC joint). Some people are born with a flat acromion and others with a curved or hooked acromion. These are known as Type I, a flat acromion; Type II, a mild hook; and Type III, a significantly curved undersurface of the acromion (see Image 91). Patients with Type II and III can be predisposed to a condition called subacromial impingement. In addition, the ligament that attaches the coracoid process to the acromion (it helps to distribute the load of the short head of the biceps and cover the front part of the rotator cuff) can calcify with stress over time. The hardened ligament can also rub against the rotator cuff, causing impingement or rubbing on the tendon and pain localized to that area.

This is referred to as "impingement syndrome." It can also occur in athletes who participate in sports requiring repetitive overhead movements (weight lifting, basketball, tennis, volleyball, etc.) or people whose work involves performing repetitive shoulder movements or overhead movements. With impingement of the tendons, overuse of the shoulder may damage the tissues underneath the bone edge (known as Acromion process).

If someone has "impingement" from an overhanging acromion, the bone edge or spur constantly rubs against the tendon. This usually presents itself as pain with overhead activity, occasional weakness with some motions, and difficulty lifting objects away from the body. The simple question is: can removing the overhang stop the rubbing? Similarly, can removing the calcified ligaments that often accompany this disorder help stop the pain? Moreover, if someone is born with a hooked acromion (Type III), can we turn it into a flat acromion (Type I)?

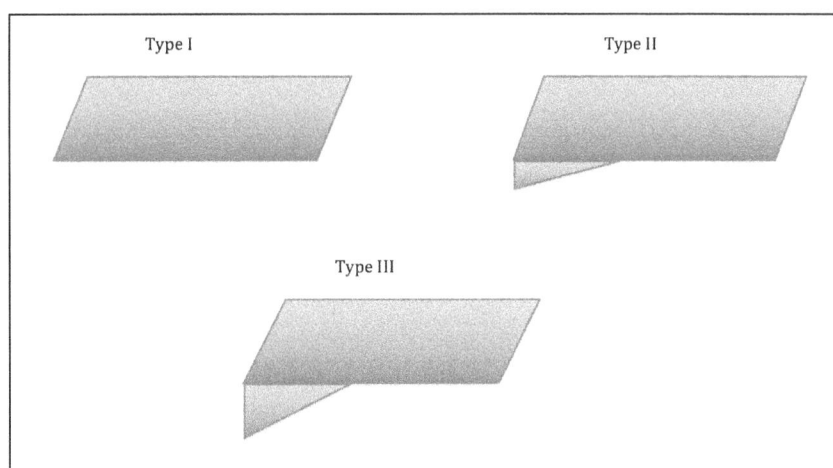

91 Three types of acromion shapes.

Luckily, the answer is yes to all three questions. When pain due to impingement fails to improve with nonoperative treatments like NSAIDs, injections, and therapy, arthroscopic surgery may be indicated. A famous shoulder surgeon, Dr. Charles Neer of New York, popularized this as an open procedure called an acromioplasty more than 30 years ago. Soon after, the concept of doing this procedure with an arthroscope started to gain acceptance in very small circles of surgeons. About 25 years ago, one of my students did one of the first summary reviews combining data (now known as a meta-analysis) ever done and showed that it was a better way to go.

Today, arthroscopic acromioplasty has come into its own as a standard treatment for impingement syndrome. In the procedure, the overhanging part of the acromion is removed to convert the curved or hooked acromion to a flat one (see Image 92). If the ligament is calcified, it can be removed with the calcium deposits. If the ligament is tight, it can be pushed back (recessed) or cut (released). Also, during the arthroscopic procedure, the rotator tendons are checked for a tear. If one or more of the tendons of the cuff are torn, the tears are treated as noted in the chapter on rotator cuff tears.

AC Joint Pain

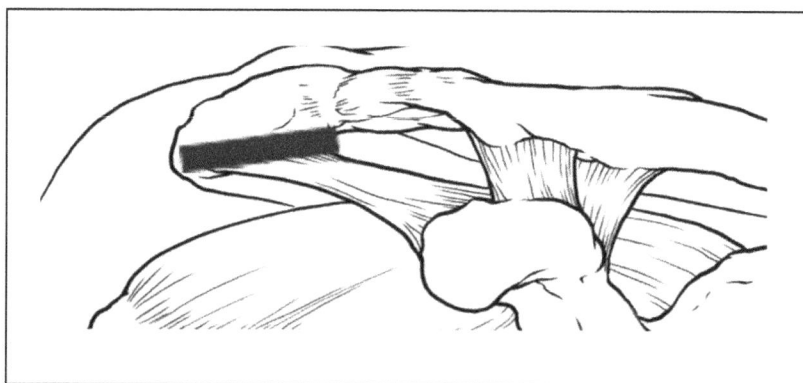

92 Diagram showing flattening the acromion shape.

In some cases, the end of the clavicle is worn down, and the AC joint is degenerated, meaning arthritic and large spurs form at the edges. Some of the spurs stick down toward the rotator cuff and impinge on its surface. This can be painful for two reasons: first, the joint itself can hurt, and second, the spurs can impinge, rub, or even tear the rotator cuff. Other times, the end of the collarbone has had small fractures, healed with scar tissue, and is very soft and painful when loaded. This is also called osteolysis of the distal clavicle (see page 127).

In these cases, when conservative nonoperative measures fail, removing the spurs and resecting the diseased bone at the AC joint is the treatment of choice. This can effectively remove the bone spurs rubbing on the rotator cuff and the AC joint pain at the same time. This resection of the end of the clavicle is also known as a Mumford procedure. If left untreated, these bone spurs rub on the rotator cuff. The friction from the rubbing weakens and damages the cuff, causes worsening pain, and, in time, can lead to a rotator cuff tear—even with seemingly minor trauma.

Shoulder Pain, or Is It?

Some patients have similar symptoms, yet no impingement signs are present during the exam. The pain is "referred" down the arm to the elbow or hand. This means that the pain starts in one location such as the neck but is felt, or "referred," to another. This is just like when someone says their back hurts when, in fact, they have a kidney stone. They don't know exactly where their kidney is. The same is true for the inside of the shoulder. When there is burning pain, spasm of the trapezius (the muscles around the lower neck), or muscle weakness or neck stiffness, we sometimes need to look elsewhere for the real source of the pain. In many cases, these patients have a pinched nerve (see Image 93).

The nerve can be trapped beneath the tight muscles, beneath an arthritic spur in the neck, a herniated disc in the neck, or in very rare instances, by an anatomic variant like an extra rib (so-called thoracic outlet syndrome).

Frequently, symptoms like burning, tingling, or numbness may be key to making the diagnosis. Sometimes, the only tip-off to this problem will be that the patient's pain is not relieved by an injection in the shoulder. To make things more complicated, both situations occur at the same time in some patients. This can be frustrating since the patient may respond only partially to the treatment of the shoulder pain and only partly to the treatment of the neck problem. In thoracic outlet syndrome, the diagnosis can be made with a very special MRI called an MRA or magnetic resonance arthrogram, which shows where the nerves and blood vessels are compressed.

Sometimes the spasms from chronic shoulder pain cause neck pain to worsen, and treatment of the shoulder can help

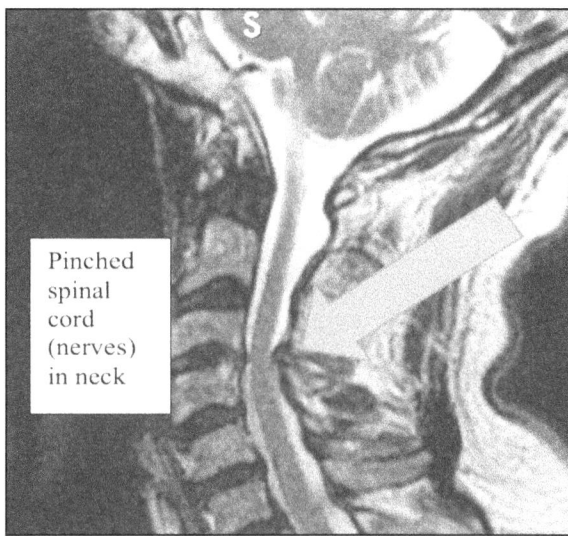

93 Neck: herniated disc causing nerve compression "pinched nerve" in the neck causing shoulder pain.

ease the pain. This is truly an individual situation for each patient, and each case is different in this respect. If the shoulder treatments, including therapy, NSAIDs, and injection fail, and X-rays or an MRI of the shoulder yield little helpful information, a thorough nerve exam should be done, and neck X-rays should be taken. In my practice, I like to add flexion and extension views to the series of films to look for abnormal motion of the vertebrae or lack of motion as a sign of significant muscle spasm or disc abnormality. If weakness and pain persist after nonoperative treatment, an MRI of the neck is indicated. If there is a disc herniation, a consultation with a spine specialist may be necessary.

Wear of the Collarbone (AC Joint Pain)

In patients who are extremely active, lift weights overhead, or perform manual labor, the end of the collarbone can develop internal swelling and microscopic fractures. This injury is like stress fractures in military recruits when they go on long marches. With repetitive impact loading of the leg in heavy boots, they get leg pain from microscopic fractures in the stressed bone. Although not cracked through and through, the bone can be as painful as a fracture. Stopping the overuse by rest, ice, and NSAIDs can help. Increased calcium and vitamin D intake can give your body the tools to heal the microfractures. However, continued lifting and repetitive stress to the bone under attack can cause the undersurface to fail due to the pressure. When this occurs, cysts form in the bone, the surface of the AC joint can become arthritic, and the distal clavicle end can widen, causing more impingement on the rotator cuff.

When the bone breakdown can be seen on plain X-rays or cysts can be seen on an MRI in the end of the bone near the AC joint, this condition is called osteolysis of the clavicle (see Image 94). When this occurs, weight lifting overhead is painful and extremely limited. Other symptoms include pain when patients cross their arms across the body. This is a so-called cross arm adduction sign. If rest does not help relieve pain and the bone is eroded, a resection of the distal clavicle (a Mumford procedure, see drawing below) works well to reduce pain and improve function. Again, this can be done either open or arthroscopically. In my practice, I prefer the less invasive arthroscopic method.

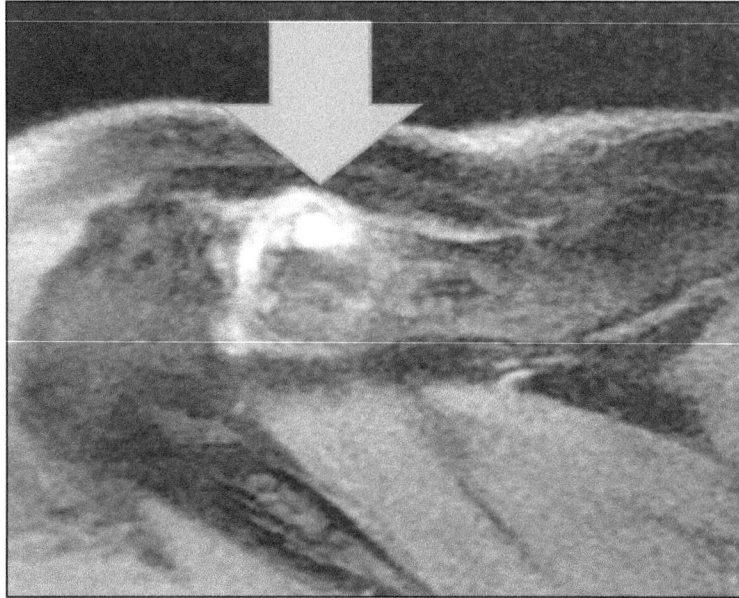

94 Fluid and cyst formation at the end of the collar bone (AC joint pathology causing pain) common in shoulder pain with overhead work or weight lifting.

19 BICEPS TENDON: TENDONITIS, PARTIAL TEARS, SUBLUXATION, AND RUPTURES

A BICEPS TENDON INJURY TYPICALLY INVOLVES A PARTIAL OR COMPLETE TEAR OF THE long head of the biceps tendon (the tendon has two parts, a long head and a short head). It is more common after age 40. Many times, it is associated with an acute injury or patients experience a painful pop, after which the muscle attached to the long head tends to "ball up" further down the arm (see Images 95-97). The short head almost always remains intact. Prior to the injury, some patients often have a long history of inflammation of the tendon, a condition known as chronic biceps tendonitis, which is usually due to years of wear and tear on the shoulder. It is often associated with repetitive lifting, chronic inflammatory tendonitis, a heavy lifting injury using the biceps muscle, falling and using the arm to stop the fall, or repetitive work trauma.

A severe, sudden traumatic injury is the cause in other patients. This is more common in younger patients, but it can occur at any age. A traumatic torn biceps muscle sometimes occurs during heavy weight lifting or from actions that cause a sudden load on the upper arm, such as a hard fall with the arm outstretched during competitive sports. Straightening the elbow against the forces of the muscles trying to hold it bent can cause this injury. A fall in a position that forces the tendon to get trapped between the humeral head (ball of the shoulder) and the sharper bone edges of the scapula or acromion can also cause a tear or rupture.

The long head of the biceps can also be injured by repetitive motion, local trauma, rapidly extending the arm, force applied while trying to flex the elbow, or during a fracture or dislocation of the shoulder. I have seen this type of injury occur when a laborer tries to catch a heavy piece of material or a large tool as it is falling, or when a nurse or nurse's aide tries to catch a patient who suddenly loses their balance and starts to fall in front of them. It can be associated with rotator cuff tears. These injuries can cause the tendon to slip out of its groove (subluxate). This problem can also be associated with tears of the anterior rotator cuff (the subscapularis tendon).

Biceps Tendon: Understanding the Biceps' Anatomy

The biceps muscle starts at the elbow, passes up the arm, and splits into two tendons, or heads. The shorter head ends at the coracoid process of the shoulder blade (the scapula), and the longer one follows a groove on the humerus (the bicipital groove) and then enters the shoulder joint. There, the longer end (the long head) attaches to the top of the socket (the glenoid) at a cartilaginous lip that covers the edge of the socket (the labrum). This is exactly where SLAP tears can occur.

To this day, the true function of the long head of the biceps inside the shoulder joint is debated in the orthopaedic and sports medicine communities. At the elbow, the long and short heads of the biceps merge, and they act in bending the elbow. The supination of the hand (clockwise rotation of the right hand and counterclockwise motion of the left hand) is aided and

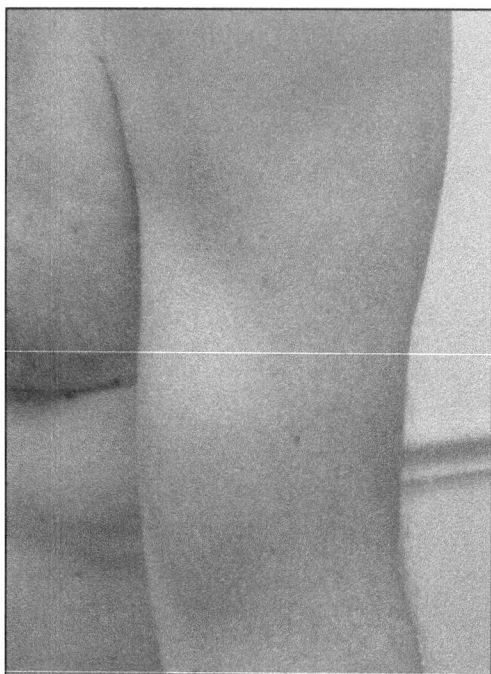
95 Torn biceps tendon.

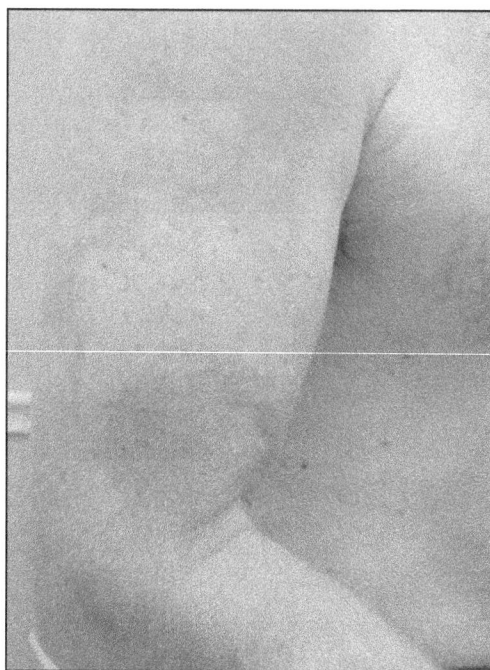
96 Normal biceps muscle.

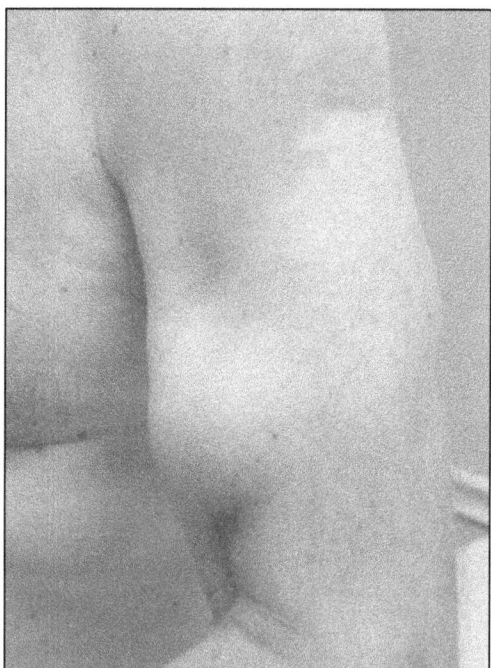
97 Torn biceps with classic "Popeye" deformity.

powered by the action of the biceps near the elbow. Therefore, the repetitive use of a screwdriver can cause biceps pain. This also explains why resisted supination of the hand (the same motion you use for turning a screwdriver) causes biceps pain when there is a biceps problem. Again, as stated before, the most common problem is biceps tendonitis in the bicipital groove.

Biceps tendonitis is inflammation of the same long head of the biceps without a tear (see Image 98). It is the most common problem seen in the long head of the biceps. It can often be treated with anti-inflammatories, ice, and rest. In more chronic cases, adding physical therapy may also be helpful.

Direct injection into the tendon covering, or sheath, may be helpful in cases that don't go away with simple treatment. I prefer to do this with ultrasound guidance to make sure I have injected the sheath—and not the tendon—in the correct spot. Occasionally, there is a structural issue and a procedure known as tenolysis (release of the tendon sheath), an arthroscopic decompression of the shoulder, or a tendonotomy (release of the tendon itself) may be required. In severe cases, moving the tendon as already described (a biceps tenodesis) may be the best solution.

Please note: This discussion is focused on injuries to the long head of the biceps, the part of the tendon closest to the shoulder joint. Tears of the biceps tendon at the elbow are a completely different problem occurring where both heads of the biceps muscle join and attach in one common location on the proximal radius. Together, they are a major flexor of the elbow, and these tears should, in general, be repaired.

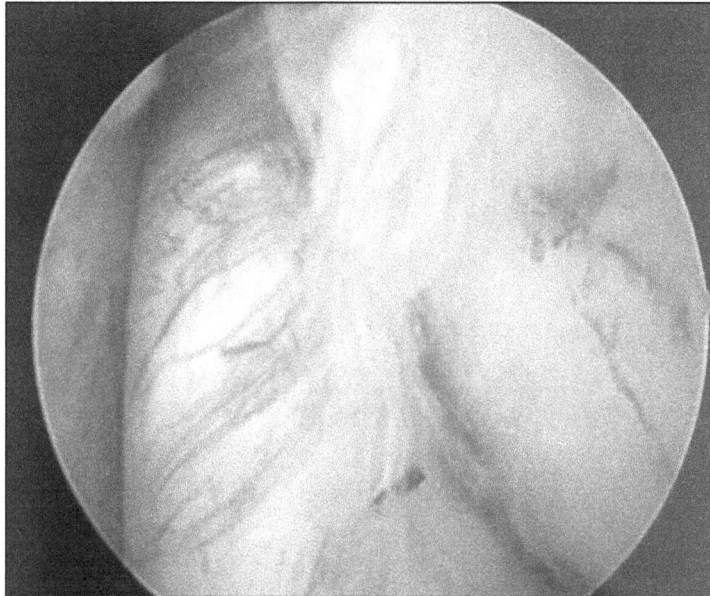

98 Arthroscopic view of inflamed biceps tendon (biceps tendonitis).

Treatment Options

Many partial and even complete tears of the biceps can be treated without surgery (see Image 99 on pg. 132). A thorough physical exam by an orthopaedic surgeon and an X-ray of the shoulder are often the best ways to determine what treatment is most appropriate. About half of all long head of the biceps tendon ruptures are associated with rotator cuff tears. Most often, the tear is of the supraspinatus tendon. If a tear of the rotator cuff is suspected, an MRI is needed to see the extent of the tear and to help determine if a repair is required. If the biceps tendon is injured and slips out of its groove, called subluxation of the long head of the biceps, it is most often associated with a subscapularis tear. Again, if there are signs and symptoms associated with a rotator cuff tear found on examination, further testing may be needed. When a patient has significant symptoms such as a torn biceps, or biceps subluxation or RTC weakness, an MRI is frequently required to diagnose the shoulder problems, like rotator cuff tears associated with a biceps rupture or subluxation (see Image 100 on pg. 132).

Surgery
When the biceps is partly torn, surgery is often reserved for patients with evidence of other accompanying shoulder problems like RTC tears or loss of function. When the long head of the biceps is completely torn, the acute soreness will resolve in weeks. After it ruptures, some patients feel better than before the injury.

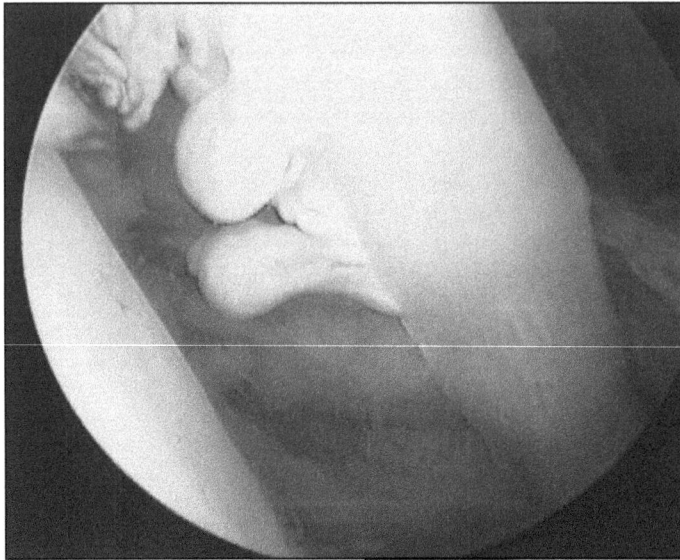

99 MRI view of partly torn biceps tendon.

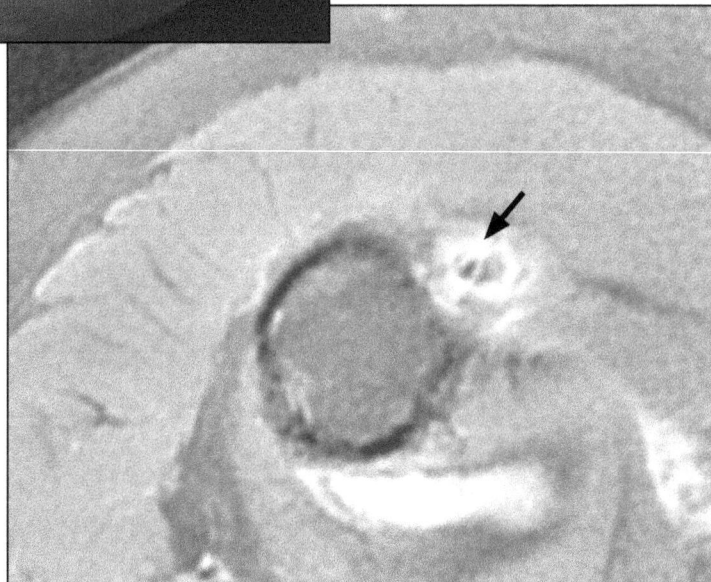

100 MRI view of partly torn biceps tendon.

If the muscle itself is painful during or after activity, the shoulder needs to be examined. If patients have weakness and pain with supination of the hand (as explained before, this is a clockwise rotation of the right hand and counterclockwise rotation of the left) after conservative measures fail, a biceps tenodesis may be required to move the tendon to a new location.

Biceps ruptures are also frequently associated with bone spurs near the tendon's path into the shoulder joint. When these are painful they must be removed, and a release of the tendon (biceps tendonotomy) may also help resolve the patient's symptoms. Once the biceps is released, the strain is off of the tendon. This is also the attachment site for the superior labrum, and if there is a SLAP lesion, it will heal better once the tendon that pulls on it is released.

The choice of procedure also depends on your age and your physical demands. Your surgeon will have to make a judgment call based on the preoperative exam and the findings at the time of surgery to determine whether surgery is needed and, if so, if a tendonotomy or tenodesis is best for you.

Biceps Tenodesis

A biceps tenodesis is a surgical procedure that anchors the ruptured end of the biceps tendon to the upper end of the humerus (see Image 101). If I suspect that a patient has a ruptured biceps, the first thing I do is an arthroscopic evaluation of the shoulder to check for other related injuries to the shoulder, especially if the MRI preoperatively showed cuff abnormalities. During surgery, once all rotator cuff related issues are treated, if a tenodesis is needed it is done through small incisions over the front of the humerus. Depending on the length and condition of the tendon, the location of the tenodesis will vary.

Arthroscopic tendon transfers are also possible in some cases; the type of procedure required will depend on your anatomy and the problem found during the surgery. When a tenodesis is performed, the tendon itself can be fixed in place with a special screw that matches the density and strength of the local bone (it is made of so-called biocompatible material), sutures, anchors, or a combination of these methods.

After using many different methods over the years, I have found that an arthroscopic release of the tendon, removing the damaged part of the tendon through the scope, and a mini-open tenodesis with a biocompatible screw yields the most predictable and effective results to decrease pain and improve overall function in the affected arm. It is done on an outpatient basis and seems to provide good pain relief shortly after surgery. Strength returns later after the tendon is fully healed in its new location.

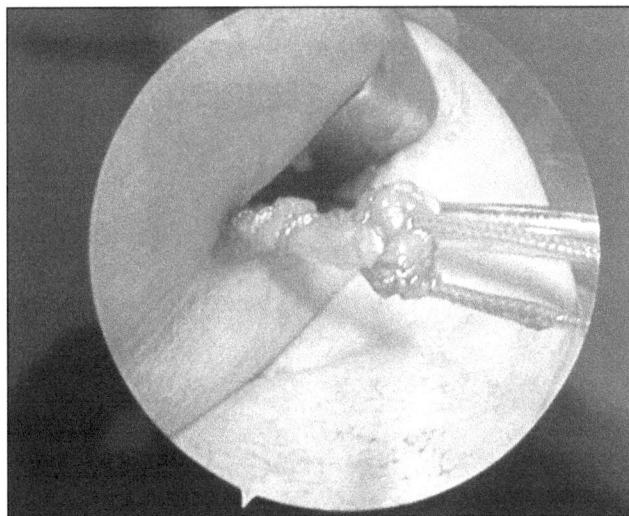

101 Sutures in place for biceps tendonitis (moving the biceps into new location to solve the pain of biceps tendonitis and partial tears of the tendon).

Biceps Tenotomy

In some cases, the biceps tendon is partially torn, which can be painful. The tendon may be swollen, worn, frayed, or inflamed in its groove. Forward flexion of the arm, supination of the hand, and pressing on (palpating) the bicipital groove is painful.

If the nondominant arm is involved, the patient is older and has a low demand occupation (no repetitive or heavy lifting or frequent use of a screwdriver), and the shape of the muscle (cosmetic appearance) is not a concern, a tenotomy (release of the tendon) can be an excellent option with good pain relief and shorter recovery time than a tenodesis. However, this procedure is not the best option for very active individuals.

THE ACROMIOCLAVICULAR **(AC)** JOINT, THE CONNECTION BETWEEN THE COLLAR-bone and the shoulder blade, is one of the most frequently injured joints during contact sports, especially football, hockey, and rugby. The main cause of injury is a fall on the point of the shoulder or onto an outstretched hand, and it also commonly occurs when someone flies over the handlebars of a bike or falls from a significant height. It can also happen during other impact injuries—for example, from skiing, slipping on ice, falling off an unprotected height at work, or during a motor vehicle accident. When the AC joint is sprung and the bones are no longer lined up, these injuries are often known as "shoulder separations" (see Image 102).

The very outer tip of the shoulder blade (scapula) is called the acromion. The collarbone (clavicle) attaches to the acromion at the AC joint. The acromion serves to protect the ball and socket joint of the shoulder. It supports the deltoid muscle and, through its connection to the collarbone at the AC joint, is the only bone directly attaching the shoulder joint to the rest of the body. The AC joint can be felt as a prominent bump or ridge at the top of the shoulder. The connection to the collarbone aids in raising the arm overhead and transfers the weight of the arm to the middle of the rib cage at the sternum.

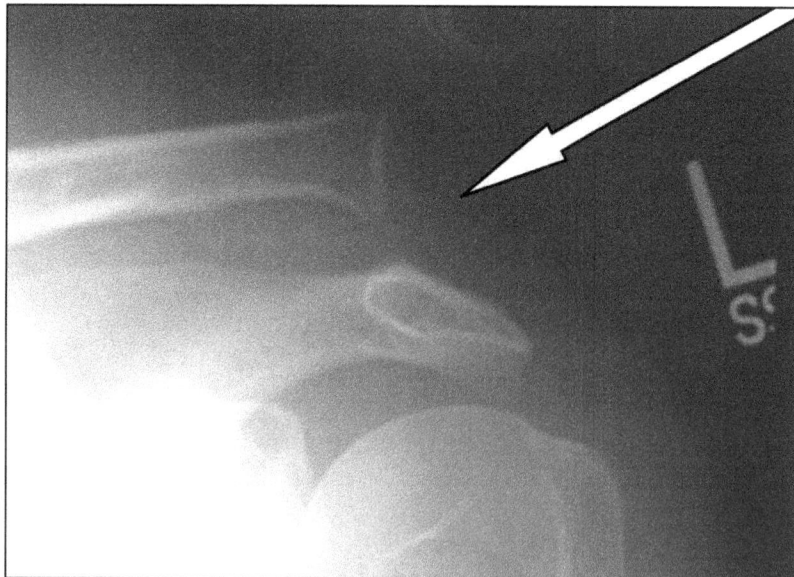

102 A severe AC joint separation of Grade 4 or greater.

AC Joint Pain

Pain in the AC joint can result from a specific injury, repetitive trauma, weight lifting, or wear and tear. A fall directly onto the shoulder can also cause the ligaments surrounding the AC joint to tear. Injuring the AC ligaments, coracoclavicular ligaments, deltoid muscle, and trapezius muscle can also result in instability of the AC joint. These injuries range from simple sprains to complete shoulder separations where the clavicle and the acromion are no longer attached.

Shoulder Separation

A shoulder separation is a sprain of the AC joint. Shoulder separations are different from shoulder dislocations, which involve the much larger ball and socket joint of the shoulder (the glenohumeral joint), which is held together by the joint capsule, ligaments, and rotator cuff muscles. A shoulder separation involves the smaller AC joint, held together by the joint capsule and strong ligaments around the capsule. The AC joint is further stabilized by strong ligaments holding the clavicle in place, called the coracoclavicular ligaments. In a higher energy accident, like a car accident, a collision in tackle football, or a fall off a mountain bike, the AC joint can dislocate just like the ball and socket of the shoulder. In more severe cases, all the ligaments holding the clavicle in place are also torn. The strong ligaments that normally hold the clavicle to the coracoid process (another bone in the shoulder) are shown in Appendix IB. Grading these tears—assessing how bad they are—helps us decide how to treat the injuries.

In patients with a shoulder separation, the injury can range from Grades 1 through 6. Grade 1 (a strain of the ligaments with no displacement of the joint) and Grade 2 (displacement less than the width of the collarbone) can be treated with rest, ice, and an anti-inflammatory medication. Grade 3 (displacement of more than one width of the collarbone, but a separation less than two widths) can also be treated nonoperatively, although there is some room for judgment based on symptoms, arm dominance, and activity requirements. Grades 4, 5, and 6 have higher degrees of displacement.

The clavicle can be displaced posteriorly (a Grade 4 injury), displaced more than two widths of the AC joint above the acromion (a Grade 5 injury), or stuck under the acromion or coracoid (a Grade 6 injury). In more extreme Grade 4 cases, the bone is "buttonholed" through the trapezius muscle, and there is visible tenting of the skin. This is irreducible and requires surgery, as do the other complete displacements of the AC joint (Grades 5 and 6).

How Do You Diagnose an AC Joint Separation?

The diagnosis of an AC joint separation is made by taking the patient's medical history and doing a physical examination. Sometimes it is obvious during the exam, like the Grade 4 separation shown in Image 103 (see pg. 136). The injury causes pain and difficulty while moving the arm, and so-called internal rotation will be painful (e.g., washing your back, taking a wallet out of your back pocket, or putting on a bra). You may have some swelling, ecchymosis (discoloration of the skin because of blood loss from a blood vessel underneath it), deformity, tenderness, or abnormal front-to-back motions or movement of the collarbone. The more unstable these injuries are, the more problematic they can become.

If the ligaments holding the AC joint in place are completely ruptured, the clavicle will move upward and backward. Patients may complain of popping, catching, or pain with overhead activities. The deformity may be obvious (a prominent bump) and disconcerting to look at, but the deformity itself is not the true indication for surgery; pain, loss of function, tenting of the skin, and instability in the dominant arm are more important factors.

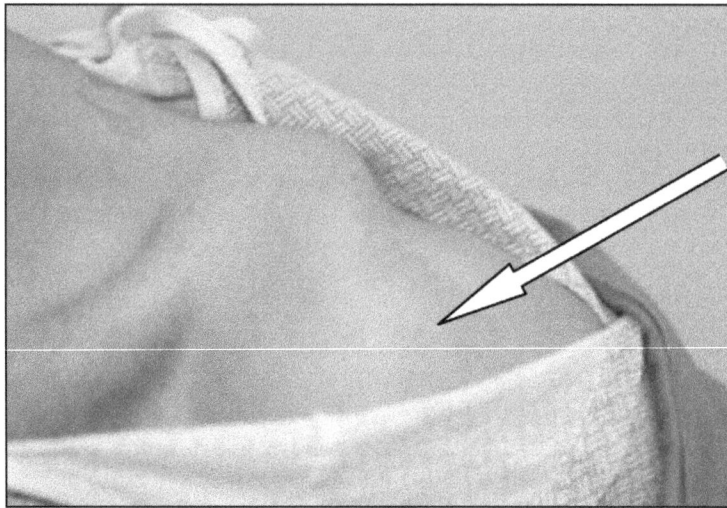

103 Clinical picture of AC joint separation.

Nonsurgical Treatment

A simple dislocation is only a sprain, and the clavicle will not move too far out of place when this occurs (Grade 1, Grade 2, and sometimes even Grade 3). It can be treated conservatively using nonsurgical treatments like NSAIDs, rest, and ice, along with wearing a sling. Certain physical therapy programs will also help. You must stop doing any painful activities or motions until the joint has formed some stabilizing scar tissue and movement is no longer painful.

Surgical Treatment

Surgery should not be performed for small separations, minimal deformity, or purely cosmetic reasons. When there is a significant deformity, as in Grades 4, 5, and 6, surgery is indicated. The surgical options vary greatly, and the outcomes were not predictable until 10 years ago. However, older procedures, like transferring a local ligament from the acromion to the clavicle (Weaver–Dunn procedure) and a screw from the top down (Bosworth screw), have been replaced by newer procedures with better results.

Dynamic muscle transfer and various combinations of the procedures in this section have also been used. Other arthroscopic procedures with novel suture anchors, washers, and loops also have been presented. These are fundamentally different ideas to try to solve the same problem. Some of the arthroscopic procedures may have a role in acute injury, and they can incorporate a tendon graft. They are technically difficult, the long-term results are not all in yet, and some nerve complications are possible because of the approach needed. In my experience, arthroscopic repairs are still not as strong as formal open repairs for chronic high-grade injuries with a lot of displacement. Again, the arthroscopic methods may be more useful in acute injuries (less than four to six weeks old), that are less displaced, and that may be too soon for some patients to decide they need the AC joint repaired.

The gold standard, in my opinion, is a procedure described by Dr. A. D. "Gus" Mazzocca, where the coracoclavicular ligaments are reconstructed with a tendon graft and locked in place in bone tunnels (see Image 104). In this AC joint reconstruction surgery, a special incision is made over the front and top of the AC joint, the collarbone is reduced into position, and the torn tendons are reconstructed with a tendon graft through tunnels in the clavicle designed to reproduce the anatomy of the torn ligaments. Small, biodegradable screws are placed, supplemented with heavy-duty sutures (Fiberwire and Ethibond). The muscle sleeve is then repaired over the reduced clavicle, reinforcing the ligament repair. In my practice, this procedure is performed under light general anesthesia. At the start of the procedure, a mixture of local anesthesia containing both lidocaine, which is a short-acting local, and longer-lasting Marcaine is injected into the area to reduce postoperative discomfort by numbing the surgical area.

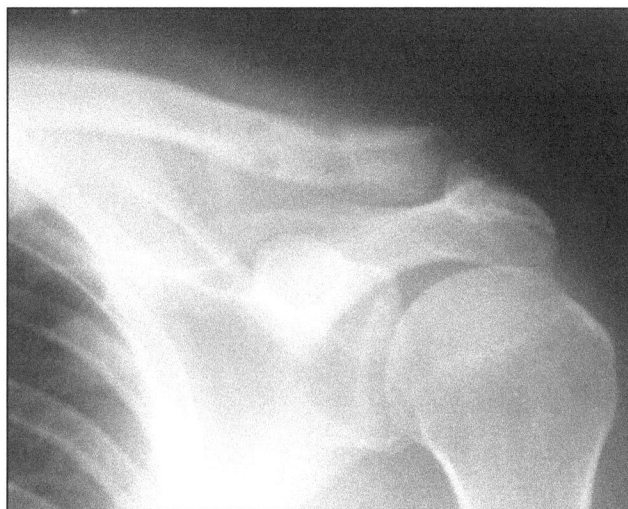

104 X-ray of AC joint repair with a ligament reconstruction.

Surgery for an unstable AC joint separation is usually very successful (see Images 105-107). However, there is always a small risk of complications, such as infection, failure of the repair, postoperative arthritis, loss of stability, or new bone formation in the ligaments (coracoclavicular ligament ossification). That's why having surgery for minor indications like Grade 1 or 2 separations is not worth the limited risk and is discouraged. Surgery for Grade 3 separations may be indicated if the patient still has pain and limitations after three to six months. Higher grades usually require repairs.

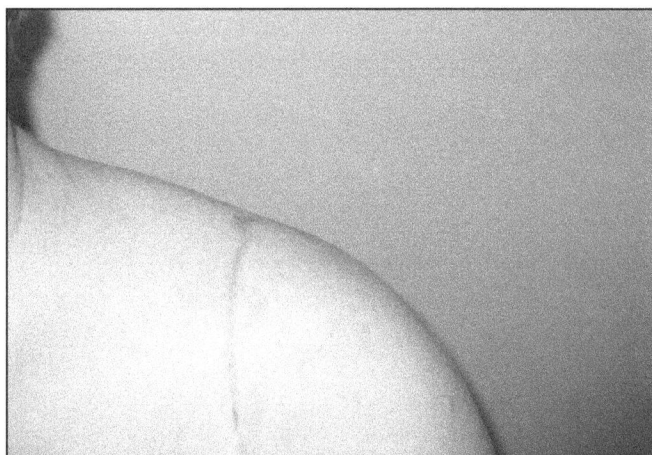

105 Post operation scar well healed.

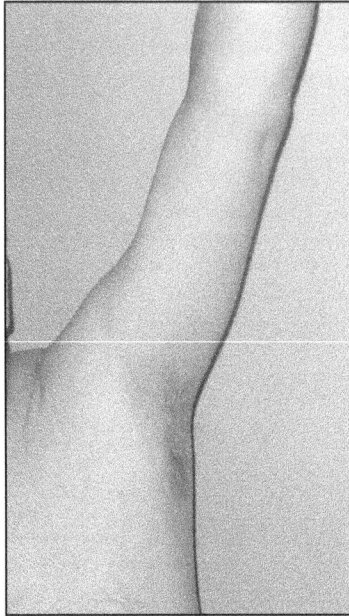

106 Full elevation after AC joint repair.

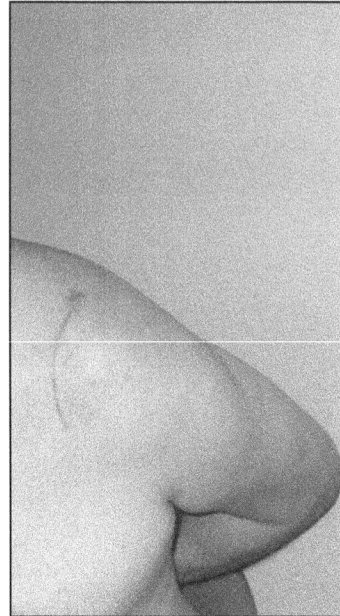

107 Full internal rotation after AC joint repair.

21 CLAVICLE FRACTURES

BELIEVE IT OR NOT, THE CLAVICLE, OR COLLARBONE, IS THE ONLY BONE CONNECTING the entire arm to the rest of your skeleton. You may wonder how this is possible since your shoulder and arm seem to be directly connected to your body. To understand this better, think of how far forward and backward your arm and shoulder can move. Think of how you can touch the middle of your back, your toes, and the back of your head. As you try these stretches, you can feel your shoulder blade move on your back, and you can tell it is not attached directly to the chest. Instead, the shoulder blade rides up and down, in and out, and over the ribs, controlled by an amazing group of muscles.

Now, feel your collarbone as you move. It is attached to the shoulder blade through a small joint near the top outer tip of the blade, just next to where the deltoid muscle (the largest muscle in your shoulder) attaches. If you follow the collarbone with your finger back toward the center of your body, you will find that it attaches to the upper part of your sternum. That joint, the sternal-clavicular joint, is the only point where your whole arm attaches to the rest of the skeleton. It's hard to believe! However, because of this single attachment, the arm and shoulder are allowed a good deal of freedom in their movement. You can touch almost any part of the rest of your body with little difficulty because the shoulder is attached at one point near the middle of the upper chest to a bone shaped like a thin stick.

Understanding that the shoulder is attached to the body only through the collarbone helps explain why it is frequently fractured during a fall. Its long, thin shape also explains why it fractures with a direct blow, as in a football tackle. Since the shoulder connects the body and the arm, it can break if the arm is used as protection during a fall. It is also frequently injured during a fall off a bike, from a ladder, down stairs, or in a motorcycle accident.

The clavicle typically breaks in the middle. These breaks can be simple (in just two pieces, with little displacement) or complex (in many pieces or displaced). They can be closed (not breaking the skin) or open (breaking through the skin). The clavicle can also break near either end. When it breaks, the AC joint or supporting ligaments could also be involved. The injury can occur in young children, teenagers, and active adults. The location of the fracture, the angulation, the displacement, the skin status, and the age of the patient are all important considerations when deciding on a treatment.

Treatment for Clavicle Fractures

Many clavicle fractures can be treated nonoperatively. If there is minimal displacement, and only a little angulation (bending), the fracture will usually heal very well. Usually, a period of rest is required with the arm in a sling, followed by slowly starting to gain mobility to avoid a frozen shoulder while allowing the fracture to heal. The fracture usually gets sticky within six weeks, but it will not be very strong, so you can't do push-ups, use a bench press, or engage in heavy activity early on. In addition, repetitive motions like using an elliptical trainer with the arm movement will cause the healing to fail under the repetitive stress. If there is shorting, or the fracture is bent (significant angulation), surgery is needed to correct the bend (restore the alignment) and correct the length of the collarbone. In the dominant arm of a throwing athlete, a surgical repair may be considered more often to restore the length when the collarbone is shortened by a fracture since a short collarbone may cause the shoulder joint to be closer to the ribs, making it harder to cock the arm back and, therefore, more difficult to throw long distances.

Indications for Operative Treatment of Clavicle Fracture

In general, non- or minimally displaced clavicle fractures are treated in a sling and do not require surgery. However, fractures that require surgery include the following:

- Fractures that break through the skin (open fractures).
- Fractures that threaten to break the skin by the nature of their sharp bone ends and how much they tent the skin.
- Fractures with muscles or soft tissues trapped between the bone ends.
- Fractures causing nerve compression.
- Fractures with overlapping fragments (shortening of the clavicle) of 2 centimeters or more and 1 centimeter in throwing athletes.

If any of these issues occur, the fracture should be surgically repaired.

Clavicle Fractures in Adults and Children

There are a few additional considerations for adult patients. One significant factor is the shortening of the fracture, which means that the bone is overlapped more than 2 centimeters or is 2 centimeters shorter than normal, which should be fixed surgically. If the fracture is angulated more than 30 to 45 degrees, it should be fixed. Also, if the shortening is in the dominant arm or occurs in a throwing athlete, no more than 1 centimeter of shortening can be accepted. In any case, patients with deformity, muscle trapped between the fragments, or the other factors noted already require surgery.

In children, as noted in the first section of this book (Image 2), many clavicle fractures heal well with very little treatment. Still, trapped muscle, excessive shortening, and significant displacement can require surgery pending the child's age. Very young children under age four can remodel and heal almost any fracture. Over age 10–12 pending the maturity of the child, many of the adult considerations come into play.

If surgery is needed, at the time of surgery, the fracture site is opened, the bone ends are realigned, and the fracture is secured in place with plates and screws or a rod. This is also known as "an open reduction and internal fixation" or "ORIF" in orthopaedic jargon. (See Images 108-122 for the steps to surgical fixation of a displaced fracture of the clavicle.)

Fractures near the AC joint or the outer end of the clavicle may require special care. The fractures that are lateral to the ligaments that hold the clavicle in place (the coracoclavicular ligaments as discussed in detail in Chapter 20) seem to heal well if the ligaments are intact. If the ligaments are torn or the fracture is close to the very strong coracoclavicular ligaments, there is a high rate of nonhealing (or nonunion) of the fractured bone. These require surgery to repair the fracture or the ligaments.

If the lateral fragment is small, the challenge is to hold the fragment in place until the bones heal. Some of these fragments are small and involve the AC joint. When this occurs and the ligaments are torn, removing the fragments and reconstructing the ligaments may be the only viable choice. However, a special type of plate has been developed to solve this complex problem. The plate has special screws in a close pattern to hold a smaller piece of bone in place. This is a big improvement over the older methods like the "hook" plate, which has fallen out of favor and is rarely used.

Fractures of the mid-third of the clavicle do well with nonoperative treatment if they are minimally displaced and not very angulated (bent), except for those in which the fracture is displaced posteriorly, or one piece of bone is behind the other piece of bone. That type of fracture can place pressure on major blood vessels and nerves just behind the clavicle, in which case an open reduction and fixation are needed.

The attachment of the clavicle closest to the body is called the sternoclavicular (SC) joint. It is where the clavicle attaches to the sternum. If it dislocates in the front of the chest, it causes a bump that may not be attractive, but it is not as problematic as a dislocation that goes behind the sternum. The same is true of medial-third fractures (fractures closer to the midline of the chest or SC joint), which can cause a compromise of the great vessels under the clavicle and above the heart. This needs close attention. Note: In children, a fracture near the SC joint may be a growth plate injury and may need to be fixed (see the "Injuries in Children" section).

Surgical Fixation of a Displaced Fracture of the Clavicle

In this section the images show the step-by-step process of fixing a clavicle fracture using a standard clavicle plating system. The plates and screws are designed to match the clavicle shape, size, and location of the fracture as well as the clavicle's thickness. Fluoroscopy is used to check the final fixation and plate position. The goal of the plate is to restore the natural length of the clavicle, align the bones, and hold them in place until Mother Nature can heal the bone. In addition to good plate fixation, the patient needs to allow the bone to heal and be well nourished with calcium, vitamin D, protein, and vitamin C.

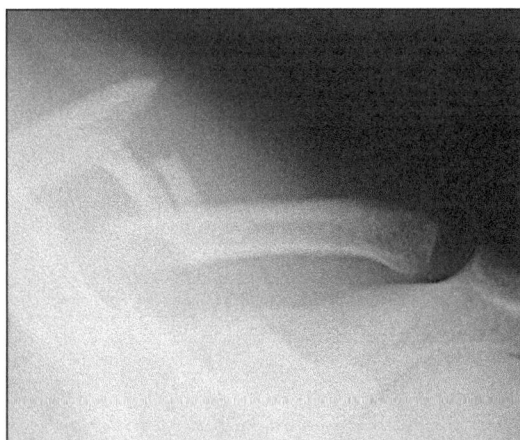

108 Clavicle (collar bone) fracture with four fragments and displacement.

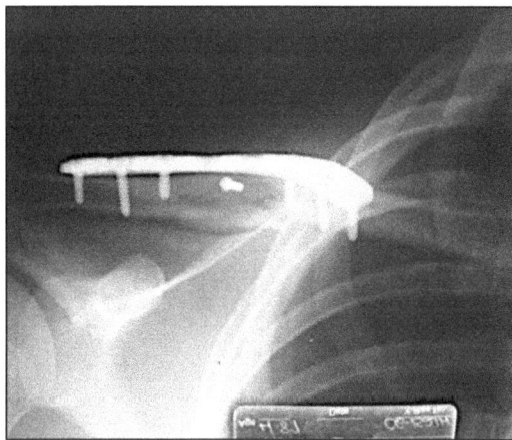

109 Plate in place.

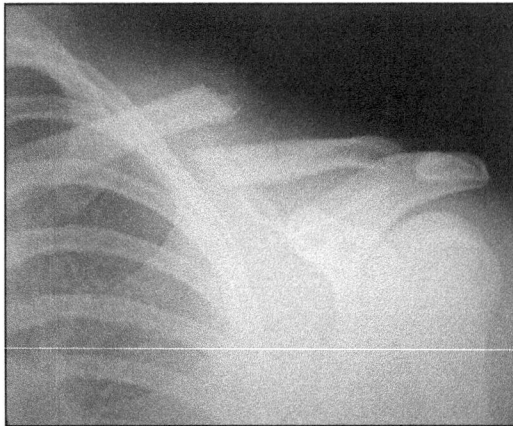
110 Transverse fracture with displacement.

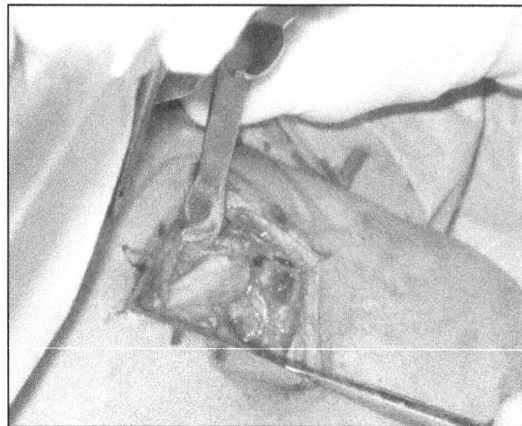
111 Open view of the fracture fragments.

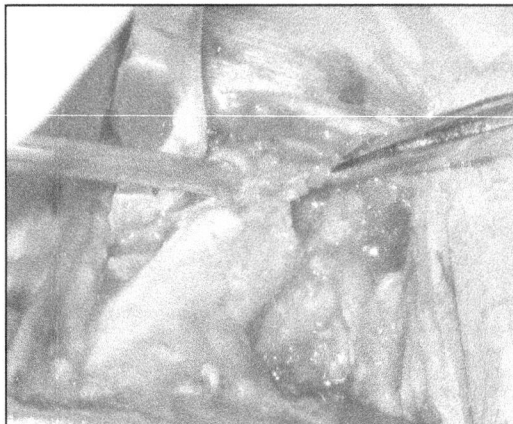
112 Cleaning the fracture edges.

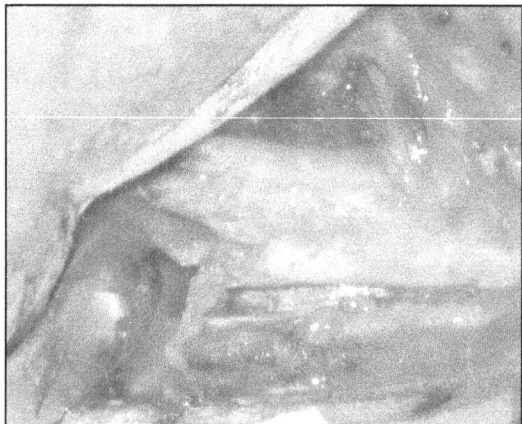
113 Fracture has popped through the muscle, explaining why it will not reduce without open reduction.

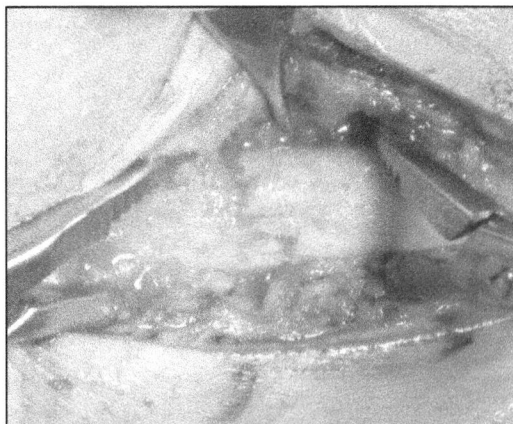
114 Fracture back in a good position (fracture reduced).

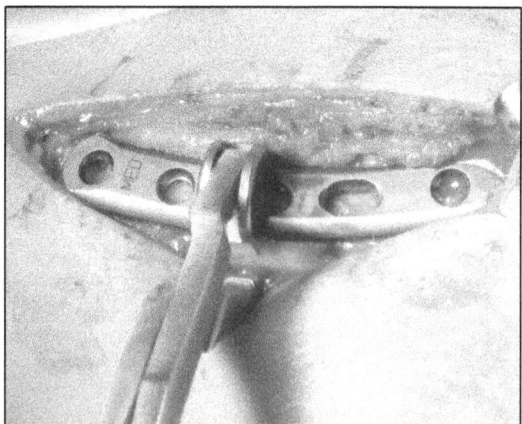
115 Plate in place without screws.

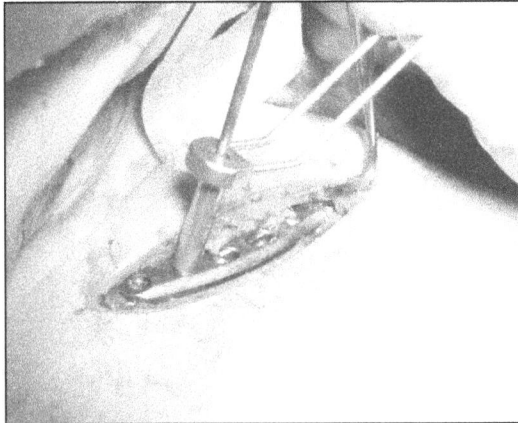

116 Drill for screw placement.

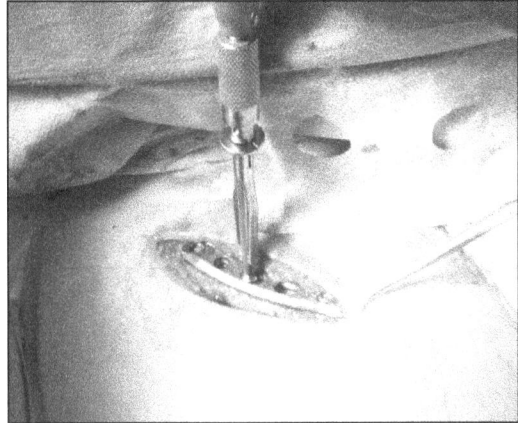

117 Screw being placed off-center to compress the fracture together.

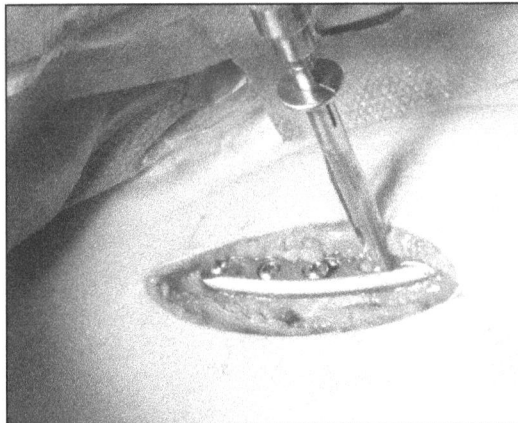

118 Additional screws being placed.

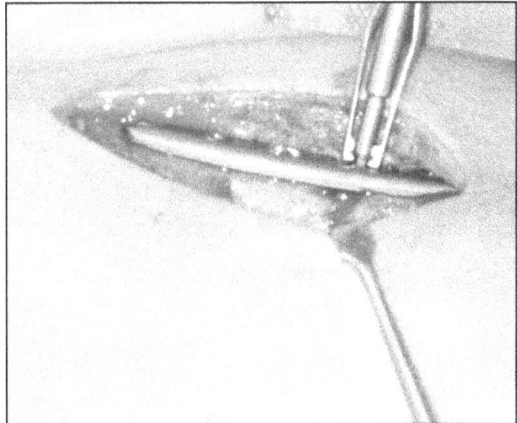

119 Final screws being placed.

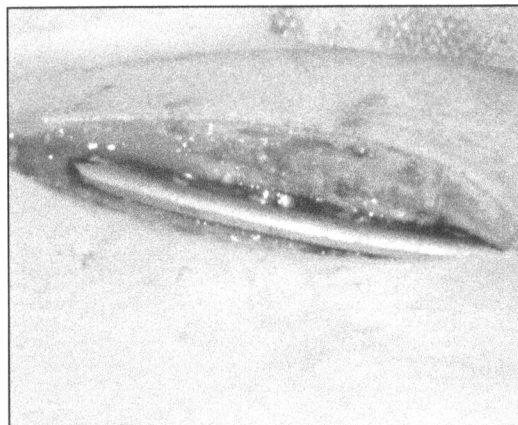

120 Final plate fixation.

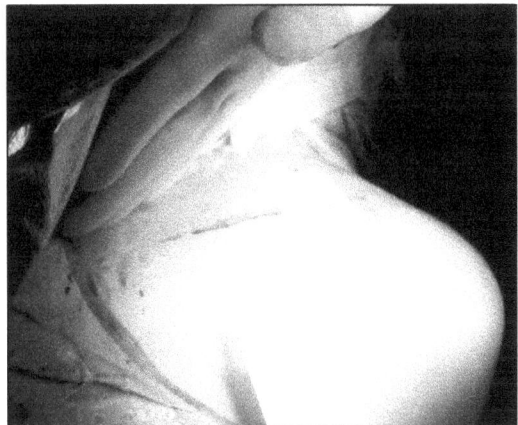

121 Incision closed with plastic closure.

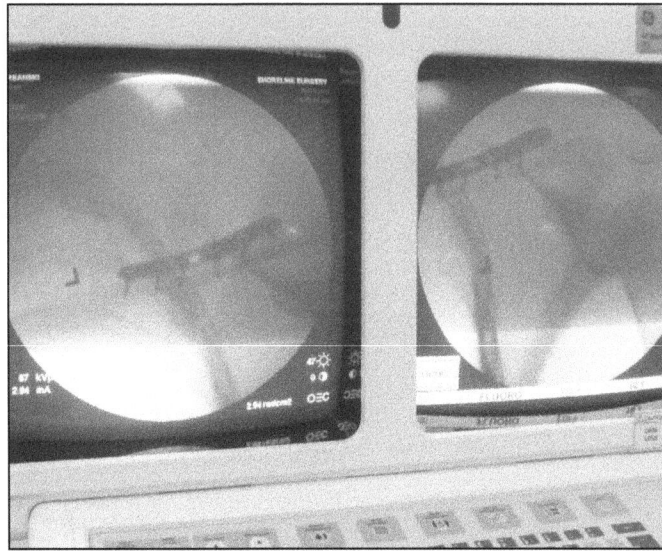

122 X-rays in the operating room of the final position confirming screw length and plate position.

Fractures of the Humeral Head

Sometimes a person falls and fractures the ball of the ball and socket. This is known as a humeral head fracture (see Image 123). Humeral head fractures most commonly occur from a simple fall and are most common in the elderly population. Many of these patients are females with thin bones (a condition known as osteoporosis). These fractures are often minimally displaced and can be treated in a sling until they begin to heal (the bones get sticky). When there is more than one piece broken into several pieces, the pieces are displaced, and if they can be put back together, they should be fixed with an open reduction and internal fixation.

Not so long ago, surgeons had to bend the flat steel plates in the operating room to fit the bone and the fracture. We used special tools, and contouring the plates to fit the bone exactly was a real surgical art form. I enjoyed the process; orthopaedic plate bending was challenging, but it took more time during the surgical procedure. Now, many orthopaedic

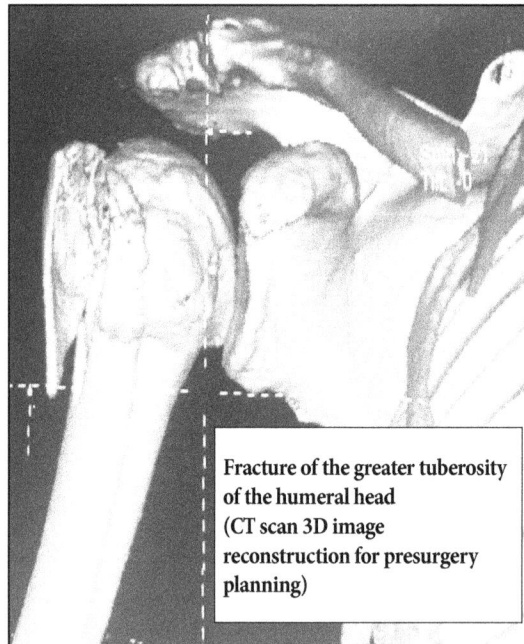

Fracture of the greater tuberosity of the humeral head (CT scan 3D image reconstruction for presurgery planning)

123 CT scan of a humeral head and a humeral neck fracture.

companies make special prebent "anatomic" plates that are made to match the anatomy and the fracture pattern based on the known shape of the broken bone. They are available for most fractures. Sometimes we still must make minor bends in these plates to match the fracture better, but it occurs less often with the newer plates.

Now I prefer the preformed anatomic plate designs with special screws that lock into the plate as well as the fracture. These make a very rigid repair and are much stronger than the older systems. I prefer these locking plates since they are the most stable once the screws are locked into the plate (see Image 124).

When the ball is fractured in many places, severely displaced, dislocated, and fractured, the ball itself may have lost its blood supply because of the injury. Most likely it cannot be put back together, and the fracture is less likely to heal no matter how you repair it. In these cases, a replacement of the ball with a new metal ball (a shoulder replacement) may be the best option.

Nonunion of Fractures around the Shoulder

Some fractures, whether treated with or without surgery, don't heal. This can happen for many reasons, and there are many ways the bones fail to heal. These include too much motion at the fracture site because of a patient's activity and non-operative treatment; the plate fixation is not strong enough to support the fracture long enough for it to heal; or sometimes, the biologic environment causes a lack of new bone formation. This can happen in patients with diabetes; poor nutrition; lack of vitamin C, D, or calcium; or other illnesses.

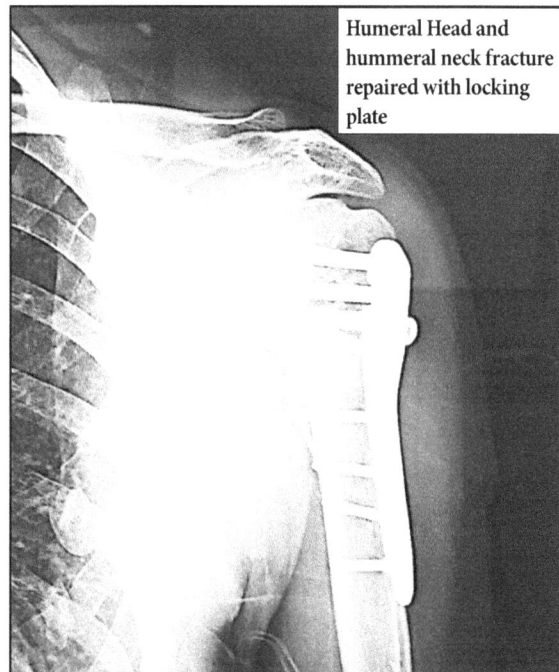

Humeral Head and hummeral neck fracture repaired with locking plate

124 Plate fixation of the humeral head and humeral neck fracture.

When a patient doesn't perceive pain at the fracture site, this can also cause a nonunion. Pain reminds us to hold the fracture still. When a person doesn't feel pain in a broken bone, they may have nerve damage in the area from the injury, or they may have diabetes and don't have good sensation because of poorly controlled blood sugars.

Nonunions can also occur when there is poor dietary intake of vitamins, calcium, and protein. In any case, the lack of pain in the area interferes with a good number of healing pathways and can lead to nonunion. We view pain as a problem in our culture, but the reality is we need it to allow Mother Nature let us know what we can and cannot do, as well as help us heal the bone. When a patient has no pain after a fracture, they tend to do too much, and I worry that they will hurt themselves again before the bone heals.

If a patient has a nonunion, I check the nutritional status (including protein levels in the blood), blood sugar level in diabetics, smoking status, alcohol use, drug dependency, and vitamin D levels to help find out if malnutrition, diabetes, or smoking are the sources of the problem. If all are negative or each one has been addressed, the immobilization and protection of the fracture itself should be reevaluated.

We must also look for signs of soft tissue trapped between the fracture fragments because muscle between the fractured pieces will also block healing. Sometimes a CT scan or an MRI is needed to see if fluid has formed between the bones with scar tissue. Sometimes the bones are moving so much that the body is fooled into "thinking" this must be a joint, so it walls off the bone ends and makes fluid between them. This has a fancy name, called a "pseudarthrosis" or "false joint." When there is muscle trapped, pseudarthrosis, nerve damage, or there are longstanding signs of nonhealing or a nonunion, it is time to consider surgery.

<table>
<tr><td>

Smoking and Healing

Fractures that fail to heal, requiring orthopaedic surgical repairs, happen much more often in smokers.

Smoking interferes with

✓ the blood's ability to carry oxygen,

✓ DNA synthesis (making new DNA),

✓ new tissue formation, and

✓ formation of the tiny blood vessels that are required for healing.

It is important to note that healing rates are lower in smokers, and complications are higher for almost all types of surgery. Smokers have delayed healing, more infections, and a higher nonunion rate (failure to unite the bones together after a fracture). For these reasons, I tell all my patients with orthopaedic problems who need surgery that they must stop smoking beforehand.

Some spine surgeons will not operate on smokers since they take three times as long to heal, and some end up with nonunions of spine fusions (a big problem after a very big surgery).
</td></tr>
</table>

Surgery for a Nonunion of a Fracture

Some of my most interesting and challenging cases have been nonunions. As a founding member of the Level 1 trauma service orthopaedic panel at Yale New Haven Hospital, I have seen my share of severe trauma, including patients with multiple bones broken at one time. It is only natural that some of these patients' fractures don't heal all at the same time, and some of them don't heal well or at all. When we have established that a bone will not heal without help, we revise the plan and fix the fracture. Sometimes that means reoperating on a fracture that was fixed already, replacing the old plates and screws with newer, more rigid fixation, and adding bone graft material to kickstart the healing. There are electric bone stimulators that can be used and biologics like BMP (bone morphogenic protein, which is meant to heal and create new bone from stem cells.)

If a bone does not heal and the patient does not have surgery, then an open reduction with internal fixation with bone graft usually works well. As in the case shown in Image 125, there was a true pseudarthrosis, a false joint between the bones. The patient had gross motion at the fracture and a very stiff frozen shoulder. She had tried to get it to heal for eight or nine months with no improvement. During the surgery the false joint and its fluid were removed, the area was cleared of all scar tissue, a plate was put in place, and bone graft was added. The patient was placed on vitamin D, vitamin C, and calcium supplementation.

The patient's range of motion at the shoulder joint was returned to 75% of its normal movement, and the fracture was 80% healed four months post-op. Her healing and range continued to improve until she became fully functional, but as expected, she never regained 100% of her full motion because of her age and the size of the fracture.

The patient was able to return to all her activities of daily living like dressing, showering, and grooming herself—things that were nearly impossible with the unstable fracture in her dominant arm. Since her arm with the pseudarthrosis was virtually useless before the surgery, she was very pleased with her results.

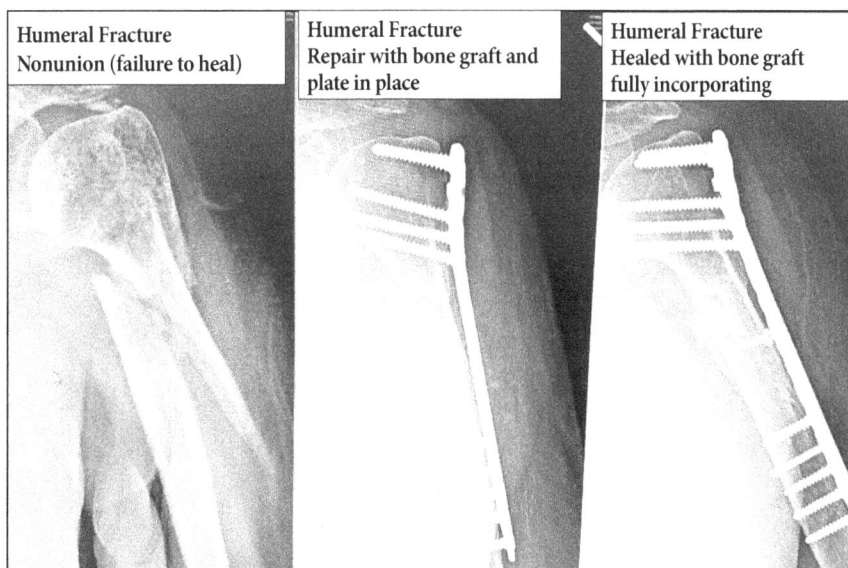

| Humeral Fracture Nonunion (failure to heal) | Humeral Fracture Repair with bone graft and plate in place | Humeral Fracture Healed with bone graft fully incorporating |

125 X-ray of a fracture that did not heal with nonsurgical methods (a nonunion), plate fixation, and bone grafting to help healing and final healing of the fracture.

PART FOUR

SPORTS TUMORS, BONE HEALTH, AND GENERAL INJURY PREVENTION

In any situation there are several overarching factors that can make a dramatic difference in our ability to restore function. The most important is not missing a diagnosis that can be life threatening like a malignant tumor or cancer that can become more serious if missed. It is every radiologist and orthopaedic surgeon's nightmare: a tumor that is missed because the patient complained of a sports injury that had nothing to do with the real problem than may have been there for months before the injury. I call these phenomena sports tumors because it's not that the sports injury caused the tumor, it is the fact that many children or young adults with tumors blame their pain on the last injury they recall. They don't present "I think I have a tumor"; they present as, "I hurt myself months ago and the swelling did not go away." Or, more simply, "I hurt myself playing a sport." It is very important that we listen carefully and sort out the differences in the stories we are told and the clinical findings. There are two examples presented here to help make this point clearer.

In this section we will also discuss injury prevention and bone health. Both are equally important. If the bone is weakened, it will fracture with less serious trauma. Lastly, if we don't pay attention to preventable injuries, we will have more of them.

THERE ARE A SMALL NUMBER OF TIMES WHEN A GROWTH OR OTHER ABNORMALITY presents as a sports injury or problem. The common sports injuries in all age groups are very common, and the tumors are very rare. It does not mean that if the injury is related to sports there cannot be something else going on. A swollen knee, for example, can be any number of mechanical problems related to an injury: everything thing from an ACL tear to a loose body, fracture, or torn meniscus. A swollen knee can also be inflammatory arthritis, gout, or Lyme disease. This chapter has everything you would want to know about figuring out such possible causes.

What happens if the injury is none of those previously listed in this book? It would be wrong to write off an injury as something simple when it was not, and it is way too easy to do just that. Physicians know that most people would prefer to believe that a football injury caused the swelling; or that it is not as big as it was last week when in fact it is bigger; or worse, that even though it has been getting bigger for months, it may still just go away by itself. This is when physicians must be vigilant for those "bad" things we wish we did not have to consider or hope our patients don't have.

This is where the idea of "sports tumors" gets its moment. It is why when there is a simple injury with more swelling, more pain, or a bigger deformity than expected we must think twice about the diagnosis. If the knee is swollen and it feels harder than just fluid or the patient's mother says it has been looking funny to her for months, our "index of suspicion" must go up. In these cases, a plain X-ray is the best place to start. If there is something there, more advanced imaging may be needed.

Sometimes the X-ray confirms that the swelling is just fluid. Other times it is Osgood-Schlatter's disease or a calcium deposit. For things that are near the skin, or "superficial," sometimes the look and feel of the swollen area helps us. For example, is there a fluid-filled sac possibly a swollen bursa or cyst? Ultrasound as an in-office image is great to see if the swelling is just fluid, in which case it could be a cyst, or normal fat, in which case it could be a benign lipoma.

Over the years, I have seen several patients with popping around the knee with locking, only to find an osteochondroma (a type of benign tumor) on an X-ray that was large enough to rub on a nearby tendon, like the hamstrings, as the cause of the popping. Most recently I had a teenaged wrestler present with the complaint of an inability to squat and get into the ready position. The patient went to physical therapy and the therapist could not improve the range of motion. In fact, during my exam I found a hard mass in the back of the knee (see Image 126a) and a stop or end point that the knee would not pass (see Image 126b). X-rays showed the bone growth behind the knee (see Image 127). This is very characteristic of an osteochondroma. This benign tumor is a growth of cartilage and then classically normal bone underneath it. An MRI can confirm the diagnosis and the treatment is removal (see Images 128a-c).

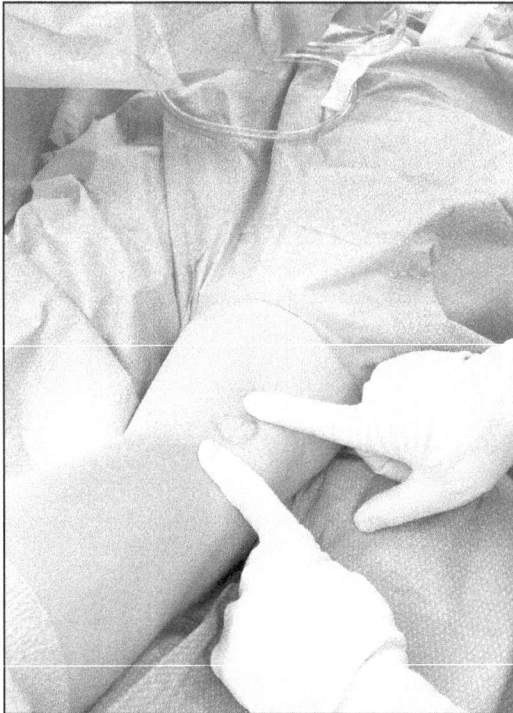

126a: The growth or tumor can be felt behind the knee as a hard mass between the fingers.

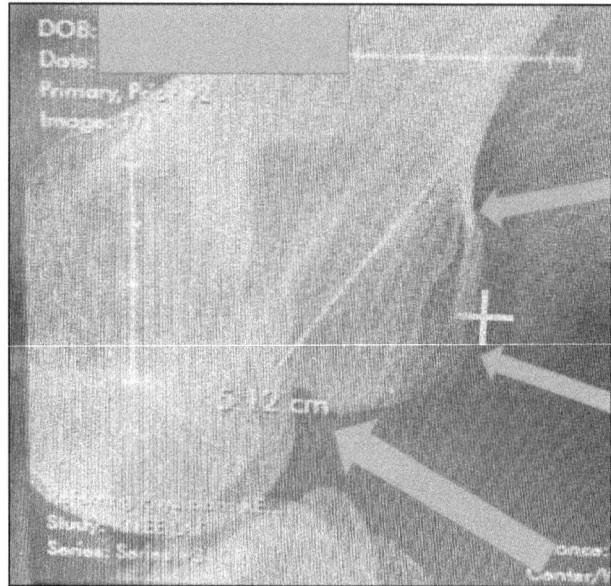

126b: The growth or tumor blocks knee motion at 90 degrees of flexion (bending).

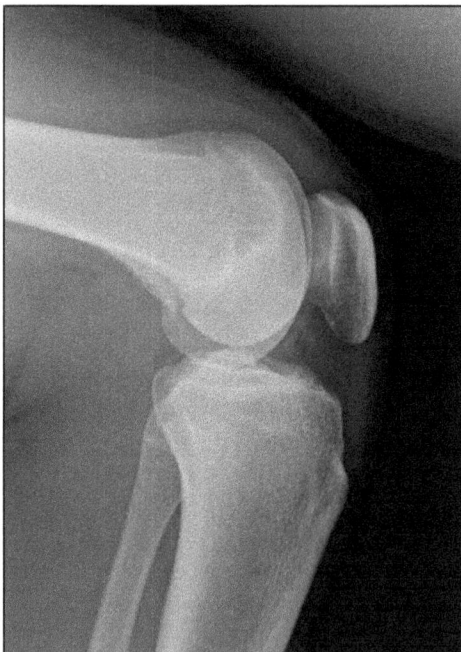

127 Plain X-ray of the normal knee for comparison. Note no bone growth on the back of the femur.

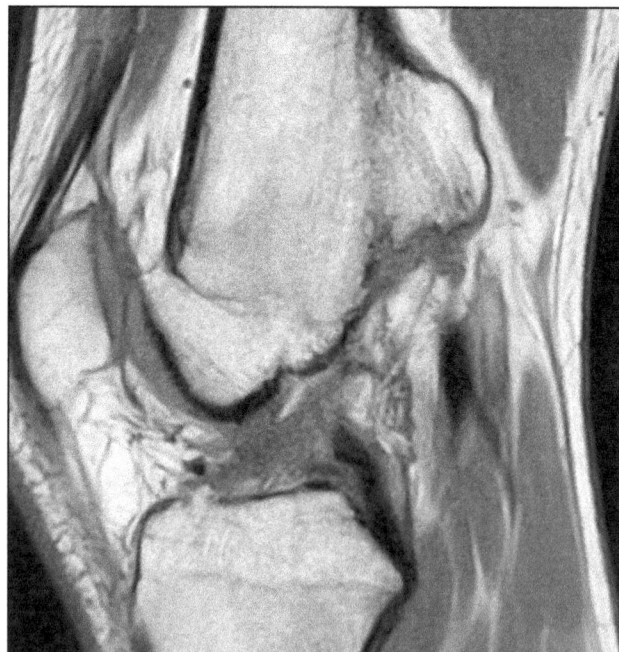

128a: MRI shows the lesion or tumor has a base of normal bone and a cartilage cap. This is consistent with a large but benign osteochondroma.

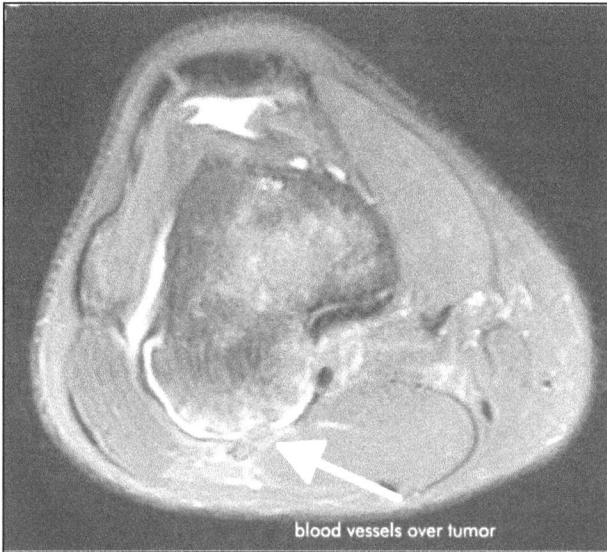

128b: The growth on MRI with a nerve and blood vessel sitting on the surface.

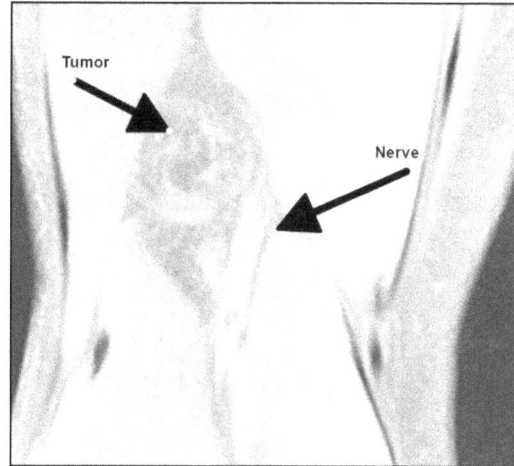

128c: The peroneal nerve on MRI (dark structure crossing the center of the image as a straight line) going around the tumor.

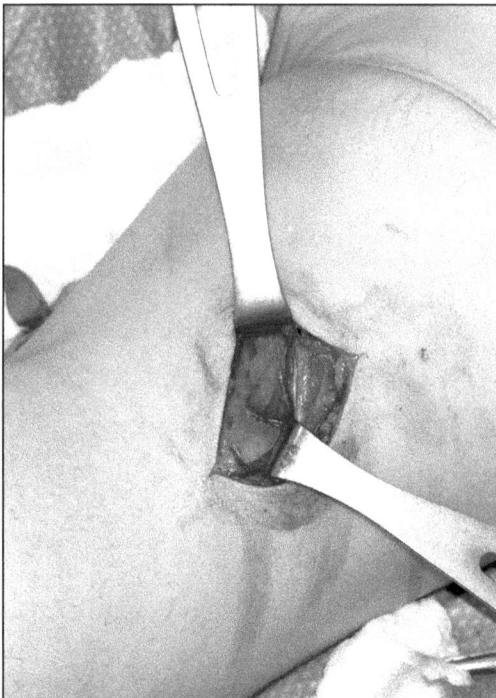

129 The tumor exposed with two veins sitting on its surface.

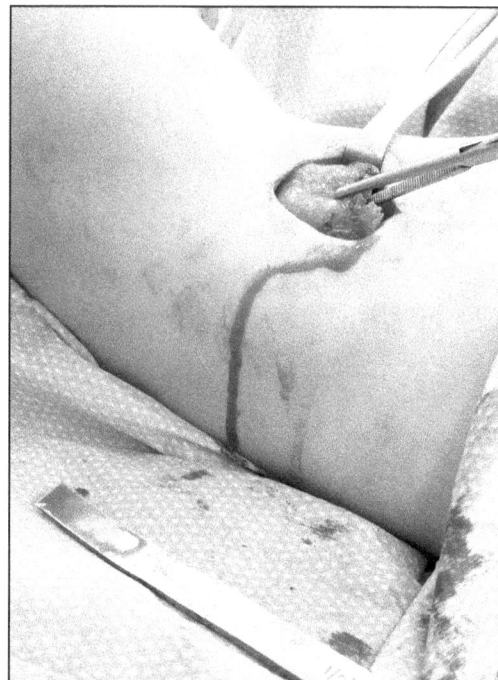

130 The tumor outlined and resected at the normal margins before being removed.

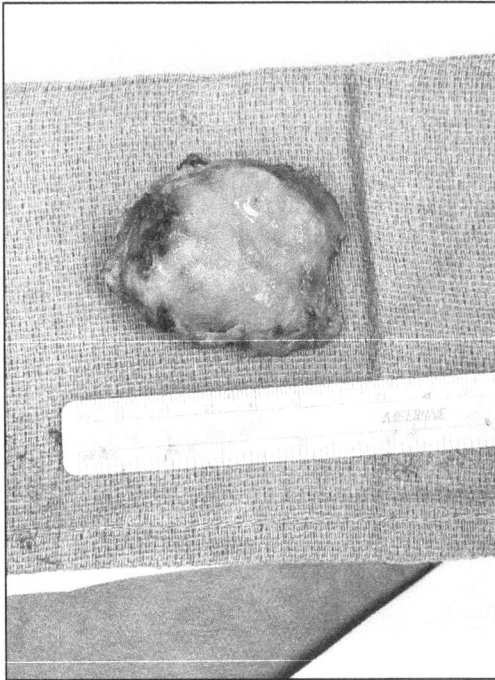

131 The tumor removed.

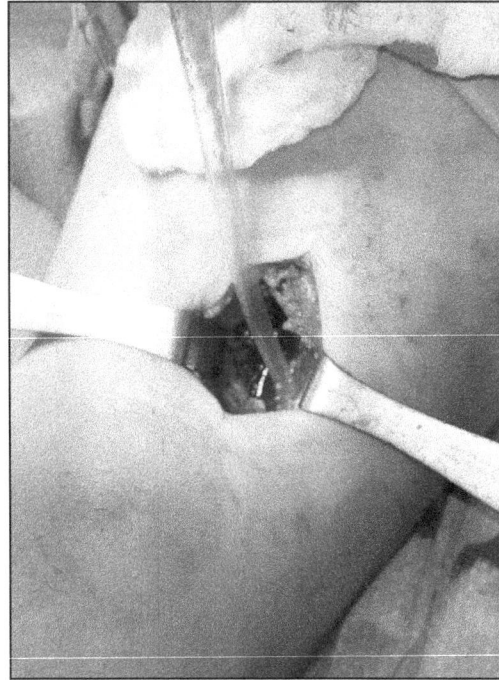

132 The remaining normal bone at the base of the lesion.

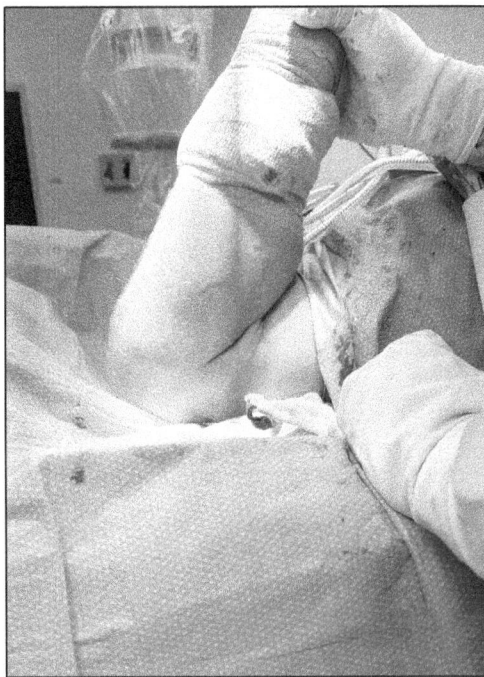

133a The knee bending (flexion) is restored after the tumor is out.

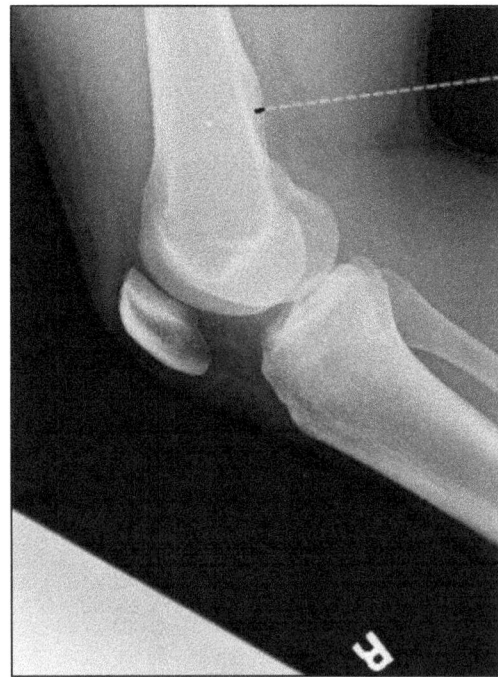

133b Post-op X-ray after removal of tumor.

Here an open approach is used to expose the growth (image 129), remove it (image 130), the lesion itself out of the body (image 131), the defect left behind (image 132), and the restoration of normal motion after the abnormal bone growth was removed (image 133a).

Other sport tumors can present as a fracture—most classically a humeral shaft fracture (in the upper arm) through a unicameral bone cyst. The bone is eaten away by the cyst wall (the pathology is the cyst itself) and when the hole in the bone is bigger than 50% of the diameter of the bone it can break with a simple fall or sports injury. Here too, a plain X-ray makes the diagnosis. Be aware that aggressive bone tumors or metastatic tumors can be seen as eating away the bone and they too can cause holes in the bone. These also can break in a simple fall or while playing sports and the X-ray, in these cases, reveals more that a simple fracture.

Other tumors have a classic appearance on an X-ray. These can be diagnosed from the X-ray. If there is a tumor, more studies are often needed to stage the tumor. A biopsy can then make the final diagnosis and help to complete the treatment plan. In a child, when the tumor is benign in nature, treatment of the fracture, removing the tumor from inside the bone, and bone grafting the defect is a fairly routine treatment and does not require a special tumor expert.

When there are more serious tumors, more aggressive types, and/or metastatic disease, these patients often will require a team approach in a cancer center. The tumor case described above is a benign tumor with classic X-ray appearance. It is so classic the diagnosis is almost always made by the X-ray's appearance alone and confirmed by MRI and/or CT scan. These simple, benign, or low grade tumors (like the osteochondroma in this particular case) can be removed with a margin of normal tissue and bone around it. They most often can be completely removed and cured with excellent long term outcomes.

The Role of X-rays, MRIs, and CT Scans

Almost everyone thinks an MRI is the answer to every question they have. It is understandable to believe the most expensive test is the best. This is just not true in real life and an MRI, like all tests, has some real benefits and important limitations. Most initial diagnoses can be made by listening carefully to the patient's story and considering things like just how this occurred, how long it has hurt, what the pain is like, what helps, and what makes it worse. Does the injury cause a specific mechanical problem like locking, buckling, or giving way? (See more about what these terms mean in the knee section of the book.) A good exam is critical and that is usually followed by plain X-rays if needed. Most of the time your doctor will have a good answer with the three main pillars of medical diagnosis: a history, an exam, and a plain X-ray.

Providing there is not an urgent situation like a fracture, for an unstable, locked knee or dislocated joint, nonoperative treatments are next and most prudent. An MRI is reserved for surgical planning in a soft-tissue injury or problem we think will need surgery or a potential tumor (or a sports tumor), but it is not always the best next test. For many fractures, the X-rays may provide enough information alone. In some fractures a CT scan gives far superior detail and is the best test for surgery planning, not an MRI. So, there are pros and cons to both MRI and CT scans. Remember, some patients with electronic implants like a pacemaker cannot have an MRI. In those cases, a CT scan may be the only choice.

MRIs Can Fool Us

An MRI is fantastic in picking up and seeing water where it should not be. So swelling is very clearly shown on an MRI. Early after an injury many things that are swollen will "light up" brightly on an MRI. Many of these structures may heal with time by themselves. So it is common to see "too much" on an MRI that is done right after an injury, and the injury may seem worse than it is. This is why many insurance companies have started to deny payment for an MRI unless simple treatment has been done first. Sadly, this takes the choice out of your doctor's hands, but it has some validity in many cases. In other cases, it can delay treatment for things we know from the patient's history and physical exam will not get better. There is no perfect answer for each case, so insurance companies tend to deny more than they should. This can be frustrating to both the patient and the treating physician.

MRIs and Sports Tumors

In the case described in this section of the book, both an MRI and a CT scan were done before surgery. This particular tumor, an osteochondroma, has the classic finding of normal bone under an abnormal cartilage "cap." The tumor's cap is almost always normal cartilage growing in an abnormal direction and normal bone fills in behind it. If the cartilage cap is too big (thicker than 1 centimeter), there is a higher chance it is a low-grade malignant tumor. Therefore, in this case both tests are needed to see if the bone is normal and the cap isn't too thick before it is removed.

I have had another case where the MRI showed what looked like a cyst on the shoulder near the AC joint in a weight lifter in their late twenties. It is common enough at the AC joint, is associated with swelling at the top of the joint, and it looks a lot like the MRI pictures I saw, a simple AC joint cyst. Another doctor tried to aspirate it (remove the fluid with a needle) and nothing came out. Still, the reading on the MRI was a cyst.

The normal treatment for a cyst arising from the AC joint would be address the injury source (damage to the AC joint) and remove the cyst. Still, I had a funny feeling there was something not right going on. In the operating room, I had second thoughts about addressing the AC joint problem before removing it. Instead, the first thing I did was a wide local resection of the "cyst." After taking it out it was clear the cyst was in fact a solid tumor. Not the best of diagnoses.

The good news was the AC joint was left untouched before the tumor was removed. It was not the problem, and the correct approach was not to go into the joint and possibly spread the tumor. In this case, the tumor had a high signal on the MRI, very similar to water, and was thought to be fluid by the MRI's appearance. The "cyst-tumor" was sent to the pathology lab. The pathology confirmed it was a soft-tissue sarcoma, a very aggressive tumor. If treated incorrectly (like cutting into another joint nearby) it could have cost this person a limb or their life. Also, it had a chance to spread if it was not completely removed. At the time of writing this, the person has been tumor free for four years after removal. It turns out the initial MRI was very misleading. This case is a very important reminder that MRIs are not always 100% correct. They can fool the best radiologists and orthopaedic surgeons. At times, they can simply be misread, and that could change the treatment plan at the time of surgery. The good news is the patient had a sarcoma and has had a complete recovery. The five-year followup tests were all clear, and she has not had any recurrence.

23 BONE HEALTH AND GENERAL INJURY PREVENTION

THERE IS THE EXPRESSION, AND I AM PARAPHRASING IT HERE, THAT IT IS NEVER GOOD enough to close the barn door after the horse has escaped. For knee and shoulder problems, understanding all the things that can go wrong and how to fix them is great, yet prevention is always preferred. The first step in prevention is listening to your body. There are so many examples of patients ignoring the signals of impending injury that there is an old joke just for them, and it's the oldest doctor joke I know:

> Patient: "Doc, if this hurts what should I do?"
> Doctor: "Don't do it."

This turns out to be very good advice.

Using Pain as a Guide

If 10 reps of an exercise hurts, 20 reps will hurt more, not less. So many of the injuries I see are purely from overdoing it. Many others are due to poor form while doing an activity that is "good." I golf, and at one point I began to have some minor issues with my own shoulder. The problem turned out to be a swing change I had imposed on myself to improve my distance. The new swing was just not good for me, and it, not my shoulder, needed to be fixed. A few golf lessons and I was better in no time.

Tennis players with tennis elbow may need to work on their backhand form, decrease the racket's string tension, increase their grip, or add antivibration sponges to the racket. Balance for throwing sports is equally important. In all these cases pain is the tip-off to poor form and future injury. Prevention can be as simple as listening to your own body tell you what is wrong.

Bone Health

Bone is a fantastic living substance that has many functions. Our blood cells are made in the marrow. Bone supports the muscles and the ends of our joints. If the bone is not healthy, other things go wrong. People with fair skin color (indicating lack of enough sun exposure needed to make vitamin D), who avoid milk, cheese, and dairy typically have some deficiency in calcium intake and lack vitamin D and vitamin C. We need 2000 mg of calcium a day for growing healthy bones and 1000 mg per day for good bone health. If we have a fracture, we need 2000 mg per day to help heal that fracture. I also recommend 1000 mg a day of vitamin C for healing and at least 2000-3000 units of D for healing.

Bone is our storehouse for calcium, and as such, we add calcium in our younger years and remove some as we need to in our older years. As we get older, the bones usually have thinner or weaker walls and are more prone to stress injury and fractures if we fall.

If a person has lactose intolerance or any gut absorption problems, getting the building blocks for good bones (vitamin D and calcium) can be difficult, and if the bone is injured, it will be harder to heal it. If you or someone you know is at risk, getting a vitamin D level and a bone density check may be beneficial in preventing poor bone health in the future and possible fractures in later life.

Weight-bearing exercises are also extremely important. It is well known that without walking and some light weight lifting it is hard to maintain good bone stock. The fact is that when astronauts are in complete weightlessness, they lose 1000 mg of calcium per day from their bones. There is no question that gravity is a prime driver of bone mass. When weightless, the body knows it does not need the bone mass and becomes more efficient by making the bones lighter. Therefore, when we see the astronauts on TV they are exercising on treadmills with straps over their shoulders. The straps hold them down and add weight to the legs. This is one of the ways they can simulate weight-bearing. The alternative is the astronauts will lose more and more bone each day. It follows that back on earth if we don't move enough and never lift any weight, we will lose bone mass quickly. As doctors, we also see this after long hospitalizations from a serious illness or major surgery. Placing people at complete bed rest, causes them to lose both bone density and muscle mass quickly.

Hormones can affect bone health as well. Chronic steroid use, poor nutrition, anorexia, chronic gastrointestinal problems, bypass surgery, inflammatory bowel disease, mal-absorption syndromes, hypothyroidism, hyper-parathyroidism, and lack of estrogen for women and testosterone for men can all cause a decrease in bone health. Bone marrow tumors can eat away at the bone in a general sense and an unexplained low trauma fracture may be the first sign of the disease. Metastatic tumors can also destroy bone locally and cause pathologic fractures.

Balance, Balance, and Balance

There are three words to remember here: balance, balance, balance. Balanced diet, balanced exercises, and balance on your feet all prevent injury.

Balanced Diet

A balanced diet prevents nutritional conditions. It's hard to maintain bone health if there is no calcium absorbed from the diet. Vitamin C is required for muscle and tendon healing. Muscle cannot grow if there is not enough protein. (This can be checked with an albumin test—low albumen correlates well with poor protein intake and poor general nutrition.) A vitamin D level is also helpful. Other issues that are related include low estrogen in women and hyperparathyroidism (high parathyroid hormone levels and low thyroid levels). Your doctor can test for all of these.

Balanced Exercise

Check your exercise program. Does it include a range of activities, not just one single form of exercise each day? Strength in only one exercise does not always mean your body is in good shape. Runners need rest days and upper body exercises to balance things out. Muscles set themselves to the optimum length for the specific exercise done. If it is always the same, you may lack good function of other muscle groups or suffer the consequences of tight muscles that are not used frequently and be at risk for strains and sprains as a result. Naturally, exercises like yoga, tai chi, and many martial arts clearly cover the entire body by design for the same reasons. These also focus on balance very nicely.

Balanced Gait

Good old-fashioned balance is at the root of most injury prevention. If you start to fall and can catch yourself, you can prevent many injuries. Being steady on our feet as we age prevents hip fracture. In sports, good hip balance and muscle control help move the ground force up the legs to the arms to create stronger throws, better catches, quicker turns in skiing and hockey, stronger soccer kicks, and the ability to break a football tackle. I do a simple test in the office that you can try at home. Stand on one leg and do a one-legged squat. See if you can keep your balance. Do you drift from one side to the other? Do your legs scissor together to stop you from tipping over? If so, you may need a balance training program with physical therapy to improve your playing level and to prevent injuries. It is that simple. There are more details on this in my book, *I've Fallen and I Can Get Up*. In that book I review all the medical issues that cause falls or unsteady gait with the idea that fall prevention is better than a broken leg.

Body Mass Index

Body mass index (BMI) is a calculation of mass-to-surface ratio that gives us a direct measure of relative obesity. Both high (>40 is too high of a weight) and low (<19 is too low of a weight) BMI have been shown to increase risks and worsen surgical outcomes. The data on the issues for high and low BMI continue to confirm this finding. More and more doctors and hospitals will not operate on high BMI patients because of the added risks and poor outcomes. Also, it is very important to remember that being overweight does not by itself mean you are well nourished. There are overweight people who are malnourished (low protein levels, poor vitamin intake, and missing vital nutrients). BMI is only one measure of relative body weigh and a blunt measure of health. Some people look more at ratios of muscle to fat, fat under the skin (pinch test), and bone density, as well as other blood tests like vitamins B and D, albumen levels, liver functions, cholesterol, lipids, blood sugar, A1c, and thyroid function as a better way to make a nutritional health assessment.

High Blood Sugars (Diabetes) and High Blood Pressure

When the blood sugars are high, there is reduced healing and increased numbers of infections. Chronic elevated sugar levels in diabetics destroys the eyes and kidneys as well as other organs. It decreases bone healing and increases overall complications. If the longer-term measures of high sugars, like an A1C levels over 8 or fructosamine levels over 293 are relatively strong contraindications (along with high BMI over 40 or low BMI under 18) to many orthopaedic procedures. Similarly high blood pressure can cause heart strain, heart attacks, and strokes. Stress of surgery and postop pain can add to the base line pressures and increase the risks of all three.

"WHY AM I IN PAIN?"

For anyone contemplating either what they'll feel if they get an injury or what they'll feel with surgery, one of the greatest fears is how much pain they will feel. However, as hard as it may be to believe, pain can be a necessary, protective, and valuable part of our experience as human beings.

24 WHY AM I IN PAIN?

HOW DO YOU KNOW NOT TO TOUCH A HOT STOVE OR THAT YOU NEED GLOVES WHEN it's cold out? The not-so-surprising answer is pain. Often a prior experience of pain and the desire to avoid that pain again drives the behavior. Pain teaches us how to navigate the world and the lessons are long-lasting. As a result of the pain experience, you pull your hand off a hot pot before a bad burn occurs and come in from the cold before frostbite sets in. Pain also tells you when you have a cut or a broken bone or you ate something that went bad days ago. These events "hurt," and we don't forget it.

Nerves "Feel" Pain

Mother Nature has created nerves that "feel" pain. These special nerves are called "pain fibers." Pain is the way your brain understands the signals from those specific nerves. Your brain then stores these memories to stop you from repeating the painful event. So, there is a learned reason for pain every time you experience it. From the time you are a baby, you are constantly learning what hurts and what doesn't. Hence, the old joke—and it's true—you say, "It hurts when I do that." And your doctor says, "So don't do it."

Pain Has Many Benefits
It helps the body release special chemicals that are needed for healthy healing. Pain also tells us when we are overdoing it. In addition, pain is an early warning system for most medical complications. Using too much pain medication can override Mother Nature's messages. Therefore, masking pain completely with a drug is never ideal. It can lead to failure of fracture repair, increased swelling, and delayed healing and make your doctor miss potential complications of an injury or surgery. So pain can be very helpful in healing properly.

When you are injured, the pain should be addressed by first fixing the reason for the pain: stop the activity that hurts, cast the fracture, stitch the cut, fix the bone, or start an antibiotic. Then we can use treatments to decrease the pain at the source, like anti-inflammatories for inflammation or elevation and ice for swelling. Narcotics are never the only treatment for pain, and narcotic medications should never mask pain so completely that your own body's ways of helping you heal cannot work properly. A dog never walks on a broken paw until it stops hurting. Only people take possibly addicting medications so they can walk, run, work, or drive while having a painful limb that is still broken.

Still, after an injury or surgery, pain medications are often prescribed to soften the pain experience while allowing for healing. Pain medication can help get people moving after an injury, and often guided movement has great benefits. Therefore, we don't want to have too much pain and at the same time no one wants their doctor to miss the early signs of a preventable complication because of too much medication.

Anxiety, stress, fear, muscle spasm, swelling, and not resting or elevating an injured body part can all worsen pain. Fortunately, stress, anxiety, and muscle spasm can be treated with nonnarcotic medications. For each problem, the full choice of treatments should be considered before increasing or continuing a narcotic in place of solving the real problem. This is call "multimodal pain management." Loosely, it means approaching pain from many directions.

Whether the patient is an adult or a child, it is important to have family or friends become part of the team to help you deal with pain from an injury or surgery. When you go to a medical appointment, bring someone along to make the plan with your doctor, and to help you stick to the plan once you are home.

As doctors, our goal is to help Mother Nature do its job and not help our patients hurt themselves more by overmedicating them. Always choose appropriate treatments over narcotic pain medicine as a first choice, and help us stop the national narcotic addiction epidemic! We can only do it together.

Opioids or Narcotic Pain Medications

Here are some examples of so called opioid or narcotic pain medications: morphine, Vicodin (hydrocodone), Percocet (oxycodone), codeine, Oxycontin, Dilaudid, Tylenol with codeine, tramadol, and others. Approximately 100 people die in the US per day from drug overdoses. Sometimes patients use alcohol, THC (marijuana products), and/or sleeping pills at the same time. This also increases the risks of an overdose.

Not using these medications when they are not the best choice for a problem is our first step to saving these lives. The US uses the vast majority of the world's oral narcotic (opioid) medications, and we are only 5% of the world's population.

---

25 WHAT TO TELL YOUR MD AND WHY

HELP REDUCE YOUR RISKS OF COMPLICATIONS DURING AND AFTER SURGERY.
Sometimes, despite your best efforts to maintain bone health and avoid injury, you may find yourself with a problem that can't be fixed by any treatment except surgery. You can take an active role in the surgery planning process by providing your doctor with the details of your medical history. If you are about to have surgery, consider making this simple **ABCD** list on paper based on your medical history and bring it to your pre-op appointment. **It will help you and your doctor avoid unwanted complications.**

Think of A, B, C, and D:

There are many things that are critical to know before you have surgery and all of them are for your safety. Prior problems with breathing, asthma, or sleep apnea are important to note if the anesthesiologist is to help you breathe while you are sleeping. In short, your airway is very important if you are going to be under anesthesia for the procedure.

Your doctor needs to know if you have a bleeding issue or a clotting problem. Your heart must be in good condition to pump blood and medications to the parts of the body that need them. It is important to know your medications and your drug allergies. Lasty, we need to know if you are at risk for not healing because of poor nutrition. To help my patients, I have a simple A, B, C, and D mnemonic to remember all of these important issues.

- "A" is for Airway and Allergies.

- "B" is for Bleeding or forming Blood clots too easily.

- "C" is for Cardiac and Circulation.

- "D" is for Drugs and Diet—the drugs you take every day even if they are "over the counter" or "natural" supplements, as well as your overall nutritional status.

"A"—Airway and Allergies

Patients don't always remember to share relevant information in this category because asthmatics often don't think of themselves as being sick, sleep apnea patients often don't like using their CPAP machines, and smokers often are not aware how that habit affects post-op healing, infections, or lung complications. However, sleep apnea can be made worse by narcotics, and the risk of **serious breathing problems** (even some rare but avoidable post-op deaths) is heightened with the combination of sleep apnea, narcotics, and obesity. Your doctor needs to know if you have any of these issues.

Make sure you tell your doctor exactly what happens with a medication you think you may be allergic to. Remember, **reactions or side effects** and **allergies** are not the same. Total body hives and difficulty breathing are commonly results of a true allergy; stomach upset, dizziness, being tired, and constipation are not. For example, one of my patients had written down they were allergic to calcium. The reason was that they became constipated after taking it. But we all know there is calcium in every bone in your body, making it extremely unlikely (actually it's impossible) that this was a true allergy.

When we ask for a history of allergies, our patients' answers range from "none" to a good number of medications, foods, and other items. For your doctor's purposes, we are interested in those things your immune system reacts to strongly. The reason for our concern is the body's ability to release factors that can close your throat, block your breathing, and put you in real danger. If a medication gives you an upset stomach or a yeast infection, that is an important fact. However, these are still just adverse reactions, not true allergies.

Another common complaint is the patient's belief that they have a Novocain allergy. This is the result of a reaction that includes palpitations (an increased heart rate) or a red, warm, and fully flushed face after use of Novocain at the dentist's office. The palpitations happen because there is epinephrine in the preparation the dentist uses to make the Novocain last longer. The epinephrine will increase your heart rate if injected near a blood vessel. Epinephrine is the same as adrenaline and can be used to save your life if your heart stops or your pressure drops during surgery. Also, epinephrine is the drug of choice for an acute allergy that antihistamines cannot control. This is why children with allergies to bee stings or peanuts usually carry "Epipens." Here too, because of the important medical uses of epinephrine, there is a very good reason to distinguish between a reaction like palpitations or flushed face with adrenaline use and a true allergy.

"B"—Bleeding/Clotting Issues

Do you have a history of bleeding problems, with both easy clotting and easy bruising or not clotting, especially during a prior surgery? A family history of easy bleeding or one of forming too many blood clots can be equally important. There are genetic disorders like hemophilia and von Willebrand's disease that prevent clotting. Other disorders, like factor V Leiden and protein S deficiency, cause too many clots. Surgeons tend to lump bleeding problems and risk of blood clots together. This confuses some patients. We always worry about the more common problems of blood clots, vein clots in the legs, and preventing fatal embolisms and, as a result, we often spend less time on the history of too much bleeding than talking about too much clotting. Your doctor needs to know about both types of problem. Patients with a history of cancer or who are undergoing cancer treatment also have bleeding issues. Those with low platelet counts can bleed more easily, and some cancers can increase clotting risks.

"C"—Cardiac and Circulation

These include problems and medications including treatment for high blood pressure or hypertension (HTN), abnormal heart rhythms, heart failure, prior cardiac surgery, various veins, or phlebitis. To confuse things more, your MD may ask a question that could have two meanings. For example, sometimes we ask, "Do you have high blood pressure?" and the patient say, "No" because their pressure is normal at that moment. But we notice Lopressor, a medication used to treat high blood pressure, is in their history intake form. When asked again, the patient will say, "I used to have high blood pressure, but my doctor has treated it, so I don't have it now." Your doctor should know all of the conditions you are being treated for, even if the symptoms are treated, controlled with medications, and you are currently not having problems or symptoms (asymptomatic).

"D"—Drugs and Diet

Your doctor should know the drugs you take every day, including "natural" products, hormones, insulin, steroids, and thyroid replacements. As strange as this sounds, in my office patients have written down on their medical history form that they are diabetic, but don't indicate they need insulin daily. Asthmatics use inhalers for breathing but don't think that the contents of the inhaler are medications since they are not in pill form. Thyroid replacement is just a hormone to some. To these patients, and many others with chronic diseases, using "natural" substances like thyroid replacement and insulin are just part of routine life. In any case, your doctor still needs to know you are using them.

Diet represents a window into your overall ability to heal, so your doctor should also know your nutritional status. Patients with poor nutrition and low body weight cannot make all the proteins needed for healing and are at higher risks for infection, bruising, slow wound healing, or an inability to heal from surgery. Similarly, those with high body weight are also at risk for more complications, including prolonged healing time, risks of not healing, lung infections (pneumonia), water on the lungs (atelectasis), wound infection, and blood clots.

Diabetes and Diabetic control are also important when thinking about reducing risks of complications, wound healing, bone healing, and infection rates. Blood sugars should be well controlled and A1C should be under 8 (some researchers say even less than 7.4) and fructosamine, if measured, should be under 293 to reduce these risks.

So, the best advice to all patients before surgery is to take some time before your pre-op exam and think about some simple A's, B's, C's, and D's for good measure. Look at the list and write the answers down. Bring it to the appointment and share it with your primary provider, your surgeon, and their medical staff. The small changes your doctor may make by knowing something important on this list can make a difference.

APPENDIX IA: KNEE ANATOMY

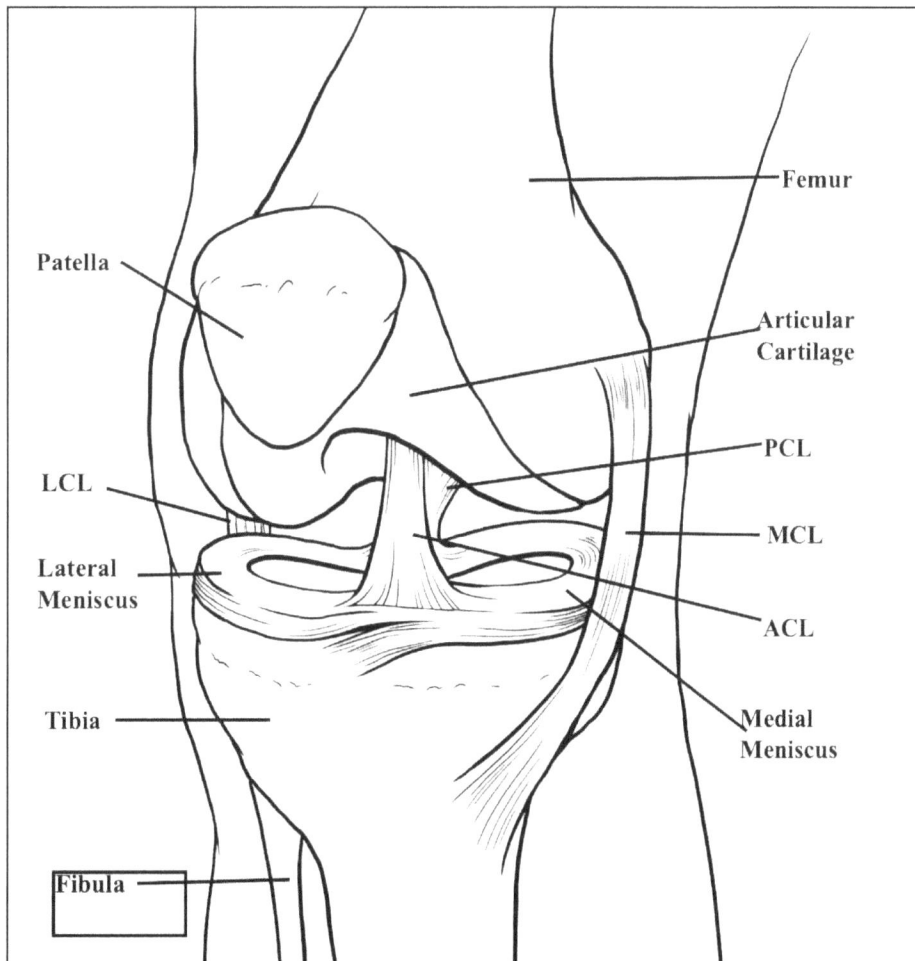

A1.1 Knee Anatomy

APPENDIX 1B: SHOULDER ANATOMY

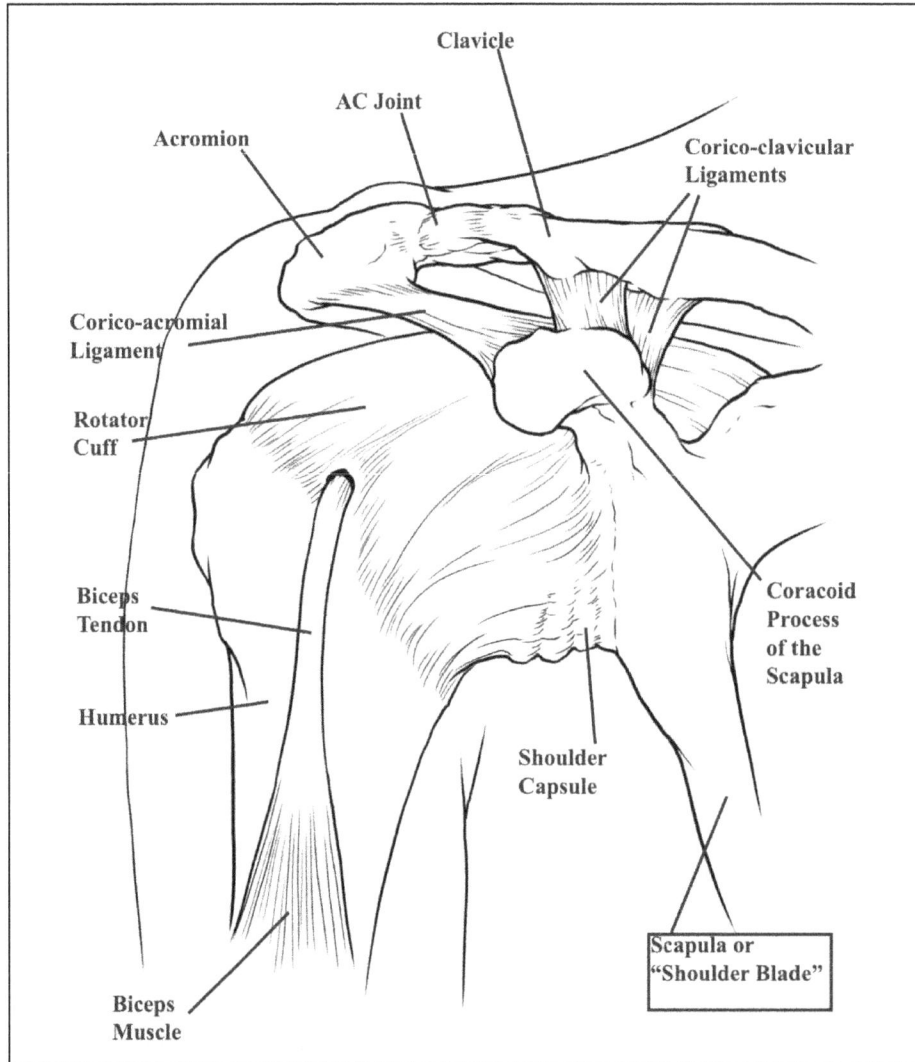

Clavicle

AC Joint

Acromion

Corico-clavicular Ligaments

Corico-acromial Ligament

Rotator Cuff

Biceps Tendon

Humerus

Biceps Muscle

Coracoid Process of the Scapula

Shoulder Capsule

Scapula or "Shoulder Blade"

A1.2 Shoulder Anatomy

APPENDIX II: PHYSICAL THERAPY

Most conditions result in some weakness and most surgeries require restoration of muscle tone after a repair of any type. There are many specific therapy protocols that are designed for non-operative treatment of many common problems (tendonitis, bursitis, tennis elbow, kneecap pain, and muscle weakness). After surgery the physical therapy is much more specific. Here are some simple, safe exercises that can be used early on after many surgeries or for simple problems in the knee and shoulder (like quads weakness after a knee contusion or sprain, and range of motion for mild frozen shoulder or tendonitis).

Leg Exercises

These are simple exercises to start with right after surgery. The goal is to decrease swelling, wake up your muscles, prevent too much scar tissue from forming, and prevent blot clots. Many of these can be done two to three times a day.

Ankle Pumps
Pump your ankle up and down for one minute as if you were pressing down on the gas pedal of a car. Switch to the other ankle (see Images A2.1 and A2.2 on page 172). Please do ankle pumps (a set of 10 reps) each hour while you're awake. Alternatively, if you're watching TV, do them during every commercial break. This exercise will help decrease swelling, increase circulation, and reduce your risk of developing a blood clot. You cannot overdo ankle pumps.

Straight Leg Raises (and Quad Sets)
While lying flat on your back, bend the good leg to protect your lower back and tighten your quadriceps on the injured side (the muscle in front of your thigh), and then raise your straight leg 8 to 12 inches off the bed (or the floor if you do these on the ground) (see Images A2.3 and A2.4 on page 172).

It's important to know that your brain naturally and subconsciously shuts the quads off to protect the knee. Waking up the quads muscle is key to a faster recovery. It is important to tighten the quads first by using them to pull your kneecap up toward your hip before doing the leg lift. This will remind the muscle how to work more normally. If you cannot recall what your knee should do (this happens all the time—the protection instinct is so strong in some people), work the quads on the uninjured side first, do a set of 10, and then alternate sides. Do three sets of 10 on each side.

Range of Motion
Sit on a chair. Place your foot on the floor (remove your immobilizer and set aside). Place the uninjured foot under the ankle of the surgical leg. Letting the uninjured side do the work, bring your leg into a straight position. Then, from that position, gently bring the foot down, bending at the knee. Again, do three sets of 10.

Knee Bends/Heel Slides
Lying flat with your heel on the bed, bend your knee while sliding your heel toward you (see Images A2.5, A2.6, and A2.7 on page 173). At first, the bending may be 20-0 degrees, but in time

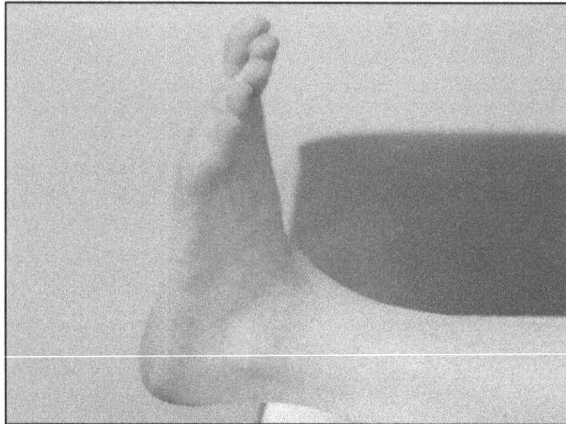

A2.1 Foot ankle pumps foot flexion

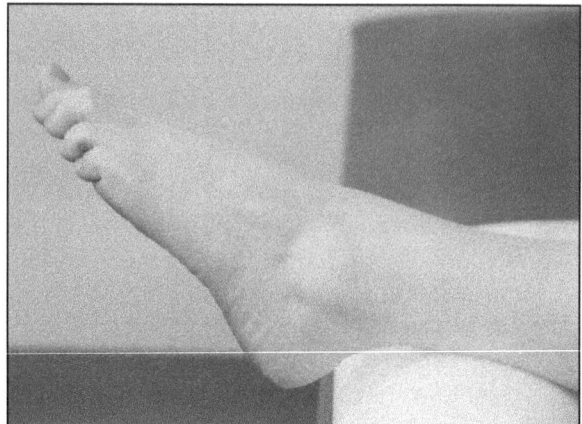

A2.2 Foot ankle pumps foot extension

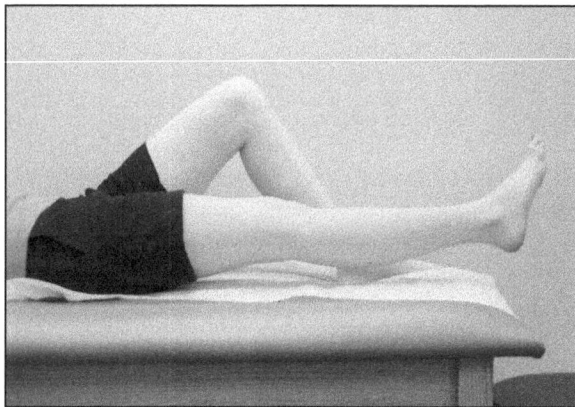

A2.3 Leg lift (straight leg raise) low position

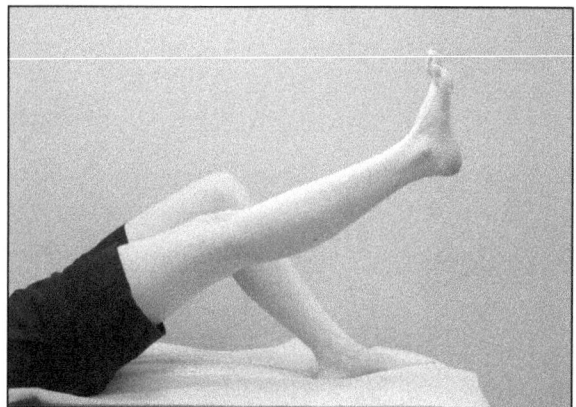

A2.4 Leg lift (straight leg raise) high position

it will increase as pain and comfort allow. Do these 10 times, rest for a minute, and repeat two more times.

Leg-ups

Lie on your back, lift your leg, and flex your hip 90 degrees. You can use your hands to stabilize your thigh when the hip is at 90 degrees (the whole leg is pointed to the ceiling). Let the leg bend at the knee as far as it will go comfortably and then slowly kick the lower leg back upwards, straightening the knee without moving the hip (see Images A2.8 and A2.9). As you move from a bent knee with the hip flexed to a straighter knee with the hip flexed, your hamstrings will act as resistance for your quads (just like a Bowflex machine). Go as far as comfort allows and repeat for 10 reps. Do the other side and alternate for three sets on each side.

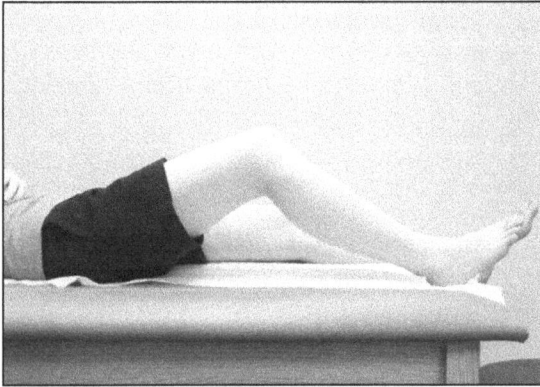
A2.5 Heal slide starting position

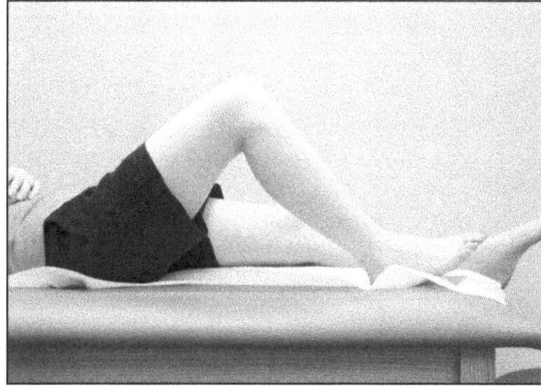
A2.6 Heal slide mid position

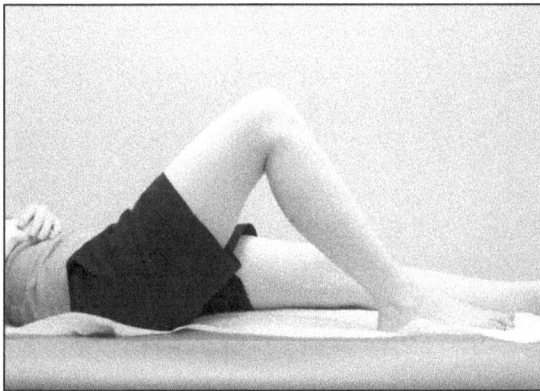
A2.7 Heal slide full bend

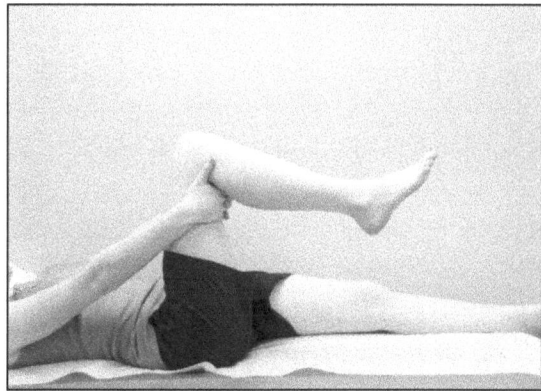
A2.8 Leg up starting position

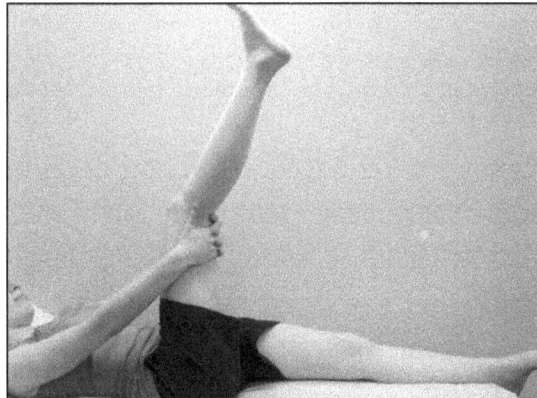
A2.9 Leg up elevation position

Arm Exercises

These are simple exercises to start with right after surgery to decrease swelling, wake up your muscles, and prevent too much scar tissue from forming. Your shoulder can get stiff in the post-operative period, so simple motion early on (depending on the surgery done; for example, larger rotator cuff repairs need to start moving more slowly in a limited way) can help avoid stiffness and a frozen shoulder after surgery. Many of these can be done two to three times a day.

Hand Squeezes/Grip Strengthening

Using a small soft rubber ball or soft sponge, squeeze your hand. When in the shower, you can use a sponge filled with water. Three sets of 12 works nicely. If this is too easy, you can try using a grip strengthener (see Images A2.10 and A2.11).

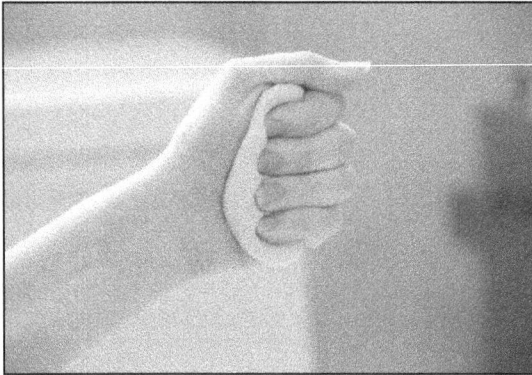

A2.10 Squeezing soft sponge or foam ball

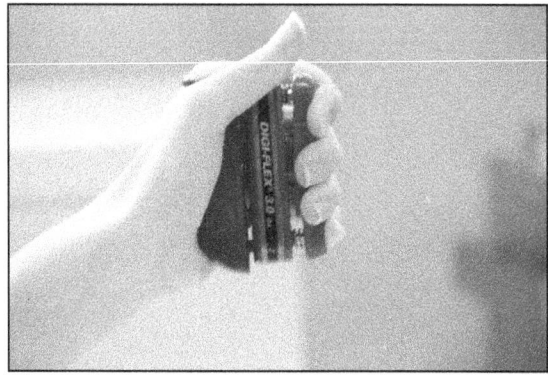

A2.11 Grip-strengthening device

Wrist Range of Motion

Roll your wrist in circles for 30 seconds after each round of grip exercises. Do this on each side three times a day.

Elbow Range of Motion

Turning your palm inward, toward your stomach; flex and extend the elbow as comfort allows (see Images A2.12 and A2.13). This will decrease pain and prevent elbow stiffness. Do three sets of 10.

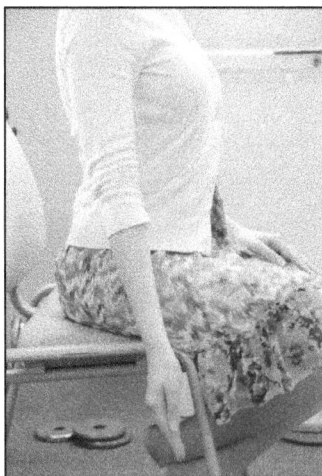

A2.12 Elbow ROM extension

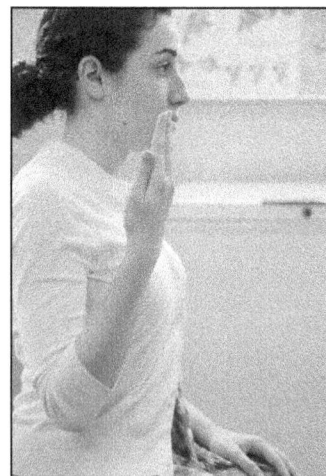

A2.13 Elbow ROM flexion

Pendulum Exercise

Holding the side of a table or chair with your good arm, bend over at the waist, and let the affected arm hang down. Swing the arm back and forth like a pendulum. Then swing in small circles and slowly make them larger (see Images A2.14 and A2.15). Do one direction for a count of 10 Mississippis, then the other direction. Do three times in each direction.

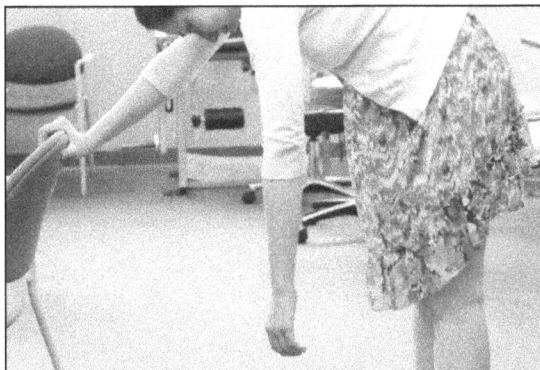

A2.14 Pendulum exercise

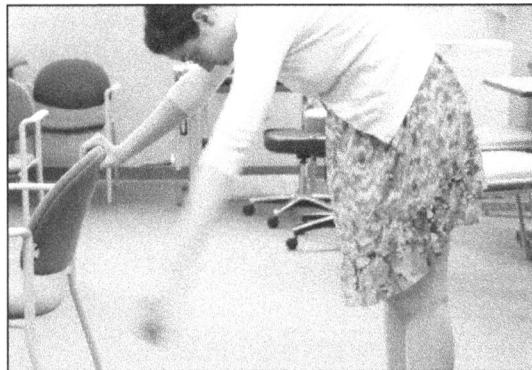

A2.15 Pendulum exercise

Wall Walking

Stand facing a blank wall with your feet about 12 inches away. "Walk" the fingers of the affected hand up the wall as high as comfort allows (see Images A2.16 and A2.17). Mark the spot and try to go higher each time. Facing the wall first and with your body close (12–18 inches away), try to do it five times up and down the first day, then add a rep each day until you do 10 reps.

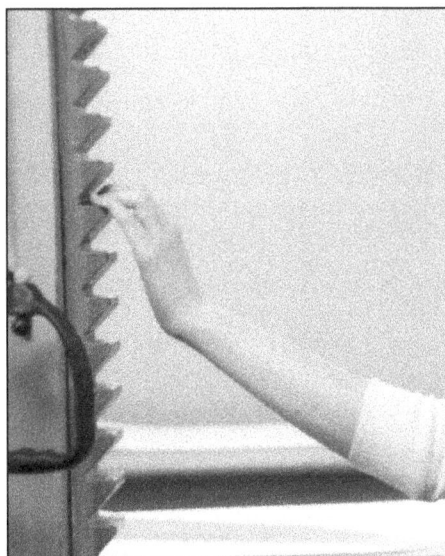

A2.16 Wall walk ladder to help with elevation of arm and protect rotator cuff repair, low position

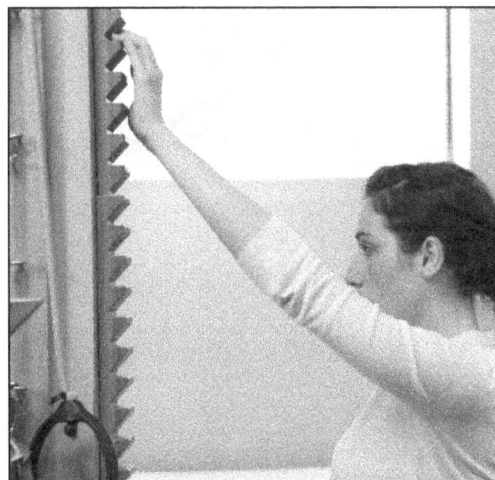

A2.17 Wall walk ladder to help with elevation of arm and protect rotator cuff repair, high position

When you feel more comfortable and are stronger (not before three weeks), do these exercises further from the wall. Then eventually do them while standing sideways to the wall, with the affected side facing the wall.

Do not let the hand drop down from the wall—you must walk your fingers down as well as up. Dropping the arm will strain the repair and be painful. If you feel weak on the way down, feel free to use the other arm to help move it down slowly in a controlled way.

Biceps Curls

Curl the arm up and down 12 times; rest for one minute and repeat for a total of three sets of 12. When comfortable, try it while holding a very small can. In a few days, you can increase the size of the can, but only as comfort allows. This exercise should not be painful. If painful, decrease the size of or eliminate the can.

Wrist Flexion and Extension

Flex and extend your wrist to reduce stiffness and decrease arm swelling (see Images A2.18 and A2.19). Do this whenever you think of it. Stretch your fingers, too. If the hand is swollen, use a hand cream and massage the swelling out at least once a day.

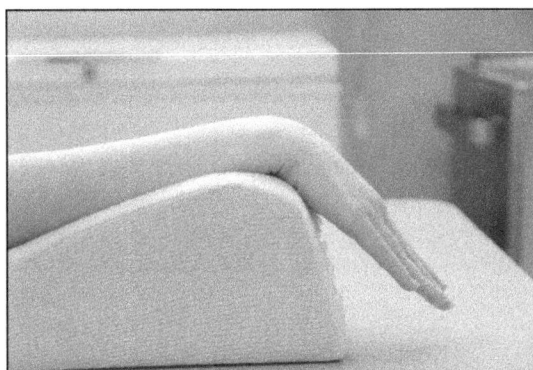

A2.18 Wrist flexion

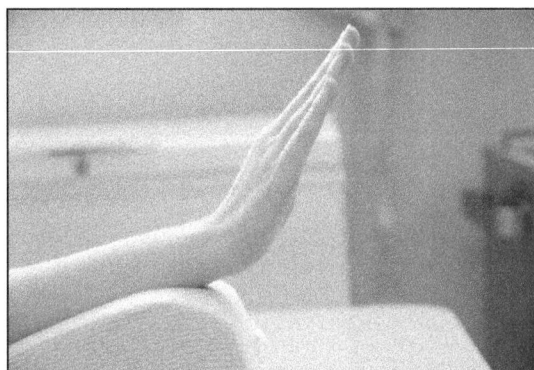

A2.19 Wrist extension

APPENDIX III: Q&A WITH DR. REZNIK

Having an orthopaedic problem requiring surgery is not an everyday event for most patients yet preforming surgery is very familiar to your doctor. Sometimes we take this fact for granted. At the same time, missing an opportunity to ask important questions is an equally common problem. When you are told you need surgery, the brain just turns off. Worse, some patients have asked so many questions before surgery they don't remember the answers. Later, patients recall all the questions they wanted to ask. Many of my patients have found ways to ask these questions. An equal number of other patients are afraid to ask them. This is when giving a written version of frequent Q&As to the patient helps.

How do I know when it's time to see a doctor?
When there is persistent pain with activity; an acute injury with any deformity at all; recurrent swelling of any joint; locking, buckling, or giving way; or an inability to use the limb.

Is surgery always the best option?
No. Many times nonsurgical treatments can solve the problem, even those that seem complicated. A good diagnosis (knowing exactly what is wrong) is very important.

Is surgery painful?
When surgery is needed, it is done with an anesthetic, so there is no pain during surgery. After surgery, Novocain, ice, and pain medication should help you throughout the early post-op period and while you are doing physical therapy. Pain at times stimulates an inflammatory response that is required for healing. It also stops us from doing too much after surgery. To better understand the natural function of the postoperative pain response, read the section on why we have pain.

Will there still be pain after surgery?
At first, there is always postsurgical soreness, stiffness, and swelling. Following your doctor's instructions is very important. Elevating the limb means keeping it above the heart, and using crutches means using crutches all the time when up and about. If you cheat on the instructions, you only cheat yourself of the value of your doctor's experience. In other words, you can't outsmart Mother Nature.

What time is my surgery?
The surgical facility decides the schedule. This is usually done on the day before surgery, and surgery times are set up to accommodate special medical conditions. Therefore, people with medical conditions and small children usually get earlier operating times.

Will I have to stay overnight?
Most arthroscopic surgeries are done on an outpatient basis. This means you will go home the same day if your procedure can be done arthroscopically (as the majority of procedures described in this book are done).

Will I be awake during the surgery?
Most surgeries are done under light general anesthesia along with a local anesthetic to the operative area. (This will help provide comfort after surgery.) Therefore, you will not be truly

awake during surgery. Some patients' surgeries can be done with sedation and a local anesthetic. Many of these patients will be awake and even talking during the surgery. Alas, many of the anesthetic agents affect short-term memory, and patients cannot remember a word of what they said or the procedure itself. Even if you were "awake" for your surgery, you may still be drowsy upon discharge and will need someone to drive you home. You cannot drive yourself under any circumstances.

Should I take my daily medications the morning of surgery?
If your primary care physician decides that you should take your medication in the morning, you may do so with a tiny sip of water. Please check with your doctor at your pre-op clearance exam. This is particularly important for patients with high blood pressure (also called hypertension, or HTN) or diabetes. People with high blood pressure should, as a rule, take their medication. Diabetics will not be eating before surgery and typically don't take their medications before surgery, but this is decided on a case-by-case basis.

When can I shower?
I let my patients remove the dressings and shower after 48 hours with most arthroscopic surgeries. Patients with larger incisions, such as those who have had an ACL reconstruction, Fulkerson procedure, AC joint reconstruction, or clavicle repair, will have the dressing removed at their first physical therapy appointment. Those patients can shower after the dressing is changed but need to keep the incision dry.

When can I drive?
In general, you must be off all pain medications and be able to bear full weight on the affected leg if you had knee surgery before you can drive a car. If you've had shoulder surgery, you must be completely out of the sling and be able to easily place your hands at the 12:00 position on the steering wheel and move them freely from the 9:00 to 3:00 positions.

When do I start physical therapy?
Physical therapy generally starts the third to fifth day after surgery. You should schedule the first several physical therapy appointments at your pre-op appointment with your doctor.

When can I return to work?
It will depend on the type of surgery that you had, as well as the type of work you perform. Your doctor will review your work status at your first post-op visit.

How soon can I return to sports after surgery?
For meniscal injuries, it depends on if you are having a repair or removal of a torn fragment. For repairs, I usually don't let patients return to competitive sports for at least four months, and then only if they wear a brace; the repair takes at least four months to be 80% healed. If the cartilage was removed and not repaired, then it's usually okay to exercise after six weeks, but a lot of prep is required before you play soccer. Remember, soccer, football, rugby, and basketball are the toughest sports on your knee after surgery.

When can I return to sports after ACL reconstruction?
For ACL tears, this is one of the most asked questions, and no one likes the answer. The ACL is reconstructed using a tendon graft from any number of sources. The key word here is "reconstructed." The tendon is moved to the site, and once harvested, the graft tissue has no blood

supply. Therefore, the body must heal the tendon to the bone and then grow new blood vessels into the new ligament. The bone may heal to the tendon in two to three months, but the creation of new blood vessels takes much longer. In fact, the tendon graft gets softer as this occurs, and you are at a higher risk of reinjury between three and six months after the surgery.

If all pain and swelling is gone, patients can start with a fast walk at six weeks, and soon after, a light jog, and can run in a straight line with no cutting (no sharp turns) on a soft track. I let my patients use a bike, swim (with no whip kick), use an elliptical trainer, and treadmill after three months. Some can go back to light sports with a brace on after six months.

In general, ACL patients must wait nine months or more to play heavy sports (soccer, basketball, football, etc.). At nine months, they can start sports-specific training, and at one year, they can usually return to a full competitive or contact level. This sounds long, but cheating this time line creates a high risk of reinjury and the need for a second surgery.

How can I prevent reinjury?

For patients with ACL tears, the fear of reinjury is probably the second biggest concern. To prevent this, many of my patients return to play with an ACL brace on, even after the ACL is reconstructed with a good clinical result. Many will give up the brace in time, but some need the extra comfort and use a custom ACL sports brace for all sports and heavy activity.

Patients with poor jumping style (known as a valgus collapse; described in the section on ACL tears) or poor hip control/balance need to work on these skills before returning to any sport.

Is it better to repair or cut out the torn part of my meniscus?

It is better to save the parts of the meniscus that can be repaired. In general, it is best to repair the menisci of younger patients with tears in the zone with the best blood supply.

There is a balance between saving the meniscus and the success of the repair. If a repair has a 90% chance of failing, it should not be done and vice versa; if there is a good chance the tear will heal, it should be repaired.

Will my meniscus ever grow back?

The meniscus does not truly grow back; although some scar will form at times, it never has the weight-bearing capability of the original meniscus.

More Frequently Asked Surgery Questions

Many other questions pertaining to planning for surgery are more specific to the actual procedure, preoperative evaluation, and some logistical details. Here are some more common questions.

Where will my surgery be performed?

With minimally invasive techniques, modern anesthesia methods, and local anesthesia for postoperative pain relief, most of the procedures in this book are done on an outpatient basis in a hospital or surgery center. A surgery center is the most frequent location for arthroscopic surgery.

Will I have to stay overnight?

Almost all arthroscopic surgeries are done on an outpatient basis. This means that you will go home the same day, usually within hours after the procedure. If you go to a hospital for a larger procedure like a total knee replacement and are healthy, frequently you will go home the same day.

What if I have a lot of anxiety about having surgery and cannot sleep?

To be a little anxious before surgery is normal. Yet, if dreadful thoughts cause you to lose sleep, you should talk to your doctor. Some people associate surgery with a prior bad experience or even a bad outcome within their own family. Some people have had more major procedures and have "sailed through them" only to be a nervous wreck for something more minor. Some people let the tension build up to the point of added stress. Think about why you feel this way and ask questions about the concerns. If you need some help reducing the anxiety and know why you have it, medications can be used before surgery to help. Anxiety also increases pain perception, so if you are less anxious, you will have less pain after surgery.

What time is my surgery?

The surgical facilities usually decide the schedule. This is done the day before surgery, and surgery times are set up to accommodate any special medical condition. Small children and people with diabetes get preference. Sometimes special equipment is required, and the surgical timing may be related to the availability of the equipment.

Do I need to see my primary care physician before surgery?

At many surgical centers, if you are over 40 years old or have any health problems, you will need to have a pre-op clearance exam with your primary doctor. This will include a physical exam and a review of any current medical conditions and medications. An EKG, chest X-ray, and bloodwork will also be done. Patients under age 40 who are in good health will often only need simple bloodwork done.

Advise your surgeon of all medical conditions and medications you may be taking prior to surgery (see the section on what to tell your doctor and why on page 178). If you have a history of diabetes, smoking, sleep apnea, or abnormal bleeding or clotting, you must tell your surgeon before surgery. No one wants to be surprised in the operating room about something you have been ignoring and hoping will just go away.

What should I wear/not wear to surgery?

You should wear loose-fitting, comfortable clothing that will fit over bulky dressings—loose, elastic-waist shorts, baggy gym pants for knee surgery, and a loose-fitting, button-down type of shirt if you are having shoulder surgery. Do not wear jewelry, fingernail polish, or contact lenses.

Can I eat or drink anything before surgery?

Many hospitals and surgery centers have varying rules about when to stop eating and drinking before surgery. Many online advice websites say its ok to eat or drink something before surgery and then give a set of rules to follow. It's been my experience that few patients get this right. A mistake leaves the patient with acid in their stomach and an increased risk of aspiration of those acids into the lungs. These patients have their surgery cancelled that day for their own safety. Plans were all in place and now everyone is upset. The simplest rules for eating are the best. Except for absolutely required medications, DO NOT have anything to eat or drink after midnight. This means nothing, no coffee, milk, juices, or water. (Most surgery centers will call you before surgery to review your medications, health issues, the medications you should take the day of surgery, and the ones you should not take the day of surgery.)

Should I take my daily medications the morning of surgery?

If your primary care physician advised you to take your medication in the morning, you may do so with a tiny sip of water (the only exception to eating and drinking the day of surgery). Please check with your doctor at your pre-op clearance exam. This is particularly important for patients with high blood pressure (hypertension) or diabetes. Many centers will have a nurse call you to review these medications and point out which are needed before surgery and which ones to avoid until after surgery.

When can I shower?

You may remove the dressings and shower after 48 hours after most arthroscopic surgeries. Surgeries with larger incisions such as an ACL, a Fulkerson procedure (tibial tubercle transfer), or a clavicle repair will have the dressing removed at their first physical therapy appointment. Those patients can shower after the dressing is changed but need to keep the incision dry.

When can I drive?

In general, you must be off all pain medications. For knee patients, you must be able to bear full weight on the affected leg. You have to be able to step on the brake without hesitation. If you cannot, you can be held liable in an accident. For shoulder patients, you must be off pain meds and completely out of the sling and can easily place your hands at the 12:00 position on the steering wheel and move your hands freely from the 9:00 to the 3:00 position without pain or hesitation.

When do I start physical therapy?

Physical therapy generally starts the third to fifth day after surgery. Some more complex procedures may be braced, slinged, or splinted for a week, three weeks, or more before therapy starts.

When can I return to work?

It will depend on the type of surgery that you had as well as the type of work you perform. Your doctor should review your work status at your first post-op appointment.

APPENDIX IV: MAKING THE MOST OF YOUR OFFICE VISIT

We all know that a visit to the doctor is not always a stress-free experience. Doctors are busier than ever these days, and it sometimes takes a while just to get an appointment. Patients are much busier too. We respect that you have less time to spend waiting to see the doctor, and it can be hard to find a good time for the visit. Still, the office is a tricky and unpredictable adventure. No matter how hard we try to get it just right, we can be ahead or behind schedule in an instant.

For instance, there is an accident on the highway that clears. Three people now are late, three come early, and in a matter of minutes we are five or six patients behind. A patient goes to the wrong office by mistake, and we try to add them back in for an appointment because they took the day off. Sometimes a little kindness is great but that can delay others. **A patient has forgotten to say something medically important until the visit is nearly done or introduce a new problem that is more serious when the visit is just ending.** They don't know that it changes the entire plan and that may need a much bigger discussion.

Of course, people never break a bone or tear something on a schedule, so there are always emergencies to be added in. We leave time for these, but the accidents don't always match the slots. Nonetheless we do the best we can, and those of you who have received a courtesy or two over the years understand how helpful it was for us to be a little flexible on our end. We only ask you to remember that we are always trying our best to help people in a timely way when we are ahead or behind or ask you to move an appointment to help accommodate an emergency surgery or make both our days smooth.

Once you arrive for your appointment, you will frequently find the waiting room a busy place. Many times, there is more than one doctor working, there is physical therapy going on, and there is the occasional person there to meet with our business staff. The waiting room often does not match up with your doctor's schedule, so don't panic. In addition, there are usually several forms you will need to complete, including a patient medical history form and insurance information. Sometimes you can do a number of these online before you come. That helps, too. Remember, if you need the information sent to an outside person you will need a HIPAA release form signed at the front desk when you make that request. Without the signed release form, we cannot send it. It is the law!

OK, So Relax!

All things considered, my nurses and medical assistants will tell you that patients who prepare for their visits seem to have a better overall experience. Planning in advance can save you time and make your visit more pleasant.

Here are some tips to make your visit less stressful and more productive:

- When making your first appointment with the doctor, ask if the new patient forms can be faxed or mailed or emailed to you, or see if you can do them online so you can complete them at home prior to your visit. Check out our website (www.ct-ortho.com) to see the type of information available to help you with your first visit.

- Sometimes if you make an appointment for a new problem or after a long absence (more than one year), you will be asked to complete a new medical history form, even if you are not a new patient. Some patients find completing these forms inconvenient, but they play an important role in your visit.

- If you are not able to fill out the forms ahead of time, try to arrive 15 minutes early for your appointment so you can complete the paperwork (or now computer/tablet work) without feeling rushed.

- If you find the waiting room full when you arrive, don't be afraid to ask if the doctor is running behind or how long you may be expected to wait. The doctor may have had an emergency or several unexpectantly complicated patients that have put him behind schedule. We understand that you may be on a time constraint and will do our best to adhere to the doctor's schedule. If you have a particular issue, like a child waiting at home or getting out of school soon, let the staff know.

- Be sure to fill out the medical history form completely. Some of the questions might seem irrelevant to you, such as, "Are you right- or left-handed?" "What is your height and weight?" (Many patients leave this one blank!) and "What are your occupation and job duties?" However, all this information is important when the doctor needs to determine things like your ability to return to work or school, appropriate medication dosages, an so forth.

- List all telephone numbers where you can be reached, as well as an emergency contact number. It is important that we have a way to reach you in case we have a question or concern.

- Be sure to note if you have any allergies. This is extremely important if the doctor needs to order any medications for you. Make sure they are allergies and not just adverse reactions like stomach upset with antibiotics; yeast infections after antibiotics; nausea, sleepiness, or dizziness after narcotics; or a racing heart rate in the dentist's office after Novocain is used with epinephrine (a heart stimulant that makes the injection last longer). These are not allergies! Hives, itching with hives, swelling in your throat, or shortness of breath requiring a trip to the hospital are true allergic reactions.

- Know what medications you are currently taking. Saying that you take "something for blood pressure" or "two small red pills" does not provide the doctor with enough information. If you can't remember, bring the medication with you, or write down the name and dosage of each medicine before you leave home.

- Please include all over-the-counter medications as well. The doctor and nurse need this information when prescribing any new medications to avoid any interactions. It is helpful to list the name and telephone number of your pharmacy in case we need to call or fax any prescriptions for you.

- What are your symptoms? Include when your symptoms began and what you were doing at the time. Be as specific as you can. Saying that you have had pain "for a long time" can mean several days to one patient and several years to another. Have you ever felt these symptoms before? What makes them better? What makes them worse? Are they better or worse after working? After waking up? Have you ever had surgery on the affected body part in the past? All this information gives the doctor important clues to help make a diagnosis.

■ Have you had any X-rays or MRI films done? If so, be sure to bring them for the doctor to review. This seems to be the most frequent source of frustration for our patients. They are often told that "the films will be sent to the office," and when they arrive, there is nothing here for the doctor to review. Most doctors' offices and diagnostic testing centers do not forward X-rays or MRI films/discs; they just send reports. If it is not one of your own doctor's imaging centers, you need to request a copy on a disc and take it with you when you leave the imaging facility, even if you were told the films would be sent to our office. In the digital age, facilities never send films. Usually they send just the report, although sometimes there can be a digital link for the actual studies. These are hit and miss. For the best diagnosis, I always read my own films and match my findings along with the report to patients' physical examination because the report alone is not ideal or adequate. It's like getting a second opinion that same day. So, if you are at an outside center that does not hook directly into your doctor's office or the hospital system that your doctor has direct access to, it is a good idea to ask for a disc to take to the visit.

■ If this is a follow-up visit, let the doctor know if your symptoms have improved, worsened, or stayed the same. If medications were given to you, did they help? Did you take them as ordered? Did you note any side effects? If physical therapy was ordered, did it help?

■ During your visit, don't be afraid to ask questions until you understand—medical jargon can be confusing! If your doctor suggests a test or a change in your treatment, ask why it's necessary and what the results will tell you. When does the doctor want to see you again?

■ If a follow-up visit is recommended, be sure to schedule it prior to leaving the office. This will allow you to book the appointment time and place that is the most convenient for you. Take an appointment card so you go to the correct office next time.

GLOSSARY

A

Achilles tendon—The strongest tendon in the body. It connects the calf muscles to the heel bone.

ACL (anterior cruciate ligament)—A ligament that connects the femur to the tibia. It helps stabilize the knee and stops the tibia from extending past the femur. The ligament controls rotation of the knee and is frequently injured in twisting and pivoting sports.

AC (acromioclavicular) joint—A joint made up of strong ligaments that connects the acromion to the clavicle.

acromion—The topmost point of the scapula. It supports the deltoid muscle and connects the shoulder blade to the clavicle.

adhesive capsulitis—Also known as "frozen shoulder." It causes the shoulder's ball and socket joint to progressively lose its range of motion. It is associated with an injury and is somewhat more common in diabetics. The joint lining (capsule) becomes inflamed and the joint stiffens, causing pain. In time, adhesions (bands of tissue) will develop between tendons and ligaments, restricting joint motion.

allograft (of cartilage or ligaments)—Pertains to cartilage or ligaments transplanted from a human donor. They are often frozen at very low temperatures for long-term storage before use. The donors are screened for diseases before the recipient accepts the donation. The grafts are held and not released until all tests are negative for infections or viruses.

ambulation—Walking. For example, "ambulatory surgery" implies walk-in and walk-out surgery, also known as outpatient surgery. Another use: "the patient currently ambulates [walks on their own] with crutches."

anesthesia—A drug that blocks nerve function, causing local numbness, general sedation, or loss of consciousness in a controlled way so that surgery can be performed without any pain. It can be "local," in which case the doctor uses an injection that numbs only the region being operated on. It can be "regional," meaning it numbs everything below the waist. It can also be a nerve block, like an axillary nerve block, which numbs a good portion of the arm, or a digital block, which numbs only a finger. Finally, it can be "general," where drugs and gases are used to keep the patient pain-free and asleep.

arthritis—A disease in which the joints become inflamed, causing pain and stiffness. There are many types of common arthritic conditions. The most common is degenerative, or the wear and tear seen over time with aging. Sometimes this has its own secondary inflammatory response. There are many other types discussed in the book related to diseases like rheumatoid arthritis, metabolic conditions like gout, and infections like Lyme disease.

arthrogram—Injecting a radiopaque substance into a joint to outline the ligaments, cartilage, and other structures in the joint. An MRI arthrogram is imaged with an MRI scanner after the injection. It is particularly useful when a ligament problem is suspected. A CT arthrogram is imaged with a CT scanner after the injection. It can be used in place of an MRI in patients who cannot have an MRI due to a pacemaker, metal in the body, or another reason.

arthroscopy—A minimally invasive surgery in which a physician can perform procedures by looking inside a joint with a fiber-optic scope.

articular cartilage—The cartilage that covers the bones in every joint and makes the surfaces smooth and low friction. It is composed of mostly Type II collagen, and unlike scar tissue, it is very well organized to optimize the joint function. See cartilage.

autograft (of cartilage or ligaments)—Transplanting cartilage or ligaments from one part of the patient's body to another.

B

biceps—A muscle that starts at the elbow and splits into two tendons. The shorter tendon (short head) ends at the coracoid process of the scapula. The larger tendon (long head) enters the shoulder joint.

biceps tenodesis—A surgical procedure in which the ruptured end of the biceps tendon is anchored to the upper end of the humerus.

biceps tendonitis—Occurs when the tendon itself is inflamed in the groove that it rides in as it exits the shoulder joint. Over time, if not treated it can lead to tearing or partial tearing of the long head of the biceps tendon.

blood clot—A mass of gelled blood cells that forms when the blood pools in an area of injury. Platelets and clotting factors combine to make a glue-like substance. It stops the bleeding. As the new tissues grow into the clot over time, it helps to form scabs and ultimately form scar tissues. Blood clotting is a normal part of healing. You cannot heal without it. At the same time, if a clot occurs inside a blood vessel because of injury to the vessel or blood pooling inside the vessel, it can block blood flow. If one occurs in a vein of the lower leg it is known as a DVT (deep vein thrombosis). There is a risk for these to break off and travel to the lung, which can cause a more serious condition called a pulmonary embolism (PE). We use ultrasound to check for DVTs when suspected and treat them with blood thinners to prevent a PE. If a PE is suspected, this is a much more serious problem, and a CT scan is needed to evaluate it and blood clot treatment can be more emergent.

bone bruise—An area of bone with increased water content visible on MRI. It can be associated with a stress fracture, overloading of the bone, an ACL tear, or stress insufficiency fracture (weak bone from osteoporosis overloaded over time).

bone spurs—Abnormal bone projections that grow off the edges of the surfaces or joints, or at tendon or ligament attachments. For example, AC joint spurs can occur in shoulder impingement or an Achilles tendon spur can occur in chronic Achilles tendonitis.

buckling (of the knee)—The knee folds or "gives way," causing the person to temporarily lose control of the leg.

bursa—A small, fluid-filled sac made of tissue. It creates surfaces for smooth motion. They are usually between soft tissues like tendons and skin or bone. They can be found under muscles as well.

C

calcified tendonitis—Occurs when calcium crystals form in a chronically irritated tendon. It can be associated with pain on motion and seen best on plain X-rays. It is much more difficult to see on an MRI. Some partial tears of the rotator cuff can be associated with calcium deposits in the substance of the tendon. This can be calcium hydroxyapatite crystals (most often in the shoulder), but it also can be calcium urate (gout). When seen with gout in the quads tendon, Achilles tendon, or patella tendon, there is a higher risk of rupture.

capsular shift procedure—Procedure done when the shoulder ligaments and shoulder capsule (lining) are stretched out of shape. The loose capsule causes increased instability of the shoulder and is tightened surgically with a capsular shift at the same time the ligaments are repaired.

cartilage—A type of connective tissue that covers joint surfaces, cushions the bones, and absorbs shock. It is composed of mostly Type II collagen, and unlike scar tissue, it is very well organized to optimize joint function. There is cartilage in your outer ear, trachea, ribs, and nose to add shape. This is very different functionally, but both have Type II collagen in them.

chondromalacia—Cracking, wear, or softening of articular cartilage in any joint. Grade 1: softening only; Grade 2: cracks in the surface; Grade 3: fissures and loss of cartilage but not down to the bone; Grade 4: complete loss to the level of the bone (no cartilage surface left). An arthritic joint can have areas of all four grades.

clavicle—The collarbone. The only bone between the shoulder joint and the axial skeleton connecting the shoulder blade to the sternum. It can be broken by direct trauma or a fall on an outstretched arm (going over the handlebars of a mountain bike, for example).

coracoacromial ligament—A ligament that connects the coracoid process of the scapula to the acromion, creating an arch with the acromion that covers the rotator cuff.

coracoid process—Part of the scapula that helps stabilize the shoulder joint. It is where the short head of the biceps attaches to the shoulder.

crepitus—The noise one can hear as crackling inside a joint with movement and pressure on the surface. It can be seen with wear of the kneecap (chondromalacia patella) especially when going down stairs or squatting.

D

degenerative tears—Tears that usually occur when cartilage weakens and thins over time. It becomes more prone to tear from simple motion. It's most commonly seen in the knee (as a partial tear of the meniscus) as we age.

dislocation—When a joint or bone slips all the way out of place.

DMARDs (disease-modifying antirheumatic drugs)—Drugs that can modify the natural destructive course of inflammatory arthritis and is responsible for a great improvement in the quality of life for patients with this disease.

distal—Describes something that is situated away from the center of the body, like limbs. The hand is distal to the elbow, the foot is distal to the knee, and the toes are distal to the ankle.

E

effusion (water in the knee)—Fluid made by the synovial lining when the knee is injured or inflamed. When the fluid fills the space of any joint, it becomes stiff and harder to move. Many times, we can drain the fluid to help diagnose the cause since infection, gout, rheumatoid arthritis, and Lyme disease are all causes. "Water on the knee" can refer to water or swelling in the prepatella bursa from kneeling too much (nursemaid's knee) and is different but can also be drained as part of the treatment.

Ehlers-Danlos syndrome— This is now known to be a group of connective tissue disorders (at least 13 subtypes) that cause the skin, joints, and ligaments to be more flexible. It is associated with scoliosis, joint looseness, arthritis, joint pain, dislocations, and aortic aneurysms. It is an autosomal genetic abnormality, meaning that specific genes are abnormal in the many variations and it is not sex linked. It happens in 1/5000 people and is often diagnosed when the person is a child or young adult.

epiphysis—Young cartilage cells lined up in columns. The columns get longer and then calcify from one direction. They are mostly radiolucent (dark) on X-ray as the majority of the growing bone is not calcified yet. Injury to the epiphysis comes in many forms. Most injuries involve the part that is softer and not calcified yet, making it harder to see a fracture or injury on an X-ray. Children must be accurately diagnosed when the growing bone is injured and treated to avoid growth arrest or deformity later in life.

F

femoral condyles—The two large bone projections that stem from the bottom of the femur and for the upper half of the knee joint. The major knee ligaments (ACL and PCL) are situated between the femoral condyles in the intercondylar notch. The lateral femoral condyle is toward the outside of the body, and the medial femoral condyle is toward the inside.

femoral notch (intercondylar notch)—The roof of the center of the knee, between the two femoral condyles. It contains the femoral attachment sites of the ACL and PCL.

femur—The thigh bone.

fracture—A crack or break in a bone. If the bone is fractured, it means there is damage to the bone whether it is displaced or not. Some fractures are considered "closed," meaning the skin is not broken. Others are considered "open," meaning the skin is broken and no longer fully covering the bone. The bone is said to be exposed. Infections occur more often with open fractures.

G

glenoid cavity (glenoid)—The shoulder socket.

glenoid labrum—The rim of tissues surrounding the glenoid cavity. It makes the surface of the socket of the shoulder wider and slightly deeper.

gout—A disease that causes inflammation of the joints because of periodic excessive uric acid in the bloodstream. The crystals of calcium urate are irritating. They are also impossible to digest, and the white cells often release a lot of joint toxic enzymes when trying to digest them.

greenstick fracture—Fracture that occurs in the middle of a child's bone, since their bones can bend without breaking.

growth plate—Softer, developing bone in growing children. Because growth plates are not calcified yet and therefore cannot be seen on X-rays, clinical judgment is required to make a diagnosis of injury in many cases. (See epiphysis page 188.)

H

hamstrings—Very large muscles behind the thigh, attached to the back of the pelvis and the tibia, crossing both the hip joint and the knee joint. Because they cross two joints they have multiple actions, including extending the hip and bending the knee. They are powerful muscles required for leg balance, walking, and running. When pulled (called a "hammy") they can hurt for months.

hemarthrosis—Bleeding into a joint. After an injury to the knee, it is associated with an ACL or ligament tear. If there are fat globules in the fluid from the knee that's bleeding, it is important to rule out a fracture or loose chip of bone in the knee. If there is blood in the knee after an injury, X-rays are required to check for fractures.

Hill-Sachs lesion—Damage to the head of the humerus that is associated with a dislocated shoulder, as the glenoid lip hits the back of the humeral head, denting the bone. Also, there is a so-called reverse Hill-Sachs lesion where the shoulder dislocates posteriorly.

humerus—The upper arm bone. The head of the humerus rests in the glenoid.

hyaluronate (hyaluronic acid)—An extremely large, water-loving molecule that acts as the main lubricant of all the joints. It is as if there are millions of water-coated ball bearings lubricating the cartilage surfaces in the joint fluid.

hyperextension—Extending a joint beyond its normal range. When the knee extends and bends backward from fully straight it is said to be "hyperextending."

hypertension (HTN)—High blood pressure. Normal blood pressure is 120 over 80 where the high number is when the heart pumps and the lower number is when it relaxes. When the lower number is over 90, risks of heart attack and stroke go up. The higher the numbers (higher or lower) the worse it is.

I

impingement syndrome—A condition that results from overuse of the shoulder. The tendons and bursa may thicken and pinch against the bone, causing irritation and pain. It can also occur at the AC joint.

insidious—In medical terminology, disease that develops so gradually that it is usually well established before it is diagnosed.

L

LCL (lateral collateral ligament)—A ligament that connects the femur to the tibia on the outer or lateral side of the knee. It helps stabilize the knee and stops the knee from opening up when a sideward force is applied to the inside of the leg.

labrum—The cartilaginous lip that covers the edge of the glenoid cavity. It widens the joint. When torn it is associated with different injuries. Anterior labrum is associated with anterior dislocations of the so-called Bankart lesion. Superior labrum tears are called SLAP tears. Posterior labrum tears include GLAD (glenoid labral articular dissociations or cracks between the labrum and the cartilage edge of the socket) and Kim lesions (posterior lip tears of the labrum itself).

lateral—Describes a body part that is located away from the center of the body. Can be used to refer to the side of a body part that is toward the outer side of the body. The lateral meniscus is one example.

ligament—Tough tissue connecting bones to bones. There are ligaments around every joint of the body, helping to guide them and preserve stability.

locking (of the knee)—When the knee becomes stuck in place, in either a bent or extended position. Usually, the knee is locked because the meniscus has torn, and the piece is stuck or because there is a loose body stuck in between the bones of the knee. Forcing the knee to straighten when locked is not a good idea because you can cause more damage. Using crutches to unload the knee and protect it along with seeing your orthopaedic surgeon ASAP is important if your knee is locked.

loose bodies—Cartilage fragments that detach and are loose in the knee. Loose bodies are often nourished by the synovial fluid and therefore can get larger in time, causing more difficulty like locking and giving way.

M

Marfan syndrome—An inherited collagen disorder associated with tall height, long arms, cardiac problems (heart murmurs, aortic dissections), poor eyesight (nearsightedness), flat feet, scoliosis, and dislocated eye lens.

MCL (medial collateral ligament)—A ligament that connects the femur to the tibia on the inner or medial side of the knee. It helps stabilize the knee and stops the knee from opening (the femur and tibia slightly gapping apart) when a sideward force is applied to the outside of the leg. Linemen on football teams can get this type of injury, which is one of the most common knee ligament sprains in sports. This is why it is often recommended that linemen wear braces to protect against this injury (so-called prophylactic knee bracing). Many are Grade 1 or 2 and heal with nonoperative treatment.

medial—Describes a body part that is located toward the center of the body. Can be used to refer to the side of a body part that is toward the inner side of the body.

meniscal repair—A procedure in which the torn part of the meniscus is repaired.

meniscus—Cartilage between the femur and tibia. It cushions the knee and distributes the weight from the femur onto the tibia. It helps stabilize the knee joint by converting the flat top of the tibia to a more stable, shallow socket.

microfracture technique—A procedure in which the bone surface is drilled to help blood and marrow get to the surface.

MRI (magnetic resonance imaging)—Strong magnets and radio waves used to create images of the soft tissues in the body. The pictures are clearer than X-rays for soft tissue problems but are limited when looking at bone detail (CT scan is better). There are mathematical constraints for an MRI. If patients move when in the scanner or if they have metal implants, it can cause mathematical artifacts and alter the images greatly. An MRI can be very helpful when it is indicated. Many conditions can be diagnosed with a care history, a good physical exam, and a plain x-ray (for example, Osgood Schlater's Disease or common fractures). Therefore, in many cases, MRIs are often overused, unnecessary, and, sadly, a waste of medical resources.

muscle function—Movement of the muscle. This can take several forms:

> **closed chain**—The end of the limb or extremity, called the distal end (like the food or hand), is fixed against the load. This is a more natural exercise than open chain (see below). When walking, the foot is fixed against the ground as your weigh is applied. Examples: Partial squats, wall sits, TRX, biking, elliptical, push-ups.

concentric—Shortening the muscle against tension that is proportional to the external load. The force remains constant as the muscle shortens. Example: The part of a biceps curl that is occurring as the elbow flexes.

eccentric—Lengthening the muscle against tension that is proportional to the external load. The force is intentionally resisted as the muscle lengthens. Example: The part of a biceps curl that is occuring as the elbow straightens from a bend position while controlling the weight as the arm straightens against gravity.

isokinetic—The muscle contracts at a constant velocity through varied resistance. These movements are often used to objectively evaluate muscle strength during injury rehabilitation. The force is less important than constant speed. Example: These constant speed exercises require a special type of workout equipment, like a Cybex machine. These control speed by varying the force throughout the range of motion being tested.

isometric—Constant muscle length and tension that is proportional to the external load. This can cause muscle hypertrophy (enlargement). Example: Pushing against an immovable object, as in a plank.

isotonic—Force remains constant through a range of motion. Isotonic exercise improves motor (muscle) performance. Example: Biceps curls using a cable column.

open chain—The end of the limb or extremity (distal end) moves freely as the muscle works. Example: Seated leg extensions or hamstring curls. The foot is not touching the ground (free to move) as the force is applied. Contraindicated in post-op care for many knee problems because they will stress or overload the healing tissue and bone.

plyometric—Rapid eccentric-concentric shortening-lengthening. Good training for sports that require power. Often called ballistic or explosive exercises. Example: box jumps. Not so great for the knees or the patella and not recommended for anyone with a prior kneecap injury, kneecap pain, or knee arthritis.

Mumford procedure—A surgical resection of the prominent tip of the distal clavicle.

N

NSAIDs (nonsteroidal anti-inflammatory drugs). Drugs that block inflammation and reduce bone and joint pian, such as aspirin and ibuprofen (Motrin). These are not steroids, hence the name NSAIDs. Of note, Tylenol is not an NSAID.

neuron—The smallest fiber inside a nerve. A nerve is made up of many neurons. These include both motor neurons (for muscle control) and sensory neurons (for feeling things).

O

osteoarthritis—Disease in which the joint cartilage breaks down over time. The normal wearing out of the joint can be considered osteoarthritis. Osteoarthritis can also be the result of trauma to a joint, which worsens later with wear and tear. Osteoarthritis is also associated with a deformity of the joint (varus knees/bow-legged or valgus knees/knocked knees) or a torn ligament with instability that is not treated. Correction of deformities and repair of the ligaments is thought to delay the onset of osteoarthritis in many, but not all, conditions.

osteochondritis dissecans (OCD)—When fragments of bone below a joint surface loses its blood supply, the bone fails or fractures and separates from the rest of the bone, forming a loose flap or loose body. The flap of cartilage and/or the loose body floating around in the knee can cause the knee to lock or catch. Repairing the loose flap and removing the loose body is the preferred treatment.

osteogenesis imperfecta—This is a genetic bone disorder that cause bones to be more fragile from birth and is associated with multiple fractures, blue sclera, curved chest shape, weak teeth, curved spine, and variable severity. There are eight types that range from Type I (mild) to Type III (the most severe). Individuals with the severe form have a poor life expectancy, lungs that tend to be underdeveloped, and fractures before birth. Many times, death occurs soon after birth. Individuals with the mild type have a higher fracture risk.

osteophyte—A boney growth on the edge of a joint surface. The body makes osteophytes when it tries to widen the bone to compensate for increased stress, often seen with wear or osteoarthritis. "Spurs" may be seen on an X-ray, which are called osteophytes when around the edges of a joint. When they are large, they can block range of motion.

P

PCL (posterior cruciate ligament)—A ligament that connects the femur to the tibia. It helps stabilize the knee and stops the tibia from sliding backward under the femur, especially when bent to 90 degrees. It tears when a direct force is applied to the tibia with the knee bent.

partial meniscectomy—A procedure in which the torn part of the meniscus is removed. This is done when there is a small tear that does not have the potential to heal if repaired; for example, a "white on white" beak tear in an area with little or no blood supply and a small tear in a zone that is known not to heal.

patella—The kneecap.

patella tendon—A large tendon connecting the thigh (quads) muscle and patella to the tibia. It holds the patella in place.

patellofemoral articulation—The smooth surfaces between the patella and the femur. The groove that the kneecap moves up and down in is the so-called trochlea groove. The patella rides in the groove and hence the name of this area in the knee is the patellofemoral articulation.

periosteum—The membrane that lines the outside of all bones, except for the ends of long joints. It is the source of the growth of the width of the bones in children.

proximal—Describes something that is situated close to the center of the body. For example, the hip is proximal to the knee.

Q

quadriceps—The thigh muscles of the leg. They control the movement of the patella. They consist of four muscles: the rectus, the vastus lateralis, the vastus medialis obliques (VMO), and the vastus intermedius. The VMO is often weak in patella dislocations, which is why physical therapists focus on strengthening this muscle in nonoperative treatment after a first-time patella dislocation.

R

recurvatum—Hyperextension of the knee, when it bends backward more than normal (more than 5–10 degrees). It is often associated with general ligament laxity, which may be genetic or due to a genetic disorder like Marfan syndrome or Ehlers-Danlos syndrome, which cause collagen abnormalities.

red zone (of the meniscus)—The outer third of the meniscus; there is good blood flow in this area, hence the name "red." ("White" is for areas without blood flow.) "Red on red" tears of the meniscus (in other words, blood is flowing on both sides of the tear) have the best chance of healing, as opposed to "red on white" tears; the worst kind of tear is "white on white."

RICE—Acronym that stands for "rest, ice, compression, and elevation," which is often the first treatment for an injury.

rotator cuff—Made up of four muscles and their tendons that originate from the scapula and form a single tendon unit that inserts on the upper humerus. The rotator cuff helps stabilize the shoulder within the joint, lift the arm, and rotate the humerus.

S

scapula—The shoulder blade.

scar tissue—Connective tissue forming a scar. It is composed mostly of fibroblasts and unorganized collagen that is mostly Type I in nature.

sprain—The stretching or tearing of a ligament. Grade 1: in place, not elongated; Grade 2: some fibers still intact and some torn, elongation may have occurred; Grade 3: complete tearing of the fibers.

subluxation—Popping or slipping partly out of place; a partial dislocation.

synovitis—An inflammation of the lining (the synovium) of any joint. When looking at it through an arthroscope, it appears red, swollen, and inflamed. There are many small blood vessels on the surface. There may be overgrowth of the lining, too. It bleeds easily when cut or during procedures to try to remove it to treat chronic effusions, as in an arthroscopic synovectomy.

T

tendon—Tough tissue connecting muscles to bones. Tendons are different from ligaments that are also thick and strong but connect bones to each other (like the PCL, ACL, MCL, and LCL in the knee).

tibia—The shinbone.

tibial tubercle—The bony prominence on the tibia below the patella. The patella tendon attaches here.

trapezius muscle—Muscles located on either side of the upper back. They are mainly used to stabilize and rotate the scapula.

triceps muscle—A three-part muscle that connects the back of the elbow to the bones of the humerus and shoulder; key in doing push-ups.

trochlea—the groove in which the patella glides up and down.

tuberosity—A prominence on a bone where ligaments or tendons attach. For example, the rotator cuff attaches to tuberosities on the humerus. In particular, the humeral head has greater and lesser tuberosities. The rotator cuff muscles, specifically the infraspinatus and the supraspinatus, attach to the greater tuberosity of the humeral head, and the subscapularis attaches to the lesser tuberosity of the humeral head.

V

valgus alignment—The legs bow inward; so-called knocked knees.

varus alignment—The legs bow outward; so-called bowed legs.

W

white zone (of the meniscus)—The inner third of the meniscus; there is no blood flow here and therefore very little potential for healing. White on white tears are usually removed. Red on white tears have some potential for healing in younger patients.

XYZ

X-ray (radiograph)—High-energy electromagnetic radiation that passes through soft tissue more easily than bones to create a photograph or shadow of part of a person's skeleton, which is captured on a film or digital cassette. It is used to make many diagnoses.

DR. REZNIK'S PUBLICATIONS

(See DrReznik.com for direct links to many the articles)

Anighoro, K, Reznik, AM: "Tranexamic Acid: A Paradigm Shift in Total Joint Care." *AAOS Now*, October 2022.

Reznik, AM, Barton, RS: "Modern Surgical Education and Primum Non Nocere." *AAOS Now*, July 2022.

Corbett, N, Reznik, AM: "Operative Treatment of Charcot Foot with 'Super-Constructs' Has Evolved." *AAOS Now*, April 2022.

Acquarulo, B, Reznik, AM: "Breaking Bad: A Practical Guide for Communicating Bad News." *AAOS Now*, May 2022.

Corbett, N, Reznik, AM: "Decision-making in Treatment of Charcot Foot and Ankle." *AAOS Now*, March 2022.

Weisberg, M, Reznik, AM: "Put the Flex Back in Flexing: Surgical Approaches to Biceps Tenotomy and Tenodesis." *AAOS Now*, March 2022.

Reznik, AM: "Korean Orthopaedics Association President Hee Joong Kim, MD, Discusses Orthopaedic Trends from South Korea." *AAOS Now*, February 2022.

Weisberg, M, Reznik, AM: "Put the Flex back in Flexing: The Best Treatment of Biceps Tendonitis." *AAOS Now*, February 2022.

Reznik, AM: "Medical Ethics and AI." 10th International Conference on Ethics Issues in Biology, Engineering and Medicine, November 2021.

Reznik, AM: "The Orthopaedic CMO Role During the Pandemic and Beyond." *AAOS Now*, November 2021.

Nelson, FRT, Reznik, AM: "Basic Science and Meniscus: Where Are We Now?" *AAOS Now*, October 2021.

Nelson, FRT, Reznik, AM: "It Is Time for Spine Surgeons to 'Own the Bone.'" *AAOS Now*, April 2021.

Cole, AA, photos by Reznik, AM: "Avoid Patient Harm by Improving Patient Positioning for Surgery." *AAOS Now*, February 2021.

Qaiyumi, Z, Reznik, AM: "Do Not Overlook Alternative Causes of Foot Drop." *AAOS Now*, January 2021.

Reznik, AM, Nelson, FRT: "Ethics in Artificial Intelligence: The Hidden Dangers." *Ethics in Biology, Engineering and Medicine*, Volume 11, Issue 1, 2020.

Nelson, FRT, Reznik, AM: "Most Orthopaedic Surgeons Have a Screw Loose (How Screws Loosen in Bone)." *AAOS Now*, July 2020.

Reznik, AM: "Explainable AI: How Do We Know What AI Is 'Thinking?'" *AAOS Now*, June 2020.

Samora, JB, Fitzgerald, K (Reznik interview): "Orthopaedic Surgeons Weigh In on eSports and Gaming-related Musculoskeletal Injuries." *AAOS Now*, June 2020.

Petit, L, Reznik, AM: "The 'Root' of All Evil: Mounting Evidence Supports Fixing Root Tears." *AAOS Now*, April 2020.

Reznik, AM: "Facing the Problem, not the Terminology; 'Lateral Violence.'" *AAOS Now*, March 2020.

Reznik, AM: "Evolution Versus Revolution in Artificial Intelligence: Why the Distinction?" *AAOS Now*, December 2019.

Reznik, AM: "A Top-down Approach Is Needed to Address Lateral Violence Among Residents." *AAOS Now*, October 2019.

Reznik, AM: "Long Hours, Insulated Specialties Result in Lateral Violence in Residence." *AAOS Now*, September 2019.

Reznik, AM: "Applying the Four Basic Principles of Medical Ethics to Artificial Intelligence." *AAOS Now*, July 2019.

Cravez, E, Reznik, AM: "Advances in Imaging and Treatments Mitigate Long-term Effects of Frostbite." *AAOS Now*, April 2019.

Reznik, AM: "Surgical Risk Reduction and Medical Malpractice, SRR Tool Kit." CMIC Lecture, March 20, 2019.

Cravez, E, Reznik, AM: "Prevention, Early Treatment Is Critical when Treating Frostbite Injuries." *AAOS Now*, March 2019.

Reznik, AM, Urish, K: "Natural Language Processing Provides Foundation for AI in Medical Diagnosis." *AAOS Now*, March 2019.

Ring, DC, Marks, MR, Burney DW, Jimenez, RL, Reznik, AM, Pinzur, MS, Lightdale-Miric, NR: "AAOS Patient Safety Committee Considers Ways to Avoid Harm Through Innovations in Quality and Safety." *AAOS Now*, March 2019.

Boyle, K, Reznik, AM, Pinzur, MS: "AAOS Strives to Reduce Surgical Risks with New Online Tool Kit." *AAOS Now*, February 2019.

Urish, K, Reznik, AM: "How Would a Computer Diagnose Arthritis on a Radiograph?" *AAOS Now*, December 2018.

Reznik, AM: "Kevin Shea, MD, and Jayson Murray, MA, Shed Light on Appropriate Use Criteria." *AAOS Now*, November 2018.

Reznik, AM, Urish, K: "Understanding the Impact of Artificial Intelligence on Orthopedic Surgery." *AAOS Now*, September 2018.

Duck, HL, Reznik, AM: "Debate: Are Ultrasounds Necessary for Routine Knee and Shoulder Injections in the Office?" *AAOS Now*, July 2018.

Ring, DCMD, Marks, MR, Burney, DW, Jimenez, RL, Reznik, AM, Pinzur, MS, Lightdale-Miric, NR: "Putting Yourself in Your Patient's Place." *AAOS Now*, September 2017.

Reznik, AM, Boyle, K, Pinzur, MS: "Surgical Risk Reduction Tool Kit For AAOS." *AAOS Now*, January 2018.

Ring, D, Marks, MR, Burney, DW, Jimenez, RL, Reznik, AM, Pinzur, MS, Lightdale-Miric, NR: "New Habits Can Better Serve Patients." *AAOS Now*, July 2017.

Reznik, AM: Disputant, "Medicaid Patients Are Less Successful When Scheduling Appointments Under the Affordable Care Act: A Meta-Analysis of Appointment Accessibility Audit Studies" by Daniel Wiznia, MD. Yale University Department of Orthopedics Disputations, June 2017.

Ring, D, Marks, MR, Burney, DW, Jimenez, RL, Reznik, AM, Pinzur, MS, Lightdale-Miric, NR: "Issues of Appropriateness and Patient Safety." *AAOS Now*, May 20 17.

Reznik, AM: "Advancing Your Idea (How to Get Your Surgical Inventions to Market)." Arthroscopy Association of North America Instructional Course lecture, 2014.

Reznik, AM: Disputant, "The Effect of NSAIDs on Glenoid Labrum Healing in a Rat Model of Anterior Shoulder Dislocation." Yale University Department of Orthopedics Disputations, 2014.

Reznik, AM: *I've Fallen, and I Can Get Up*. LULU Press, 2012. CT Press Club Award: First Prize Educational Book, 2013.

Reznik, AM, Reznik, JY: *The Knee and Shoulder Handbook for All of Us*. LULU Press, 2010. CT Press Club Award: First Prize Instructional Book, 2011.

Reznik, AM: Disputant, "The Distal Triceps Tendon Footprint and a Biomechanical Analysis of Three Repair Techniques" *A Cadaveric Anatomic Study and Biomechanical Testing of Three Suture and Anchor Methods of Triceps Repair* by Peter Yeh, MD. Yale University Department of Orthopedics Disputations, 2010.

Reznik, AM: "The Business Aspects of Medicine as It Is Practiced in Other Countries. A Comparison of Care, Expectations, and Costs; How It Affects Service Levels and Satisfaction." Quinnipiac University Business School, Guest Professor, 2003–2008.

Shea, KP, McIntyre, L, Blatz, D, Reznik, AM, Leger, R: "Arthroscopic Rotator Cuff Repair Using Ultrasonic Suture Welding: A Prospective, Multi-center Study." AANA Meeting, April 2006.

Reznik, AM: "Hurricane Medicine, Report on the Treatment and Status of a Displaced Population after Hurricanes in the Gulf Coast." New Haven Medical Society Meeting, November 2000.

Reznik, AM: "International Aspects of Business and Medicine." Quinnipiac University, Visiting Professor, 2008–2016 and 2022.

Reznik, AM, Sembler, R, Novak, A: "Outcome and Cost-effectiveness of Patient Controlled Analgesia in ACL Reconstruction." Hospital of Saint Raphael, 1997.

Phillips, P, Reznik, AM, Daignault, J: "Arthroscopic vs. Open Surgical Shoulder Stabilization in Patients with Traumatic Recurrent Anterior Shoulder Instability and a Documented Bankart Lesion." Proceedings of the Arthroscopy Association of North America 15th Annual Meeting, 1996.

Ryan, J, Reznik, AM: "Open vs. Arthroscopic Acromioplasty." *Physician Assistant Journal,* May 1994.

Reznik, AM, Davis, JL, Daniel, DM: "Optimizing Interference Fixation for Cruciate Ligament Reconstruction." Proceedings of the Orthopaedic Research Society 36th Annual Meeting, February 1990, 1997–2003.

Reznik, AM, Davis, JL, Daniel, DM: "Experimental Evaluation of Pin Design and Configuration for Soft Tissue Fixation to Bone." Proceedings of the Orthopaedic Research Society 36th Annual Meeting, February 1990.

Reznik, AM, Daniel, DM: "ACL Graft Placement, Tensioning and Fixation: Part II." *Surgical Rounds for Orthopaedics,* August 1990.

Reznik, AM, Daniel, DM: "ACL Graft Placement, Tensioning and Fixation: Part II." *Surgical Rounds for Orthopaedics,* September 1990.

Sachs, RA, Reznik, AM, Daniel, DM, Stone, ML: "Complications of Knee Ligament Surgery." In *Knee Ligaments Structure, Function, Injury, and Repair.* Raven Press, 1990.

Mont, MA, Reznik, AM, Sedlin, E: "Radial Head Fractures: Factors Important for Treatment and Prognosis." Presentation, American Academy of Orthopaedic Surgeons, February 1989.

Reznik, AM: Discussant for presentation on collagen-based synthetic ligaments. New York Academy of Medicine, Orthopaedic Section Annual Meeting, May 1988.

Reznik, AM, Mont, MA, Tenceiro, R, Pilla, AA, Siffert, RS: "The Effect of Differences in Osteotomy Method on Bone Healing." Presentation, Orthopaedic Research Society Annual Meeting, January 1987.

Reznik, AM: Intracapsular Hip Fractures: A Clinical Review. MD thesis, Yale University School of Medicine, 1983.

Epstein, MAF, Reznik, AM, Epstein, RA: "Determinants of Distortions in CO_2 Catheter Sampling Systems: A Mathematical Model." *Respiration Physiology,* 1980.

Reznik, AM, Epstein, MAF, Epstein, RA: "CO_2 Catheter Sampling Systems Evaluation of Distortions." Presentation, American Academy of Anesthesiologists Annual Meeting, 1979.

Reznik, AM: "A Test Drive of ChatGPT and Generative AI in Orthopaedics." *AAOS Now,* May 2023.

Reznik, AM: "ChatGPT is the Next Step in Artificial Intelligence." *AAOS Now,* March-April 2023.

WEBSITES OF INTEREST

My own website: DrReznik.com

Ortho Information: Orthoinfo.org

https://www.littleleague.org/playing-rules/pitch-count/

DR. REZNIK'S PATIENTS

10,572,556   02/25/20 Systems and Methods for Facilitating Enhancements to
Search Results By Removing Unwanted Search Results

8,568,308   10/29/13 Customizable, Self-holding, Space Retracting, Arthroscopic
Endoscopic Cannula System (device)

8,517,934   08/27/13 Customizable, Self-holding, Space Retracting,
Arthroscopic Endoscopic Cannula System (method)

8,326,862   12/04/12 Systems and Methods for Facilitating Enhancements
to Search Engine Results

8,075,520   12/13/11 Arthroscopic Fluid Control Device and Method for
Controlling Fluid Flow in Arthroscopic Procedures

7,785,287   08/31/10 Arthroscopic Fluid control (device)

7,569,024   08/04/09 Shoulder Holder for Arm Surgery (Manufacturing license
and produced by IMP)

INDEX

Italic numbers indicate photographs.

Acromioclavicular (AC) joint, 99, 134-138, *134*
    anatomy, 134
    diagnosis of separation, 135
    joint pain, 135
    nonsurgical treatment, 136
    shoulder separation, 135
    surgical treatment, 136-137, *137-138*
Adhesive capsulitis. *See* Frozen shoulder.
Airway and allergies, 165
Allografts, for cartilage replacement, 74
Anatomy
    of knee, *169*
    of shoulder, *170*
Anterior cruciate ligament (ACL) tears, 42-55
    braces, 45, *46*
    diagnosis, 42-43, *42-43*
    in female athletes, 45, *46*
    instability, 43-44, *44*
    KT-1000 testing, 47, *48*
    nonsurgical treatment, 47
    other knee ligaments, 52-55, *53, 54*
    surgical repair, 49-52, *51*
    instability, 43-44, *44*
    valgus collapse, 45, *46*
    in very young people, 52
Athletes. *See* Sports.
Arthroscopy
    of AC joint, 136
    of biceps tenodesis, 133
    of rotator cuff, 121
    of shoulder, 109-111
Autologous chondrocyte implantation (ACI), 70

Balance
    and injury prevention, 159
    of throwing athletes, 115
Bankart lesion of shoulder, 107, 109, 110, *108*
Baseball, Little League, 16-27
Biceps tendon, 129-133, *130*
    anatomy, 129-131, *130, 131*
    and rotator cuff, 131
    surgical treatment 131-132, *132*

        tendonitis, 131
        tendonotomy, 132, 134
        tenodesis, 133
        tenolysis, 131
Bleeding and clotting, 166
Blount's disease, 58
Body mass index, 159
Bone bruise, 93
Bone health, 157-159, 166
Bone morphogenic protein (BMP), 146
Braces
        for ACL tears, 45, *46*
        for bowed knees, 58
Bursitis, 98

Calcium, in bone growth, 12
        injury prevention, 12-13
Cancer, and frozen shoulder, 103
Cardiac problems, 166
Cartilage
        defects of, 70-75, 90-91, *74*
        of meniscus. *See* Meniscus tears.
        types of, 61, 70
        SLAP tears in shoulder, 113-116
Chemotherapy, and frozen shoulder, 103
Children
        ACL tears, 52
        overuse injuries, *See* Overuse injuries; Sports
        shoulder pain, 108
        and teenagers, knee pain. *See* Knee pain.
Clavicle fractures, 98, 139-147
        In adults and children, 140-141
        surgical fixation, 141, *141-144*
        treatment, 139-140
Coracoclavicular ligaments, 135, 136
Cortisone, for cartilage defects, 71-72
CT scans, of sport tumors, 155
Cysts, meniscal, 65-66

Degeneration, of meniscus, 63-64
Diabetes
        and bone health, 159
        and frozen shoulder, 10, 103
Dislocation, of shoulder, 98, 106, 111, *106-107*
Double joints, 105, 108

Ehlers-Danlos syndrome, 108
Epiphysis, slipped capital femoral (SCFE), 12
Exercise, weight-bearing, 158

Females, anterior cruciate ligament tears, 45, *46*
Femoral condyle, 91
Fibroma, non-ossifying (NOF), 12, *11*
Frozen shoulder (adhesive capsulitis), 99, 100-104
    causes, 100
    and diabetes, 100, 103
    keloid treatment, 101
    treatment, 102-103

Growth plate
    injuries in children, 11, 12
    and knee pain, 19-20

HAGL lesions, 111-112
Hill-Sachs lesion of shoulder, 107, 109, *106-107*
Humeral fracture, 144, *144*
    ACL tears, 43-44
    of patella, 81-82
    of shoulder, 98, 106, 108

Internal rotation.
    In throwing athletes, 114-115
See also Frozen shoulder.

Jumper's knee, 20-21, 84, *22, 84*

Keloid treatment for frozen shoulder, 101
Knee anatomy, *169*
Knee deformities, 56-60
    bowed legs and knocked knees, 56-58, *56-57*
    bowed or varus knees, 58-59, *59*
    knocked or valgus knees, 45, 59-60, *60*
    surgery for, 56, *57*
Knee extensor injuries, 83-89
    cartilage injury, 86
    patella fractures and tendon ruptures, 83-84, *84*
    quadriceps rupture, 84-85, *85*
    surgical treatment, 86-88, *86-89*
    tibial plateau fractures, 85-88, *86-89*
Knee pain, in children and teenagers, 19-26
    growing pains, 22
    jumper's knee, 20-21, *22*
    kneecap pain, 22
    Osgood-Schlatter's disease, 19-20, *20-21*
    osteochondritis dissecans, 22-26, *23*
    patellar tendinitis, 22
Knee replacement, 95, *96*
    and infections or tumors, 95

in older patients, 94
vs. osteotomy, 58, 59
Kneecap. *See* Patella.
KT-1000, for ACL tear, 43-44, 47-48

Ligaments, of knee. *See* ACL tears.
Loose bodies, 91-92, 94, *92*
Lubricants, for cartilage defects, 72

Marfan syndrome, 108
Meniscus tears, 61-68, *62*
    and Baker's cyst, 65-66
    cartilage repair, 67-69, *68*
    degeneration of, 63-64
    diagnosis, 65
    discoid, 64
    root tear, 68-69, *69*
    treatment of, 66-67
Microfractures, 92, 94
MACI (matrix-induced autologous chondrocyte implantation), 94
MRI
    of meniscus tears, 62, *63*
    of sport tumors, 155-156

Nonsurgical treatment
    of anterior cruciate ligament, 47
    of patella, 77-79, *77*
NSAIDs
    for cartilage defects, 70-71
    for frozen shoulder, 102-103
    for patella pain, 77
Nutrition
    bone morphogenic protein (BMP), 146
    in children, 12
    for clavicle fracture, 141
    diet, 158
    and knee deformities, 57

OATS, 94
Obesity, and bone growth, 12
Office visits, 182-184
Orthopedic questions and answers, 177-181
Osgood-Schlatter's disease, 19-20, *20-21*
Osteoarthritis
    and meniscus tears, 63, 67
    of shoulder, 99
Osteochondritis dissecans, 22-26, 70, *23*
    loose bodies, 91, *92*
Osteocondroma, and sports. 156

Osteogenesis imperfecta, 108
Osteonecrosis, 25-26
Overuse injuries
     in children, 7, 12-13
     growth plate injuries, 11
     noncancerous bone lesions, 12, *11*
     See also Sports.

Pain
     benefits of, 163-164
     and bone health, 157
     of kneecap, 76-82
See also Knee pain.
Patella
     alta, 81, *82*
     fractures, 83-84
     pain and dislocation, 76-82, *77-80*
     tendon, 20-22, 84, *21*
Patellafemoral pain, 22, 80-81
Physical therapy
     arm exercises, 173-176
     for frozen shoulder, 104
     leg exercises, 171-173
Platelet-rich plasma, 66
Popliteal cysts, 65-66
Pseudoarthrosis, 146

Quadriceps rupture, 84-85, *85*

Rheumatoid arthritis, of shoulder, 99
Rickets, and bone growth, 12
Rotator cuff tears, 98, 112, 117-128
     acromion pain, 126, *126*
     arthritis, 122-123
     arthroscopy, 121
     calcific tendonitis, 119, *119*
     collarbone wear, 127-128, *128*
     "empty can sign." 117
     ganglion cysts, 124
     nerve issues, 124-125
     impingement syndrome, 125-126, *126*
     size and shape, 119
     and SLAP tears, 113
     treatment, 119-121, *120-122*

Shoes, and knee deformities, 58
Shoulders, 98-99
     anatomy, 107-108, *107, 170*
     nonunion fractures, 145-147, *147*

HAGL lesions, 111-112

instability and dislocation, 105-112, *106, 107*

loose joints and subluxation, 110-111, *110*

rotator cuff tears, 112

SLAP tears, 113-116, *116*

treatment, 109-110, *109*

See also Frozen shoulder.

SLAP (superior labral anterior to posterior) tear in shoulder, 113-116, *116*

Sleeper's stretch, 114

Smoking, and healing rates, 146

Sports

for children

equipment, 14

exercise and form, 17-18

field conditions, 14

injury prevention, 12-13

nutrition, 12

pitching limits, 15-17, *16*

supervision, 15

weather condition, 14-15

and meniscus tears, 63-64

and patella dislocation, 78

shoulder structure, 106, 108, 110

throwing athletes, 114-115

tumors, 151-156, *152-154*

x-rays, MRIs, and CT scans, 155-156

Subluxation

of patella, 77-79

of shoulder, 98

Surgical repair

of ACL tear, 49-50

of cartilage defects, 73

of frozen shoulder, 102-103

of knee extensor mechanism, 86-88, *87-89*

of meniscus tear, 66-67

Swelling, and sports tumors, 152

Tendon, patellar, 84

Tendinitis, 98

Thyroid, and bone growth, 12

Tibia

fractures, 85-88, *86-89*

tubercle, and knee pain, 19-20, *20-21*

Tumors, and sports, 151-156, *152-154*

Valgus collapse, 45, *46. See also* Knee deformities.

Varus knee. See Knee deformities; Vitamins, and bone growth, 12

Vitamin deficiency, 58, 158

X-rays, and sports tumors, 155

AUTHOR'S BIOGRAPHY

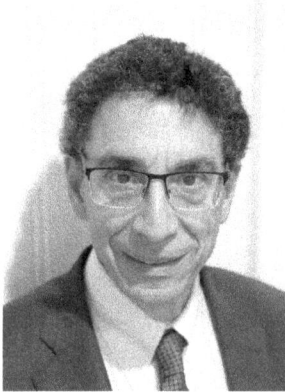

DR. ALAN REZNIK is board-certified in orthopaedic surgery, arthroscopic surgery, and sports medicine. Dr. Reznik received his Bachelor of Science from Columbia University's School of Engineering and his medical degree from Yale University School of Medicine, and he was a fellow in England at Oxford University's renowned Nuffield Orthopaedic Centre. He completed a sports medicine fellowship at the University of California, San Diego. Dr. Reznik was court physician at the US Open Tennis Tournament, on the 1995 Special Olympics Games Organizing Committee, and the team physician for the New Haven Knights Professional Hockey Team. He truly enjoys working with competitive, recreational, and weekend athletes of all ages. He enjoys golfing, kayaking, biking, and paddleboarding.

Connecticut Magazine rated Dr. Reznik as a "Top Doc" in the state numerous times based on reviews from his orthopaedic surgeon peers, physicians, nurses, and patients. Consumer's Research Council of America named him one of "America's Top Physicians." Utilizing his expertise and over three decades of experience in arthroscopic techniques for shoulder and knee repair, he has innovated many procedures, invented surgical instruments, and has been granted seven US patents.

Dr. Reznik is active locally and nationally:

- Chief Medical Officer of Connecticut Orthopaedics

- Served on several American Academy of Orthopaedic Surgeons (AAOS) Committees:

    * Communications Cabinet

    * AAOS National Patient Safety Committee

    * Council on Research and Quality as the Communications Cabinet liaison for the AAOS

    * Editorial board of *AAOS Now*, the academy's orthopaedic news journal.

- Member of the Arthroscopy Association of North America

He writes many educational articles to educate patients and physicians and has been interviewed on general media on many occasions. In addition to this book, he is also the author of *I've Fallen, and I Can Get Up*, a book that explains why we fall and how to prevent those falls. It has a fall risk checklist and a guide on how to make your home safe for everyone. He hopes his two books will help all patients live better, healthier, active lives with fewer injuries and if they do get hurt by a fall, sports participation, or another type of injury, then they will know what to do next.

www.ingramcontent.com/pod-product-compliance
Lightning Source LLC
Chambersburg PA
CBHW042338030426

42335CB00030B/3390